General Practice

For David and for Caroline.

For Elsevier:

Commissioning Editor: Alison Taylor
Development Editor: Kim Benson
Project Manager: Christine Johnston
Design: Erik Bigland
Illustration Manager: Bruce Hogarth

General Practice

Simon Cartwright
General Practitioner
White Horse Medical Practice, Faringdon, Oxfordshire

Carolyn Godlee
General Practitioner
Summertown Health Centre, Oxford

THIRD EDITION

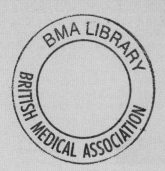

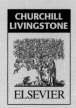

EDINBURGH   LONDON   NEW YORK   OXFORD
PHILADELPHIA   ST LOUIS   SYDNEY   TORONTO   2008

CHURCHILL
LIVINGSTONE
ELSEVIER

© 1998, Pearson Professional Limited
© 2003, Elsevier Limited
© 2008, Elsevier Limited. All rights reserved.

ISBN-13: 978-0-443-10359-9

British Library Cataloguing in Publication Data
A catalogue record for this book is available from the British Library.

Library of Congress Cataloging in Publication Data
A catalog record for this book is available from the Library of Congress.

Note
Knowledge and best practice in this field are constantly changing. As new research and experience broaden our knowledge, changes in practice, treatment and drug therapy may become necessary or appropriate. Readers are advised to check the most current information provided (i) on procedures featured or (ii) by the manufacturer of each product to be administered, to verify the recommended dose or formula, the method and duration of administration, and contraindications. It is the responsibility of the practitioner, relying on their own experience and knowledge of the patient, to make diagnoses, to determine dosages and the best treatment for each individual patient, and to take all appropriate safety precautions. To the fullest extent of the law, neither the Publisher nor the Authors assume any liability for any injury and/or damage to persons or property arising out of or related to any use of the material contained in this book. *The Publisher*

ELSEVIER your source for books, journals and multimedia in the health sciences
www.elsevierhealth.com

Working together to grow libraries in developing countries
www.elsevier.com | www.bookaid.org | www.sabre.org

ELSEVIER   BOOK AID International   Sabre Foundation

The Publisher's policy is to use **paper manufactured from sustainable forests**

Printed in China

CONTENTS

Foreword   vi

Preface   vii

Abbreviations   viii

1. Contraception   1
2. Obstetrics   21
3. Gynaecology   37
4. Urology   63
5. Men's health   73
6. Paediatrics   83
7. Endocrinology   105
8. Gastroenterology   115
9. Dermatology   129
10. Cardiology   145

11. Respiratory medicine   169
12. Infectious diseases   187
13. Ear, nose and throat   209
14. Ophthalmology   223
15. Rheumatology and orthopaedics   237
16. Haematology   257
17. Surgery   263
18. Neurology   273
19. Psychiatry   291
20. Terminal care   315

Appendices   329

Index   361

FOREWORD

In the Foreword to the previous edition of this book I said it was one of very few that is genuinely useful for GPs. This is still true. It manages to be evidence-based but concise. It focuses on questions the clinician is likely to ask and provides practical answers. It gives simple but important tips on clinical practice. It identifies the important red flag issues which need to be recognised in order to practise safe medicine in the community. It will fit easily into most emergency bags.

The book will be particularly helpful to young doctors entering general practice. I also commend it as an accessible source of useful information and a checklist of good practice for established practitioners and other members of the primary health care team.

David Mant MA, MSc, FRCP, FRCGP
Professor of General Practice, Oxford University
2007

This book was conceived during our early years in general practice when we felt the need for a concise practical text on the management of problems which presented in primary care. It was written principally to help GP registrars make sense of what GPs are expected to do for their patients, but we hoped that it would also be a useful reference book for established GPs, medical students, practice nurses and other primary care professionals. The fact that it has reached a wide readership within the profession suggests that we were not alone in feeling the need for a book such as this.

In this updated third edition we have included the latest evidence-based guidelines on asthma, diabetes, hypertension and coronary heart disease, and have added new topics, including a chapter on men's health.

No attempt has been made to discuss the aetiology or pathology of illness, or the complexities of general practice management. By focusing on the clinical and practical aspects of medical management, we have tried to clarify the steps which the aspiring GP might take to manage disease effectively in general practice.

Chapters are divided traditionally into systems of the body, for ease of organisation and reference. Most subjects within these chapters are presented either as diagnoses, such as epilepsy, or as symptoms, such as chest pain. Where clarity has demanded, some subjects are presented otherwise, such as the combined oral contraceptive pill.

The prescription form FP10 is equivalent to GP10 in Scotland and HS21 in Northern Ireland.

Two symbols have been used to draw the reader's attention to important points:

> **Tip**
> This denotes a useful tip, such as: 'The diagnosis of asthma in young children relies almost entirely on history.'

> This indicates crucial information, such as: 'Call 999 and request ambulance paramedics as soon as MI is suspected, even if this is before the patient has been seen.'

Making important decisions as a GP can be a lonely business. We hope this book helps to lessen the burden.

Simon Cartwright
Carolyn Godlee
2007

ABBREVIATIONS

ACBS	Advisory Committee on Borderline Substances	**DU**	duodenal ulcer
ACE	angiotensin converting enzyme	**DVT**	deep vein thrombosis
		E/C	enteric coated
ADH	antidiuretic hormone	**ECG**	electrocardiogram
A&E	accident and emergency	**EDD**	estimated date of delivery
AF	atrial fibrillation	**ELA**	endometrial laser ablation
AFP	α-fetoprotein	**ERCP**	endoscopic retrograde cholangiopancreaticogram
AIDS	acquired immune deficiency syndrome	**ERPC**	evacuation of retained products of conception
ALO	*Actinomyces*-like organisms	**ENT**	ear, nose, throat
ASO	antistreptolysin O	**ESR**	erythrocyte sedimentation rate
AST	aspartate transaminase	**FBC**	full blood count
ASW	approved social worker	**Fe**	iron
BCC	basal cell carcinoma	**FH**	family history
BCG	bacillus Calmette–Guèrin	**FOBs**	faecal occult bloods
B-HGC	beta human chorionic gonadotrophin	**FSH**	follicle-stimulating hormone
BMI	body mass index	**γ-GT**	γ-glutamyl transferase
BNF	*British National Formulary*	**GI**	gastrointestinal
BP	blood pressure	**GnRH**	gonadotrophin-releasing hormone
BPH	benign prostatic hypertrophy	**GORD**	gastro-oesophageal reflux disease
BS	blood sugar		
BTB	breakthrough bleeding	**GTN**	glyceryl trinitrate
BV	bacterial vaginosis	**GTT**	glucose tolerance test
CABG	coronary artery bypass graft	**GU**	gastric ulcer
		GUM	genitourinary medicine
C&Es	creatinine and electrolytes	**HAV**	hepatitis A virus
CHD	coronary heart disease	**Hb**	haemoglobin
COC	combined oral contraceptive	**HbA$_{1c}$**	haemoglobin type A$_{1c}$
CPR	cardiopulmonary resuscitation	**HCG**	human chorionic gonadotrophin
CRP	c-reactive protein	**HGV**	heavy goods vehicle
CSF	cerebrospinal fluid	**Hib**	*Haemophilus influenza* B
CT	computerised tomography	**HIV**	human immunodeficiency virus
CVA	cerebrovascular accident		
CVD	cardiovascular disease	**HPV**	human papilloma virus
CXR	chest X-ray	**HRT**	hormone replacement therapy
DMARD	disease-modifying antirheumatic drug	**HVS**	high vaginal swab
		IBS	irritable bowel syndrome
DRE	digital rectal examination	**IHD**	ischaemic heart disease
DTP	diphtheria, tetanus, pertussis	**INR**	international normalised ratio

IUCD	intrauterine contraceptive device		**SC2**	self certificate
IUS	intrauterine system		**SHBG**	sex-hormone binding globulin
IVU	intravenous urogram		**SIDS**	sudden infant death syndrome
JVP	jugular venous pressure		**SLE**	systemic lupus erythematosus
KUB	kidneys, ureters, bladder		**SLS**	selected list scheme
LFTs	liver function tests		**SPF**	sun protection factor
LH	luteinising hormone		**S/R**	slow release
LMP	last menstrual period		**SSRI**	selective serotonin reuptake inhibitor
LRTI	lower respiratory tract infection		**STI**	sexually transmitted infection
LVF	left ventricular failure		**TB**	tuberculosis
LVH	left ventricular hypertrophy		**TCRE**	transcervical resection of the endometrium
ME	myalagic encephalomyelitis		**TFTs**	thyroid function tests
MCH	mean corpuscular haemoglobin		**TIA**	transient ischaemic attack
MC&S	microscopy, culture and sensitivity		**TOP**	termination of pregnancy
MCV	mean corpuscular volume		**TSH**	thyroid stimulating hormone
MDI	metered-dose inhaler		**UPSI**	unprotected sexual intercourse
MI	myocardial infarct		**URTI**	upper respiratory tract infection
MMR	measles, mumps, rubella		**UTI**	urinary tract infection
MST	morphine sulphate		**UVA**	ultraviolet wavelength A
MSU	mid-stream urine		**UVB**	ultraviolet wavelength B
NRT	nicotine replacement therapy		**VA**	visual acuity
NSAIDs	non-steroidal anti-inflammatory drugs		**VDRL**	venereal disease reference laboratory
OCD	obsessive–compulsive disorder		**WHO**	World Health Organization
OTC	over the counter			
PE	pulmonary embolus			

Dosage abbreviations:

PEFR	peak expiratory flow rate
PID	pelvic inflammatory disease
PMH	past medical history
PMR	polymyalgia rheumatica
PMS	premenstrual syndrome
PMT	premenstrual tension
POP	progestogen-only pill
POS	polycystic ovarian syndrome
PPA	Prescriptions Pricing Authority
PPI	proton pump inhibitor
PSA	prostate-specific antigen
PU	peptic ulcer
PUO	pyrexia of unknown origin
PUVA	psoralens with UVA

bd	twice daily
im	intramuscular(ly)
iv	intravenous(ly)
mr	modified release
od	(once) daily
om	(once) every morning
on	(once) every night
po	by mouth
PR	per rectum
prn	whenever required
PV	by the vaginal route
qds	four times daily
sc	subcutaneous(ly)
stat	immediately
tds	three times daily

CONTRACEPTION

Introduction   2

Combined oral contraceptive (COC)   3

Combined contraceptive transdermal patch   8

Progestogen-only pill (POP)   8

Injectable progestogens   10

Progestogen-releasing implant (Implanon)   11

Postcoital (emergency) contraception   11

Condom   13

Diaphragm   13

Intrauterine contraceptive device (IUCD)   14

Intrauterine progestogen-only system (Mirena/IUS)   16

Natural birth control   16

Sterilisation   17

Hormonal contraception in the perimenopause   18

Postpartum contraception   19

The practice nurse with family planning training may play a significant role, e.g. diaphragm-fitting, pill-teaching and coil-checking.

Methods of contraception include: combined pills, progestogen-only pills, injectable and implanted progestogens, condoms, diaphragms, intrauterine contraceptive devices, natural methods and surgical sterilisation. Other methods, e.g. coitus interruptus, the use of spermicides alone and contraceptive sponges, are not discussed in this chapter as their failure rates are relatively high. Long-acting reversible contraceptive methods (IUD, IUS, depot injections and implants) are more cost-effective than the COC. All contraceptives, other than condoms, are available free on prescription.

Discussion of 'safe sex' and the prevention of HIV infection and other sexually transmitted infections should be part of the routine advice given to the sexually active. This is particularly important when counselling the very young. (Surveys suggest that about 50% of all under-16-year-old females have had intercourse.) 'Safe sex' means sex in which the exchange of bodily fluids is eliminated. 'Low-risk sex' means wet kissing, oral sex without ejaculation, and sexual intercourse using a condom. The use of the condom should be promoted in addition, often, to the main contraceptive. The advantages of fidelity within a sexual relationship, and, in the very young, of postponing intercourse, should be discussed in a non-judgemental way.

Always consider the possible STI risk when discussing contraception, particularly in the following situations:

- Young patient/early in sexual career.
- Emergency contraception request.
- IUCD request.
- TOP request.
- Assault.
- Patient symptomatic (pain, discharge, ulcers, intermenstrual bleeding, postcoital bleeding, breakthrough bleeding on COC, contact bleeding on taking cervical smear).
- Multiple partners or recent change of partner.
- Partner symptomatic.

FRASER GUIDELINES

A doctor must consider the following issues when the patient is under 16 years old:

- Whether the patient understands the potential risks and benefits of the treatment and the advice given.
- The value of parental support. Doctors must encourage young people to inform parents of the consultation and explore the reasons if the patient is unwilling to do so. The patient must be assured of confidentiality.

- Whether the patient is likely to have sexual intercourse without contraception.
- Whether the patient's physical or mental health is likely to suffer if s/he does not receive contraceptive advice or supplies.
- Whether the patient's best interests would require the provision of contraceptive advice or supplies, or both, without parental consent.

COMBINED ORAL CONTRACEPTIVE (COC)

STARTING THE COC

Assessment

History. Ask about/think about possible contraindications.

Absolute contraindications

- DVT or emboli.
- Heart disease (valvular or ischaemic).
- Hypertension (>160/100).
- Hyperlipidaemia.
- Focal or severe migraine/TIAs.
- Cancer of the breast/cervix.
- From 4 weeks before to 2 weeks after major surgery.
- Rare:
  - liver disease (active)
  - polycythaemia; sickle cell anaemia
  - porphyria
  - hydatidiform mole (recent)
  - hyperprolactinaemia
  - diabetic complications.

Relative contraindications

- Family history of arterial disease.
- Diabetes.
- Hypertension (>160/95).
- Heavy cigarette smoking.
- Excessive weight.
- Age. (Smokers should stop the pill at the age of 35 years; there is no definite upper age limit in healthy non-smokers.)
- Common migraine.

Examination. Check:

- weight
- BP
- smear status.

Management

The following points should be considered and discussed, if appropriate:

Failure rate. The failure rate is in the range 0.1–3/100 women-years.

How to start the COC

- Start on day 1 to 5 and no extra contraceptive precautions are necessary.
- Alternatively, start after day 5 and take extra precautions for the first 7 days. (The COC may in fact be started on any day of the cycle, provided that extra precautions are taken for 7 days, but initial bleeding will be unpredictable.)
- Take 1 tablet daily for 21 days. Subsequent courses repeated after 7-day pill-free interval.

Ovulation. The COC stops ovulation; 'periods' are light withdrawal bleeds.

Risks of taking the COC

- Smoking >15 cigarettes per day increases the risk of coronary heart disease by three times.
- Vascular disease in general is increased by about three times. (There is no statistically significant increased risk of myocardial infarction among pill users, unless they also smoke.)
- Hypertension develops in 5% of pill users after 5 years.
- There is a 1.2 relative increase of carcinoma of the breast during use and for 10 years after stopping the COC; this does not appear to be related to duration of use. It is more than counterbalanced by the protective effect against cancers of the ovary and endometrium.

Side-effects

- Breakthrough bleeding. (This usually settles within 2–3 months.)
- Nausea, breast tenderness, weight gain, PMT, bloating (fluid retention), depression, vaginal discharge (secondary to cervical erosion), headaches, reduced libido, chloasma.

Gastrointestinal upset. Vomiting and severe diarrhoea lead to reduced hormone absorption. Take extra contraceptive precautions for the period of illness and for 7 days afterwards.

Prescribing. Ideally, use the lowest strength of pill that does not cause breakthrough bleeding. The dose of oestrogen (ethinyloestradiol) should normally be no more than 20–35 μg. Ideally, a preparation with the lowest oestrogen and progestogen content which gives good cycle control and minimal side-effects should be chosen.

Low strength preparations (containing ethinyloestradiol 20 μg) are particularly appropriate for women with risk factors for circulatory disease.

Standard strength preparations (containing ethinyloestradiol 30 or 35 μg) are appropriate for standard use.

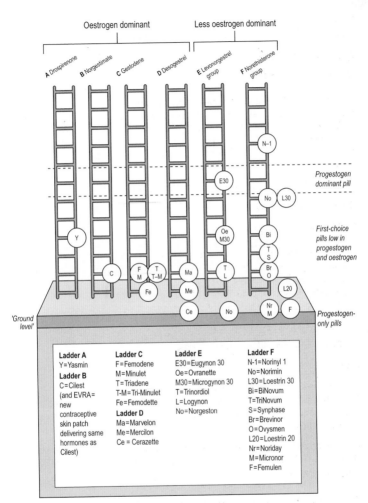

Reproduced with permission from Guillebaud J 2004 Contraception: your questions answered, 4th edn. Churchill Livingstone, Edinburgh

Phased preparations are particularly appropriate for women who either do not have withdrawal bleeds or who have BTB with monophasic pills.

Common choices for women free of risk factors for arterial disease under the age of 30 years are pills delivering levonorgestrel or norethisterone. Women with risk factors for arterial disease or those who are relatively intolerant of pills containing levonorgestrel or norethisterone may do better on a pill containing a third-generation progestogen.

Pills containing the third-generation progestogens (desogestrel, gestodene or drospirenone) can also be useful for women who have side-effects (e.g. weight gain, acne, headaches, depression, breast symptoms and BTB) with other progestogens. Desogestrel and gestodene increase the risk of DVT. In 100 000 women, the approximate number developing a DVT in 1 year is:

- for women taking a pill containing desogestrel or gestodene, 25
- for women taking one of the other COCs, 15
- for women who are pregnant, 60
- for other healthy women not taking a COC, 5.

Women with risk factors for venous disease (including women with a BMI of >30, those with marked varicose veins, those with an immobility problem and those with a family history of DVT) should not use these pills.

What to do if a pill is missed

The most risky pills to miss are those in the first or last week of the pack, as the 7-day pill-free interval is lengthened.

- If pills are missed, take the last missed pill as soon as possible and then resume the normal schedule.
- If the missed pills are in week 3, the pill-free interval should be omitted.
- If pills are missed in week 1 (because the pill-free interval has been extended), emergency contraception should be considered if UPSI occurred in the pill-free interval or in week 1.
- Use condoms or abstain from sex for 7 days if:
  - two or more 20 μg pills have been missed
  - three or more 30 μg pills have been missed.

Drug interactions. Liver enzyme inducers, e.g. phenytoin, carbamazepine, griseofulvin and topiramate, increase the metabolism, and thus elimination in the bile, of both oestrogen and progestogen. If the patient is on a liver enzyme inducer, start a higher dose pill ($\geqslant 50$ μg oestrogen). Consider 'tricycling' (i.e. taking 3 or 4 packets of monophasic tablets without a break followed by a short tablet-free interval of 4 days).

Tip

Certain broad-spectrum antibiotics (e.g. ampicillin, tetracyclines and griseofulvin) alter gut flora and reduce oestrogen absorption. Take extra precautions for the duration of treatment and for 7 days afterwards. Long-term treatment with antibiotics does not require extra precautions, as resistant flora develop.

Follow-up. The first follow-up is at 3 months. Subsequent follow-ups are at 6–12 month intervals.
Check:

- new risk factors
- smoking status
- weight change
- BP
- smear status.

Management of subsequent problems

Breakthrough bleeding

- Ask about COC compliance or vomiting (prevents COC absorption).
- Liver enzyme inducing drugs (e.g. phenytoin) can cause BTB.
- Consider pregnancy.
- Check for cervical lesions if BTB is persistent.
- (*Chlamydia* may cause a blood-stained discharge/BTB.)

If BTB persists for >2–3 months after starting the COC, try an equivalent pill with a different progestogen (see pill ladder, p. 5) or a pill with a higher oestrogen or progestogen content or change to a triphasic pill.

Absent withdrawal bleed. Absent withdrawal bleeds are harmless in themselves. Consider pregnancy. Consider changing to a pill with a lower dose of progestogen or to a triphasic pill.

Side-effects. As a general rule, for all minor side-effects, reduce the dose where possible (this usually means reducing the dose of the progestogen, as nearly all pill-takers are on 30–35 μg of the oestrogen), or change to a pill containing a different progestogen.
    The following side-effects are due to a relative oestrogen excess, and may be alleviated by changing to a progestogen-dominant pill (e.g. Loestrin 30, Microgynon 30 or Eugynon 30):

- nausea
- dizziness
- PMT
- cyclical weight gain
- 'bloating'
- vaginal discharge.

The following side-effects are due to a relative progestogen excess, and may be alleviated by changing to an oestrogen-dominant pill (e.g. Brevinor, Mercilon, Trinordiol, Logynon, Marvelon, Femodene or Dianette):

- vaginal dryness
- sustained weight gain

- depression
- loss of libido
- lassitude
- breast tenderness
- acne
- hirsutism.

If headaches occur in the pill-free interval, consider tricycling (taking 3 packs consecutively, thus avoiding the pill-free intervals).

Changing from one pill to another. If the new pill has the same oestrogen dose or higher than the old pill, start it after a 7-day gap. If the new pill has a lower oestrogen dose than the old pill, start it immediately after the previous pack without a break.

To postpone a period (e.g. for a holiday). Start the next pack immediately, without a pill-free interval. (With phased pills, except Synphase, take the extra pills from the last phase of the new pack. This will postpone the period by the same number of days as there are tablets in the last phase of the pack.)

Stopping the pill to conceive. Ideally, use an alternative method of contraception for 3 months and until one natural period has passed. Preconceptual counselling is important (see p. 22).

COMBINED CONTRACEPTIVE TRANSDERMAL PATCH

Indications (in view of expense)

- Women who comply poorly with COC.
- Women who work difficult shifts or travel between time zones frequently.

Releases ethinyloestradiol 20 μg and norelgestromin 150 μg daily. One patch per week for 3 weeks and 7 patch-free days. Similar efficacy and contraindications to COC.

PROGESTOGEN-ONLY PILL (POP)

The POP is particularly useful for the following:

- Older women – especially those over 35 years old who smoke. (In women over 40 years old the POP is as effective as the COC.) It can relieve PMT and climacteric symptoms.
- Lactating women.
- Women in whom the COC is contraindicated by e.g. hypertension, diabetes, migraine, thrombosis and embolus.

- Women with troublesome oestrogenic side-effects from the COC, e.g. fluid retention, cyclical weight gain, headache and chloasma.
- Women awaiting major surgery.

STARTING THE POP

Assessment

History. Ask about/think about possible contraindications:

- past or present severe arterial disease or an exceptionally high risk of the same
- recent hydatidiform mole
- porphyria.

> **Tip**
> There is no evidence of an increased risk of thrombosis.

Examination. Check:

- weight
- blood pressure
- smear status.

Management

The following points should be considered and discussed.

Failure rate. The overall failure rate is in the range 0.3–4/100 woman-years.

Irregular bleeding or amenorrhoea. These may occur. Most women have a cycle of between 25 and 35 days. The blood loss is light.

Drug interactions. Efficacy is reduced by enzyme-inducing drugs.

> **Tip**
> Antibiotics do not affect the POP.

How to start the POP

- Start on day 1 (the first day of the period) and no extra contraceptive precautions are necessary.
- If starting in mid-cycle, take extra precautions for the first 7 days.
- If changing from a COC, start the POP immediately, without a 7-day gap. No extra precautions are necessary.

- Take the POP regularly every day (no breaks) at the same time, within 2–3 hours. It is maximally effective 5 hours after taking it. If a couple normally have intercourse in the morning, the POP should ideally be taken in the evening.

What to do if a pill is missed

Take it as soon as it is remembered and carry on with the next pill at the right time. If a pill is taken more than 3 hours late (12 hours for Cerazette), protection may be lost. Continue normal pill-taking and take extra contraceptive precautions for 48 hours. Emergency (oral or IUCD) postcoital contraception (see p. 11) should be offered after any unprotected intercourse which occurs during the 7 days after missing 1 pill by more than 3 hours.

Complications. There is an increased incidence of ectopic pregnancies.

Side-effects. Breakthrough bleeding, nausea, breast tenderness, acne, weight gain, loss of libido, depression. These often settle after 2–3 months.

Vomiting and severe diarrhoea. In the event of these symptoms, continue normal pill-taking and take extra precautions for the period of illness and for 7 days afterwards.

Follow-up. The first follow-up is at 3 months. Subsequent follow-ups are at 6–12 month intervals.
Check:

- new risk factors
- weight change
- BP
- smear status.

INJECTABLE PROGESTOGENS

Injectable progestogens inhibit ovulation. The failure rate is 0–2/100 woman-years. The contraindications are as for the POP. They are especially useful for forgetful pill-takers in whom other methods may be inappropriate or contraindicated. The main disadvantage is that the method is irreversible for at least 3 months, and early side-effects may therefore have to be tolerated for this length of time.

The main side-effects are (as for the POP):

- breakthrough bleeding
- amenorrhoea with delay in return to fertility for up to 1 year
- weight gain.

Depo-Provera reduces bone mineral density in many women who use it. This reduction occurs in the first 2–3 years of use and then stabilises. In adolescents, Depo-Provera should only be used when other methods of contraception are inappropriate. Consider other methods of contraception in women with risk factors for osteoporosis (see p. 243). Formally re-evaluate women who have used Depo-Provera for more than 2 years.

The usual treatment is 150 mg Depo-Provera im every 12–13 weeks. The second choice injectable progestogen is Noristerat which is given every 8 weeks. The first injection should be given within the first 5 days of the cycle to give immediate contraceptive effect.

Late injections. The only reason for not giving an injection is a possibility that the woman has already conceived. Consider emergency contraception (see below), if appropriate, with the next injection. Pregnancy must otherwise be excluded before the next injection.

PROGESTOGEN-RELEASING IMPLANT (IMPLANON)

This etonogestrel-releasing single flexible rod is inserted subdermally into the lower surface of the upper arm. Special training is required, although the technique is not difficult.

- It should be inserted during the first 5 days of the cycle to give immediate contraceptive effect.
- It is effective for up to 3 years. In women with a BMI >35 it should be replaced after 2 years.
- The side-effects and contraindications are as for the POP.
- The contraceptive effect is immediately reversible on removal of the implant.

POSTCOITAL (EMERGENCY) CONTRACEPTION

Postcoital contraception is sometimes needed as an emergency measure to prevent pregnancy when unprotected intercourse has put the woman at risk.

HORMONAL EMERGENCY CONTRACEPTION

Assessment

History. Ask about:

- contraindications:
  - pregnancy
  - porphyria
- LMP
- normal menstrual cycle

- times of all unprotected intercourse during the present cycle
- present method of contraception.

For advice on when to consider postcoital contraception in a COC or POP taker, see pp. 6 and 18.

Management

Advice

> **Tip**
> Hormonal postcoital contraception is effective for up to 72 hours after intercourse, in preventing implantation (60% of pregnancies are prevented when treatment is given between 72 and 120 hours after UPSI (unlicensed use)).

- The failure rate is 1–2%.
- The sooner it is started after unprotected intercourse, the greater the efficacy.
- Nausea occurs occasionally. If vomiting occurs within 2 hours of taking it, a further dose should be taken together with an antiemetic.
- The next period may be early or late.
- Barrier methods should be used until the next period.
- Discuss future contraception.
- There is no known teratogenic effect if the method fails.
- A pill taker should continue to take her usual pills in the normal way and be warned that she may get spotting in that cycle.
- This method may be used more than once in any one cycle.
- Available OTC for those aged 16 or over.

Prescribing. Levonorgestrel 1.5 mg as a single dose. Also available OTC.

Follow-up. This is not usually necessary. It may be arranged 1 month later in order to establish that the patient is not pregnant. Discuss future contraception.

EMERGENCY IUCD

Assessment

History. Ask about:

- contraindications: the majority of general contraindications to the IUCD apply (see p. 14). However, the IUCD *can* be used for postcoital contraception in women with a past history of an ectopic pregnancy, in nulliparous women and in women with a recent history of pelvic inflammatory disease (providing antibiotic cover is given)

- LMP
- normal menstrual cycle
- times of all unprotected intercourse during the present cycle
- present method of contraception.

Management

Advice

- The IUCD can be fitted up to 5 days after unprotected intercourse or up to 5 days after the most probable calculated date of ovulation, e.g. day 19 of a regular 28-day cycle.
- It can be removed after the next period or kept for long-term contraception, if appropriate.

CONDOM

The failure rate of the condom is <1/100 couple-years if used correctly.

Management

Advice

- A condom should be used every time intercourse takes place.
- It should always be used with a spermicide.
- The base of the condom should be held during withdrawal.

> **Tip**
> The condom is the only contraceptive which effectively protects against STI and AIDS.

Administration

The condom is not prescribable on FP10 but is free at Family Planning Clinics and GP surgeries. Available OTC.

DIAPHRAGM

The failure rate of the diaphragm is about 4/100 woman-years.

At the initial fitting, check the smear status. Advise the woman to practise insertion at home and, if appropriate, to use the diaphragm during intercourse with additional contraception until the first follow-up.

Management

Advice

- Always use a spermicide with the diaphragm.
- Insert the diaphragm any time prior to intercourse.
- Insert additional spermicide (a pessary or foam) prior to each episode of intercourse taking place more than 2 hours after initial insertion.
- Leave the diaphragm in place for at least 6 hours after intercourse, up to a maximum of 24 hours.
- Check the diaphragm intermittently for holes.
- A diaphragm usually lasts for 1–2 years.

Follow-up

- This should be about 10 days or shortly after fitting, and then annually.
- Check the position of the diaphragm, after the woman has inserted it herself.
- Recheck:
  - if the woman's weight changes by more than 3.5 kg (8 lb)
  - at the 6-week postnatal check
  - after vaginal surgery.

Administration

Prescribe the device and a spermicide on FP10. The cost and administration of the diaphragm can be claimed from the PPA.

INTRAUTERINE CONTRACEPTIVE DEVICE (IUCD)

The failure rate of the IUCD is in the range 0.3–2/100 woman-years. It renders the endometrium unsuitable for implantation.

Assessment

History. Ask about/think about contraindications:

- undiagnosed irregular genital tract bleeding
- pregnancy
- pelvic inflammatory disease (within the previous 6 months)
- previous ectopic pregnancy
- distortion of the uterine cavity
- past history of bacterial endocarditis or valve replacement.
- the IUCD is less suitable for nulliparous women and those with menorrhagia or dysmenorrhoea (see IUS, p. 16).

Management

Insertion. Insertion should be in the first 14 days of the cycle and the contraceptive effect is immediate.

Women at high risk of *Chlamydia* infection should be screened (see p. 46). Take swabs for *Chlamydia* and await results before inserting IUCD, if possible. Those at high risk:

- age <25 years
- more than one sexual partner in the preceding 12 months
- emergency IUCD request
- previous STI
- symptoms of infection.

Advice

- The patient should check the threads weekly for 6 weeks, and monthly thereafter, ideally right at the end of a period.
- Warn the patient about crampy pains for 2–3 days after insertion.
- Tampons can be used.
- Irregular spotting may occur in the first cycle.
- Periods may be heavier and more prolonged.
- Any normal discharge may be heavier.
- Menstrual irregularity and pelvic pain require exclusion of an ectopic pregnancy.

Follow-up. At 6 weeks, and then annually:

- Check threads.
- Check smear status.
- Exclude anaemia, if appropriate.
- Consider replacement/alternative contraception, if appropriate.

Main disadvantages of IUCDs

- Dysmenorrhoea and menorrhagia (especially in the first 3 months).
- Pelvic infection (see p. 45).
- Perforation.
- Expulsion.
- Lost threads. If the threads are lost, exclude pregnancy and advise temporary alternative contraception. The device may be within the uterus, have perforated the uterus or have been expelled. Try retrieving the threads by inserting Spencer–Wells forceps into the endocervical canal. If unsuccessful, arrange an ultrasound. If the IUCD is seen to be in the uterine cavity and does not need changing, leave in situ. Arrange gynaecological assessment, if appropriate.
- Intrauterine pregnancy. If the IUCD is in situ, there is an increased risk of miscarriage and, therefore, of infection. The risk can be reduced if the IUCD is gently removed as early as possible. If the pregnancy is >12 weeks, refer to an obstetrician.
- Ectopic pregnancy. (1 in 10–20 pregnancies occurring with the IUCD are extrauterine.) The patient should be advised to report pelvic pain or abnormal bleeding.

Removal. All coils are licensed for 5 years' use (the T Safe 380 A is licensed for 8 years). They should be removed during a period or following 7 days abstinence or protected intercourse. If an IUCD is fitted in a woman over the age of 40, it may remain in the uterus until the menopause.

If the woman is planning a pregnancy, she should delay conception until 1 month after removal of the IUCD to allow time for normal endometrium to regenerate.

The IUCD should be removed 2 years after the menopause in women under the age of 50 years, and 1 year after the menopause in women over the age of 50 years.

Tip

If the IUCD is removed intermenstrually, alternative contraception should be used for 7 days prior to removal.

INTRAUTERINE PROGESTOGEN-ONLY SYSTEM (MIRENA/IUS)

This is highly effective, with a failure rate of 0.2/100 woman-years. It results in a lower ectopic pregnancy rate than in women using no method. It usually leads to oligomenorrhoea or amenorrhoea, and is therefore suitable for women with heavy periods. Dysmenorrhoea and the risk of pelvic infection are reduced, compared to normal. It is suitable for nulliparous women as well as those who have had children. It is effective for 5 years. Return of fertility is rapid after removal. Fitting should be in the first 14 days of the cycle. If fitted after day 7 of the cycle, condoms should be used for the following 7 days.

Insertion is more painful than with standard IUCDs in view of an inserter of greater diameter, and intermenstrual spotting is a common problem in the early months of use. Spotting may occasionally continue for up to 6 months.

The IUS can be combined with systemic oestrogen for relief of menopausal symptoms, providing endometrial protection and effective contraception for perimenopausal women.

NATURAL BIRTH CONTROL

CALENDAR METHOD

This should only be considered when periods are regular. The period of abstinence required is often long. In a 28-day cycle, ovulation is around day 14 and the fertile period is between days 8 and 17. The released ovum survives for 1 day. The sperm survives for up to 6 days within the female body.

Method of calculation

- Define the shortest and longest menstrual cycle over the previous 12 months.
- To derive the first day of the fertile period, subtract 20 from the length of the shortest cycle. (14 days = maximum length of a luteal phase; 6 days = maximum sperm survival.)
- To derive the last day of the fertile period, subtract 11 from the length of the longest cycle. (12 days = minimum length of a luteal phase; 1 day = maximum ovum survival.)

This method has a high failure rate, even with good compliance.

PERSONA

This machine is available over the counter. The woman's hormone profile is analysed using daily urine testing strips, giving an indication of the 'safe period'.

MUCOTHERMAL METHOD

Intercourse should be confined to between 72 hours following the detection of ovulation and the onset of the next menstrual period. Ovulation can be detected by:

- a rise in basal body temperature
- thinning of cervical mucus (Billing's method).

STERILISATION

Both partners must accept that surgical sterilisation should be considered to be irreversible. Sterilisation should not be performed immediately postpartum or post-TOP, as regret is more likely if the decision is made at a time of stress.

The failure rate of sterilisation is about 0.2/100 woman-years.

Assessment

History. Ask about:

- the age of the man and the woman
- the number and ages of their children, and their health
- the menstrual history
- present contraception
- relationship stability.

Discuss:

- the irreversibility of sterilisation
- alternative forms of contraception

- the pros and cons of male versus female sterilisation
- complications (these should be discussed by the surgeon).

Laparoscopic sterilisation is usually performed as a day case under general or local anaesthetic. It may require 1 week off work.

Vasectomy is usually a local anaesthetic outpatient procedure. Sperm clearance takes about 20 ejaculations. It takes two sterile semen specimens, 4 months after vasectomy, 2 weeks apart, to confirm its contraceptive effect.

Examination. Examine the male genitalia for vasectomy.

Administration

The patient should sign a consent form, as appropriate.

HORMONAL CONTRACEPTION IN THE PERIMENOPAUSE

Contraception should be continued for 1 year after the LMP in women over the age of 50 years, and for 2 years in women under the age of 50.

THE COC

Women who smoke and those with other cardiovascular risk factors should stop the COC at the age of about 35. Fit, normotensive non-smokers with no family history of cardiovascular disease may continue the COC until the age of 50 (consider a 20 μg oestrogen pill, as the absolute risk of cardiovascular disease and breast cancer increases with age).

Synthetic oestrogens in the COC reduce perimenopausal symptoms.

THE POP

The POP does not usually disguise the menopause. Vasomotor symptoms may occur while taking it and the serum FSH may be raised. The failure rate in older women is minimal and is equivalent to the COC in younger women.

In order to establish whether or not natural periods have ceased, stop the COC/POP and use non-hormonal contraception:

- The onset of vasomotor symptoms together with amenorrhoea indicates the menopause, and contraception only needs to be continued for 1 year if over 50 or 2 years if under 50.
- If periods return, the COC/POP may be resumed. (Whether amenorrhoea occurs or periods return, HRT may be started with non-hormonal contraception, if appropriate.)
- Two FSH levels of >30 IU/l, 3 months apart, indicate the menopause.

POSTPARTUM CONTRACEPTION

No contraception is necessary for the first 25 days postpartum. If breast-feeding, avoid the COC, as oestrogen may inhibit lactation.

When to start

- COC and POP: can be started at 21 days postpartum.
- IUCD/IUS: can be inserted at 6 weeks (postnatal check) or at 12 weeks after a caesarean section.
- Diaphragm: can be fitted at 6 weeks (postnatal check).

CHAPTER 2

OBSTETRICS

Preconceptual counselling   22

Booking visit   23

Subsequent antenatal visits   25

Prenatal screening and
diagnosis   25

Bleeding in early pregnancy
(<14 weeks)   27

Bleeding in later pregnancy   28

Nausea and vomiting   28

Heartburn   28

Swollen ankles   29

Varicose veins   29

Glycosuria   29

Proteinuria   30

Anaemia   30

Rhesus-negative mothers   31

Pre-eclampsia   31

Abnormal lie   32

High head   32

Back pain   32

Postpartum bleeding   32

Postpartum pyrexia   33

Postnatal depression   33

Postnatal check   34

Breast-feeding   35

PRECONCEPTUAL COUNSELLING

Preconceptual counselling ensures that the woman is fully informed about measures which may be taken to protect herself and the developing foetus during any future pregnancy.

Assessment

History. Ask about:

- past medical and obstetric history, family history and social problems
- present contraception.

Examination

- Check the pre-pregnancy blood pressure.
- Perform a cervical smear, if due.

Investigations

- Rubella antibodies should be checked before the first pregnancy. If the woman is non-immune she should be vaccinated and should avoid conception for 1 month.
- If the woman has had a previous large baby (>4.5 kg), consider performing a fasting blood glucose and a modified GTT.
- Arrange haemoglobin electrophoresis to exclude thalassaemia trait in those from southern Europe, the Indian subcontinent and the Far East, and sickle cell trait in Afro-Caribbeans. All pregnant women and partners of carriers should be offered screening. Refer couples who are both heterozygous.

Management

Advice

Smoking and alcohol. Women should be advised to stop smoking and to reduce their alcohol intake to a minimum.

Diet and nutrition

- Advise a well-balanced diet.
- Advise a diet rich in folic acid (green vegetables, bread, potatoes, fruit and fortified cereals). Advise all women to take supplements of folic acid, 400 mg per day, from before conception to 12 weeks of gestation. This may reduce the risk of neural tube defects. (Folic acid can be prescribed on FP10 or bought OTC.)
- To minimise the risk of listeriosis, avoid unpasteurised soft cheeses, cooked chilled foods, prepacked salads and pâtés.
- To minimise the risk of toxoplasmosis, avoid undercooked meat, wash all vegetables and fruit prior to consumption, and avoid handling soil or cat faeces.

- Avoid high vitamin A intake.
- Avoid peanuts.
- Advise a high-calcium diet or calcium supplements for women who may require it, e.g. grand multiparous women or those who are socially deprived.

Contraception. If oral contraception or an IUCD is being used, one natural period without contraception should ideally be allowed before conception.

Referral

Obstetric problems

- Previous miscarriages: if the woman has had three or more miscarriages, refer for assessment of, e.g. cervical incompetence (which tends to cause mid-trimester miscarriages) or chromosomal abnormalities.
- Previous still births, foetal abnormalities or a family history of foetal abnormalities: refer for genetic counselling where this is likely to be beneficial. Advise, where appropriate, on antenatal screening and diagnosis. If the patient has a previous history or family history of a neural tube defect, advise her to take folic acid 5 mg daily from 1 month prior to stopping contraception to 12 weeks of gestation.

Medical problems

- Hypertension: refer for assessment. Methyldopa and some beta blockers, e.g. propranolol, are known to be safe and effective in pregnancy.
- Diabetes: refer for assessment. Perinatal mortality is around 10%, even with excellent control of blood sugar, which is crucial. The incidence of congenital abnormalities can be significantly reduced by good blood sugar control both before and during pregnancy. HbA_{1c} levels should be checked before stopping contraception.
- Epilepsy: refer for assessment. Congenital abnormalities are more than twice as common as usual. All anticonvulsants increase the incidence of foetal abnormalities to varying degrees, and this has to be assessed against the risk of untreated epilepsy and convulsions during pregnancy.

BOOKING VISIT

The booking visit is ideally between 8 and 14 weeks, and usually requires a 20–30 minute appointment.

Diagnosis

Pregnancy can be confirmed by home or laboratory testing of an early morning urine specimen taken after a missed period, measuring urinary HCG.

> **Tip**
> A diagnosis of pregnancy can usually be made on the history alone.

History. Ask about:

- LMP (and degree of certainty of that date), and calculate EDD
- age, occupation, race of both patient and partner (if appropriate), medical and obstetric problems (see p. 23), socioeconomic background, family history, alcohol, smoking and dental hygiene.

Examination

- BP
- weight
- heart
- lungs
- legs (for varicose veins)
- abdomen.

Vaginal examination is unnecessary.

Investigations

- Urine: check for protein and sugar and send an MSU.
- Bloods:
  - Hb
  - ABO and rhesus groups and antibodies
  - VDRL and hepatitis B status
  - HIV status (this is now routinely checked with patient consent)
  - rubella antibodies
  - consider testing for haemoglobinopathies (see p. 22)
  - arrange serum AFP and a 'triple test'/integrated test if required at appropriate times (see p. 26).
- Ultrasound scan (see p. 26): consider
  - a dating scan at 7–11 weeks
  - a nuchal scan at 10–13 weeks
  - an anomaly scan at 18–20 weeks.

Management

After assessing risk factors, discuss the most appropriate form of antenatal and intrapartum care. The usual options are 'shared care' (the patient's care is shared between hospital doctors and GPs/midwives, and the mother is delivered by the hospital team) and community care (involving the GP and the community midwives with delivery in hospital, community units or at home). Arrangements and criteria for low-risk community units will vary according to the locality. Refer as appropriate.

Advice

- Discuss diet (see p. 22).
- Discuss prenatal screening and diagnosis (see p. 25), as appropriate.

- Discuss the woman's concerns and expectations with regard to the pregnancy and delivery.

Administration

- Complete form FW8. This authorises free prescriptions and dental care throughout the pregnancy and for 12 months after delivery.
- Complete the relevant maternity hospital registration form.

SUBSEQUENT ANTENATAL VISITS

Follow-up intervals vary. Normal multigravidae require at least six antenatal check-ups at 12, 16, 22, 30, 36 and 40 weeks. In addition, normal primigravidae require check-ups at 26, 34, 38 and 41 weeks.

History. Ask about:

- general health
- gestation.

Examination

- Blood pressure.
- Look for oedema.
- Fundal height.
- Foetal presentation (from 32 weeks).
- Foetal movements/foetal heart (Doppler, e.g. Sonicaid, can detect the foetal heart from 12 weeks of gestation).

Investigations

- Urinalysis for protein and sugar.
- At 28 and 34 weeks re-check Hb and ABO and rhesus groups.
- Prenatal screening (see below), as appropriate.

Administration

Complete form Mat B1 at 26 weeks, if appropriate.

PRENATAL SCREENING AND DIAGNOSIS

SCREENING TESTS

All women may be offered ultrasound, serum AFP and the triple test or integrated test as part of routine screening. Discussion of the pros and cons of these tests must take account of the patient's feelings regarding termination of pregnancy. False-positive results can cause considerable unnecessary anxiety. Diagnostic tests are necessary to confirm a positive screening test.

Ultrasound

- Dating scans: estimation of gestation is more accurate early in pregnancy, from 7–11 weeks. Helpful if the LMP is uncertain. Often now routine if screening tests are to be accurately timed.
- Nuchal scans: performed at 10–13 weeks can detect 80% of Down's syndrome babies (only available privately in some areas).
- Foetal anomaly scans: best performed at 18–20 weeks and usually organised routinely. Various abnormalities can be detected, including:
  - cranial and neural tube defects
  - abnormalities of the heart, chest and abdominal organs
  - cleft lip and palate.

Serum AFP. This is performed from 15 weeks. A high level indicates a higher risk of neural tube defect, or twins. A low level indicates a higher risk of Down's syndrome.

Triple test. This is a blood test, performed between 15 and 21 weeks and in some areas only available privately; it estimates the risk of Down's syndrome and neural tube defects. The estimated risk of Down's syndrome is based on serum AFP, HCG and unconjugated oestriol, as well as maternal age. The risk of a neural tube defect is based on AFP alone. It is particularly helpful for older mothers. (The risk of Down's at age 35 years is 1:400, while at age 40 it is 1:100.)

Integrated test. This is the best available screening test. It involves:

- a 10–13 week nuchal scan
- a 10 week assay of serum pregnancy associated protein A
- a 14 week quadruple test (serum AFP, B-HCG, unconjugated oestriol and inhibin-A).

The measurements are integrated into a single screening result, taking account of maternal age. The test detects 92% of Down's syndrome babies, with a false-positive rate of only 0.9%. Other tests involving a nuchal scan and blood tests are also available. In most areas they are only available privately.

DIAGNOSTIC TESTS

Chorionic villus biopsy. This is performed at 8–12 weeks, allowing termination in the first trimester if an abnormality is confirmed. It enables early detection of chromosomal abnormalities and other rare genetic diseases. There is a 1–2% miscarriage rate. Limb deformities are a rare risk of this biopsy.

Amniocentesis. This is performed at 15–16 weeks, allowing termination before 20 weeks if an abnormality is confirmed. The miscarriage rate is 0.5–1%. It detects Down's syndrome, X-linked disorders (e.g. haemophilia and Duchenne muscular dystrophy) and some inborn errors of metabolism (e.g. Tay–Sachs disease). Results of fluid analysis for AFP usually take 1 week, while cell culture for karyotype or biochemistry takes 3 weeks. Anti-D is given if the woman is rhesus negative.

BLEEDING IN EARLY PREGNANCY (<14 WEEKS)

Diagnosis

History. Ask about:

- the extent of the bleeding, including the presence of clots, and whether or not pelvic pain is present
- rhesus blood group.

Examination. This is not necessary if the bleeding is slight and there is no pain. An open cervix, confirmed on vaginal examination, suggests an inevitable abortion and a non-viable pregnancy.

Investigation. Arrange an urgent ultrasound scan to assess foetal viability.

Management

For vaginal spotting without pain:

- Telephone advice is usually adequate.
- Advise to rest at home.

For vaginal bleeding with pain:

- Mild discomfort and light bleeding can usually be managed at home.
- Worsening pain usually suggests the need for admission, especially if it is associated with the passing of clots.
- An open cervix confirms the need for admission. If the bleeding is heavy, remove any products of conception, with a gloved hand, and give syntometrine im, 1 ml.

Tip
Vaginal bleeding at >12 weeks in a rhesus-negative woman requires an injection of anti-D 500 IU im within 72 hours of the start of bleeding. At <12 weeks, anti-D only needs to be given if the bleeding is heavy, e.g. ERPC is required.

If the miscarriage is complete (i.e. products have been passed and the pain and bleeding have settled):

- Advise rest at home and arrange early review.
- Tell the patient to contact the doctor if bleeding recurs.
- Give an explanation, as appropriate:
  - the likely cause is foetal abnormality or implantation failure
  - investigation is not useful in first-trimester miscarriages unless there have been three or more.
- Bereavement counselling is often important.

If the pregnancy continues and the symptoms settle:

- Review. If not already performed, arrange an ultrasound scan to exclude a missed abortion.
- Explain that bleeding in pregnancy does not increase the risk of foetal abnormalities.

BLEEDING IN LATER PREGNANCY

After 14 weeks, admission should be arranged when bleeding occurs, with or without pain. Bleeding with severe pain is likely to be due to placental abruption. If the woman's blood group is rhesus negative, she requires an injection of anti-D 500 IU im within 72 hours of the start of bleeding.

Do not perform a vaginal examination after 14 weeks in case of placenta praevia.

NAUSEA AND VOMITING

Vomiting in pregnancy can be extremely debilitating and the patient often requires considerable support and reassurance.

Management

- Explain that the symptoms are likely to resolve by 14–16 weeks.
- Encourage fluids (carbonated drinks can be helpful) and frequent, small, plain meals.
- Consider drug treatment if the symptoms are severe, e.g. promethazine 25 mg mane, 50 mg nocte.
- Consider admission if vomiting is prolonged or dehydration is a concern.

HEARTBURN

Heartburn usually worsens as pregnancy progresses. It can be exacerbated by oral iron.

Management

- Recommend frequent small meals.
- Prescribe an antacid with a low sodium content, e.g. Maalox 10 ml after meals or prn.

SWOLLEN ANKLES

Swollen ankles are common in pregnancy.

Management

- Exclude pre-eclampsia. (Check for more generalised oedema, hypertension and/or proteinuria.)
- Advise the patient to avoid long periods of standing. If oedema becomes uncomfortable, advise her to sit with the ankles above the level of the hips when resting, and to wear support stockings or tights (see below).

VARICOSE VEINS

Varicose veins tend to worsen with each pregnancy.

Management

- Avoid long periods of standing.
- Advise the patient to sit with the ankles above the level of the hips when resting, and to wear support stockings or tights. Support stockings are obtainable on FP10 in three grades. Support tights are usually more comfortable, but are only available OTC. Support hosiery should ideally be put on before getting out of bed in the morning.
- Surgery should be avoided until the woman has completed her family.

GLYCOSURIA

Misleading detection of postprandial glycosuria can be avoided by testing an early morning specimen.

Modified glucose tolerance test

After two episodes of glycosuria a modified glucose tolerance test should be performed:

- Measure fasting blood glucose.
- Give a 75 g oral load of glucose (e.g. 350 ml of Lucozade).
- Measure blood glucose again after 2 hours.

Management

Fasting values of >5.8 mmol/l or 2-hour values of >9.5 mmol/l suggest gestational diabetes, and the patient should be referred urgently.

PROTEINURIA

A trace of protein in the urine can be ignored.

Management

- Check the blood pressure to exclude pre-eclampsia.
- Arrange an MSU to exclude a UTI.
- If the MSU is negative, exclude any underlying renal disease by checking serum creatinine and 24-hour urinary protein. (Proteinuria in pregnancy is defined as >300 mg/l.)
- Refer as appropriate.

ANAEMIA

The importance of severe anaemia during pregnancy is that perinatal mortality is increased and postpartum haemorrhage may become life-threatening.

Haemoglobin is measured routinely at booking, and at 28 and 34 weeks. The Hb concentration falls during pregnancy due to haemodilution. A low to normal Hb (10–11 g/dl) with a normal MCV and MCH suggests simple haemodilution. A pregnant woman is anaemic if the Hb is <10.

Management

Mild anaemia can initially be assumed to be secondary to iron deficiency and treated with, e.g., Pregaday, one tablet daily (100 mg elemental iron as ferrous fumarate and 350 mg of folate). Check the Hb 2 weeks later. It should rise at the rate of 0.5 g/dl per week. If the response is poor, or if the anaemia is more severe, double the dose of Pregaday. Check 2 weeks later, and refer if the haemoglobin is <9.

Iron prophylaxis

This should be given to those at high risk of deficiency, e.g. those with:

- a poor diet
- closely spaced pregnancies
- a past history of iron deficiency anaemia.

Folate prophylaxis

This should be given to all mothers at a dose of 400 mg per day up to 12 weeks of pregnancy. A higher dose of 5 mg per day should be given to mothers with a previous spina bifida child or a family history of spina bifida, as well as to mothers with:

- a past history of folate deficiency
- malabsorption
- haemoglobinopathies
- anticonvulsant therapy, e.g. phenytoin
- multiple pregnancies
- grand multiparity.

RHESUS-NEGATIVE MOTHERS

Fifteen per cent of women are rhesus negative. If the baby is rhesus positive and foetal red cells cross into the maternal circulation, maternal antibodies are produced. These cross back to the foetus, causing haemolysis.

Management

- Take blood at booking, and at 28 and 34 weeks to screen for rhesus antibodies.
- Anti-D may be administered routinely to rhesus-negative mothers at specific times in the pregnancy (e.g. primips at 28 weeks, 34–36 weeks and at delivery). Check the local protocol.

Give 500 IU of anti-D immunoglobulin to all rhesus-negative women after:

- spontaneous abortion (if >12 weeks)
- termination of pregnancy
- amniocentesis
- ectopic pregnancy
- antepartum haemorrhage
- delivery.

PRE-ECLAMPSIA

Pre-eclampsia occurs in 2–3% of all pregnancies. Its detection is the most important aim of antenatal care in general practice. It is suggested, after >20 weeks, by a BP above 140/90 or a rise in diastolic pressure of more than 20 mmHg from booking. The presence of proteinuria is an additional indication of pre-eclampsia. Pretibial or generalised oedema may also be present.
   Risk factors include:

- PMH or FH of pre-eclampsia
- diabetes
- primips and twin pregnancies
- maternal age >40

- diastolic BP >80 at booking
- increased BMI at booking.

Women should be aware of the early signs and symptoms including headaches, abdominal pain and vomiting.

Arrange urgent hospital assessment. If the mother is not admitted, the hospital will advise on frequency of follow-up.

ABNORMAL LIE

An oblique or transverse lie or breech presentation should be referred for hospital assessment from 34 weeks for discussion of possible trial of external cephalic version and/or mode of delivery.

HIGH HEAD

A 'high head' (i.e. one that lies totally outside the pelvis) is of less significance in a multiparous woman who has already experienced a vaginal delivery than in a primiparous woman. Before making this diagnosis, ensure that the bladder is empty. It is useful to ask the patient to lift her upper body onto her elbows. This may cause the head to descend. Refer primiparous women at 34 weeks for consultant assessment, and arrange an ultrasound to assess placental position. Multiparous women should be referred at 38 weeks for assessment of placental position, if not already known.

BACK PAIN

Back pain in pregnancy is usually lumbar, secondary to ligament laxity.

Management

- Advise on posture: try to eliminate, as far as possible, the lumbar lordosis when standing and sitting.
- Avoid heavy lifting.
- An elastic back support may be helpful (obtainable OTC or from the maternity physiotherapy department).
- Consider referral to maternity physiotherapy.

POSTPARTUM BLEEDING

> **Tip**
> The lochia usually disappear by 6 weeks. However, they may persist for some further weeks, and as long as they are decreasing and fading to pink or brown the patient can be reassured.

If the lochia remain red but bleeding is mild, consider using oral ergometrine 500 μg tds for 3 days. Co-amoxiclav 1 tds for 7 days may be useful in suspected endometritis (see below).

If bleeding is excessive (especially if there are clots present) or if the patient is pyrexial, admit with a view to ultrasound and/or ERPC.

POSTPARTUM PYREXIA

UTIs, DVTs and breast infections may present with pyrexia. Patients with endometritis (fever, foul discharge and low abdominal pain) should be admitted with a view to ERPC and/or intravenous antibiotics. (Foul lochia without fever can be treated at home with amoxicillin and metronidazole, or co-amoxiclav.)

POSTNATAL DEPRESSION

The maternity blues are considered to be normal. They are experienced by one-half to two-thirds of mothers, and usually occur in the first week. Postnatal depression, however, affects 10–15% of mothers, usually within the first 3 postnatal months.

Diagnosis
As with other forms of depression, the patient is not always aware that she is depressed, and diagnosis can be difficult. The Edinburgh Postnatal Depression Questionnaire is a useful screening tool which can be completed by all mothers. Women who score >9 should be assessed further.

Check for a physical cause, e.g. anaemia or hypothyroidism.

History

Risk factors for postnatal depression

- A past history of depression.
- A family history of depression.
- Problems in the early relationship between the patient and her own mother.
- Marital problems.
- Stressful life events.
- Emotional problems during the pregnancy.
- A first pregnancy.

Management

- The health visitor can play an important role in non-directive counselling. Encourage women to discuss their own needs separately from those of the baby.

- Antidepressants play an important role. Most are secreted in breast milk. Lofepramine 140–210 mg daily in divided doses is safe for breast-feeding mothers. The higher dose is often necessary.
- Consider involving other social support agencies, e.g. a social worker.
- Refer for counselling or to a psychiatrist, as appropriate.
- See depression (p. 292).

POSTNATAL CHECK

This takes place at 6 weeks. It is often the first time that the GP and the mother meet after the immediate postnatal period. It is a particularly important time to assess maternal mood.

Assessment

History. Ask about:

- any continuing vaginal bleeding (persisting brown lochia is neither uncommon nor abnormal; see also p. 32)
- feelings about the birth and postnatal period
- sleep, mood, perineal discomfort, incontinence and breast- or bottle-feeding
- contraception
- rubella status.

Examination

- BP (especially if raised in pregnancy).
- Weight (if appropriate).
- Abdomen for muscle laxity. When divarication of the recti muscles is significant (i.e. three or more fingers' breadths can be inserted between them), consider referral to a maternity physiotherapist.
- Breasts, especially if there are specific problems, e.g. sore nipples.
- Perineal wounds. Intercourse may already be pain-free, but there is often residual perineal soreness and tenderness.
- If a cervical smear is due, it is ideally delayed until about 3 months postpartum.

Management

- See sections on breast-feeding (p. 35) and postnatal depression (p. 33), if appropriate.
- Discuss the importance of long-term abdominal and pelvic-floor exercises. Consider referral to a maternity physiotherapist if pelvic-floor weakness is significant.

BREAST-FEEDING

Many early breast-feeding problems, e.g. mastitis, sore nipples and infant colic, are likely to be due to a failure to position the baby correctly on the breast. Therefore, always ensure a good feeding position. The midwife and health visitor are best placed to advise. Encourage unrestricted, demand feeding in order to stimulate lactation, and advise the mother to avoid giving the baby additional water or supplementary feeds, if possible.

SORE OR CRACKED NIPPLES

- Check positioning: the nipple should be in the roof of the baby's mouth, thus avoiding friction from the tongue.
- Encourage continued suckling as far as possible.
- Creams, ointments and local treatments are probably not effective.
- Apply breast milk to sore nipples and allow them to dry.

ENGORGEMENT

- Check positioning.
- Encourage continued suckling.
- A good supportive bra is helpful.
- It is often helpful to express engorged breasts gently before feeds. This may be more comfortable in a warm bath.
- Cold compresses between feeds may be soothing.

BLOCKED DUCTS (causing tender lumps)

- Check positioning.
- Feed on the tender breast first.
- Gentle massage of a hard lump while feeding may be helpful. The milk should be smoothed towards the nipple.

MASTITIS

- A segment of the breast is usually red and tender and the patient is often pyrexial.
- 50% of cases may be non-infective, i.e. related to poor positioning, engorgement or localised obstructions (see above).
- If appropriate, treat with flucloxacillin 500 mg qds for 5 days (or erythromycin if the patient is allergic to penicillin). Antibiotic treatment will alter the taste of the milk and may cause the baby to develop mild diarrhoea.

SUPPRESSION OF LACTATION

- Lactation is naturally suppressed within 5 days of the cessation of breast-feeding.
- Advise simple analgesia and good breast support only.
- If lactation needs to be stopped more quickly, e.g. after stillbirth, prescribe bromocriptine 2.5 mg daily for 3 days and then increase to 2.5 mg bd for 2 weeks.

CHAPTER 3

GYNAECOLOGY

Premenstrual syndrome   38

Intermenstrual (or postcoital) bleeding   39

Postmenopausal bleeding   40

Irregular periods   40

Dysmenorrhoea   40

Menorrhagia   42

Amenorrhoea   43

Pelvic pain   44

Vaginal discharge   45

Sexually transmitted infections   46

Urethral syndrome   48

Hirsutism   48

Polycystic ovarian syndrome   49

Breast screening   50

Breast awareness   50

Breast cancer   51

Breast lumps   51

The menopause/climacteric   51

Hormone replacement therapy (HRT)   52

Cervical cancer   58

Infertility   59

Termination of pregnancy request   60

PREMENSTRUAL SYNDROME

Diagnosis

The diagnosis of premenstrual syndrome requires that the symptoms occur only in a particular phase of the ovarian cycle, nearly always at some time between ovulation and the onset of full menstrual flow.

> **Tip**
> The distinction between PMS and psychological disorders that become worse in the premenstrual phase is often difficult. Examination is unnecessary.

Management

Advice

- Support and reassurance are vital, as there is undoubtedly a strong placebo effect.
- A menstrual diary, kept for at least 3 months, is useful.
- Exercise should be encouraged. (Increased endorphin release may improve symptoms.)
- A healthy, well-balanced diet should be encouraged in order to maintain steady blood glucose levels.

Prescribing

- NSAIDs are useful for pain symptoms and often improve mood and bloating.
- Pyridoxine (vitamin B_6) 10 mg per day from day 14 to the onset of menstruation is often used initially. Its efficacy is in doubt. It is prescribable on FP10, and available OTC.
- Evening primrose oil (gamolenic acid) as a daily dose may be recommended. It is available OTC.
- Oestrogens may be used. (The rationale for their use is that cyclical ovarian activity is necessary for the symptoms of PMS, and oestrogens may suppress ovulation.)
  - The COC may be given. (Symptoms occasionally become worse.)
  - Transdermal oestradiol patches ($25–100 \mu g$) may be used twice a week, or consider an oestradiol implant (100 mg). Give concomitant treatment with a progestogen, e.g. norethisterone, 5 mg per day from day 19 to day 26, to prevent endometrial hyperplasia. Sequential combined oestrogen/progestogen patches are available.
- Progesterone and progestogens are often used, but there is no evidence of benefit. Treatment is given during the luteal phase only.

  – Natural progesterone has poor oral absorption and is therefore given PR or PV, 100–800 mg daily.
  – Synthetic progestogens (oral), e.g. dydrogesterone 10 mg bd or norethisterone 5 mg tds may be given. (The POP may be helpful.)
- SSRIs often help to relieve all aspects of PMS.
- Diuretics can be helpful for fluid retention in the luteal phase.
- Bromocriptine 2.5 mg od in the luteal phase can be helpful for cyclical breast pain.

INTERMENSTRUAL (OR POSTCOITAL) BLEEDING

Single episodes of non-menstrual bleeding are often innocent; the patient can usually be reassured and reviewed if the bleeding is persistent.

> **Tip**
> Persistent non-menstrual bleeding suggests a carcinoma until proven otherwise.

Diagnosis

History. Ask about:

- the duration of symptoms
- the amount and pattern of bleeding, e.g. postcoital, sporadic or regular
- contraception: if the woman is on the COC or the POP, query her compliance
- the possibility of pregnancy.

Examination. Examine the cervix and perform a smear and bimanual examination.

Investigations. Arrange a pregnancy test, if appropriate.

Management

- Ask about STI risk factors (see p. 2) and consider chlamydia screening (see p. 15). (Infection with chlamydia may cause a blood-stained discharge.) Consider referral to a GUM clinic.
- If the woman is on the COC and she has experienced breakthrough bleeding for more than 3 months, consider changing her pill to one with a higher progestogen content.
- If there is an IUCD in situ consider removing it if the symptoms persist for more than 3 months.
- Spotting may occur for up to 6 months after IUS insertion.

- Cervical erosions, if symptomatic, e.g. causing postcoital bleeding, can be treated with a silver nitrate stick, prescribable on FP10, or referred for treatment.
- Cervical polyps can be twisted and avulsed and sent for histology. Silver nitrate may be used on the resultant raw area. Always consider referral, especially if the base of the polyp is endocervical.

 Women over 40 should always be referred, unless the bleeding settles after removal of the presumed cause, e.g. a polyp. All women should be referred if the bleeding is persistent.

POSTMENOPAUSAL BLEEDING

Postmenopausal bleeding is any bleeding which occurs 1 year after the LMP.

Examination. Examine the vagina for, e.g. atrophic vaginitis (see p. 54), and the cervix, and perform a bimanual examination. Take a cervical smear, if appropriate.

Management
Women taking HRT should be referred for any significant unscheduled bleeding or consider review after stopping HRT.

Always refer to exclude malignancy, unless the bleeding is due to vaginitis which improves with treatment.

IRREGULAR PERIODS

Irregular periods are almost always a non-pathological variant of normal. They are most common at the extremes of reproductive life. The patient can usually be reassured. Irregular periods are a feature of POS (see p. 49). This symptom may progress to amenorrhoea (see p. 43).

DYSMENORRHOEA

Dysmenorrhoea, or painful menstruation, is common and can be severe, causing absence from school or work. It is usually fairly easy to differentiate between primary and secondary dysmenorrhoea.

PRIMARY DYSMENORRHOEA

(That is, there is no pelvic pathology.)

Diagnosis

History

- It is common in young girls.
- It usually appears within 12 months of the menarche.
- Pain tends to occur within the first 2 days of the period.
- Enquire into factors that have been associated with dysmenorrhoea: smoking, overweight, alcohol and stress.

Management

- Prostaglandin synthetase inhibitors, e.g. mefenamic acid 250–500 mg tds or naproxen 250–500 mg bd are usually helpful.
- The COC is especially useful, particularly when contraception is required.

SECONDARY DYSMENORRHOEA

(That is, the dysmenorrhoea is associated with pelvic pathology, e.g. endometriosis, pelvic inflammatory disease or adenomyosis.)

Diagnosis

History

- The dysmenorrhoea usually starts several years after the menarche.
- There is often a clear change in the degree and timing of the pain.
- The pain often starts well before the period and may continue throughout the period.
- Discuss the significance of the dysmenorrhoea and the effect of the pain on the patient's lifestyle, e.g. time off work.

Examination. Perform a speculum and bimanual examination to exclude any obvious pelvic pathology.

Management

- Consider removing an in situ IUCD.
- If the symptoms are suggestive of PID, see p. 44.
- Patients should be referred in order to exclude pelvic pathology.

ENDOMETRIOSIS

Endometriosis is a common cause of dysmenorrhoea, dyspareunia, pelvic pain and menorrhagia. Diagnosis is by laparoscopy. Women with infertility and worsening symptoms should be referred. Hormonal treatment aims to suppress ovulation for 6–12 months, during which time the lesions atrophy. Endometriosis usually resolves at the menopause. Pelvic pain may be treated with:

- prostaglandin synthetase inhibitors, e.g. mefenamic acid 250–500 mg tds, prn
- the COC (usually one with a high progestogen content, e.g. Eugynon 30), prescribed either with a pill-free break or continuously
- progestogens, e.g. norethisterone 10–15 mg daily on a continuous basis
- danazol 200–800 mg daily, adjusted to achieve amenorrhoea (inhibits gonadotrophin release). The dose can be titrated by balancing symptom control against side-effects, which are mainly androgenic
- GnRH analogues, e.g. buserelin nasal spray 300 µg tds for a maximum of 6 months (produces a reversible artificial menopause)
- surgery, e.g. local excision/diathermy of endometriotic tissue, or total hysterectomy and bilateral salpingo-oophorectomy.

MENORRHAGIA

Menorrhagia (regular heavy periods) is common at the extremes of reproductive life. Regular bleeding is relatively unlikely to be due to pelvic pathology.

Diagnosis

History. Ask about:

- the passing of clots
- symptoms of anaemia.

Examination and investigations

- Check the haemoglobin.
- Perform a bimanual examination to exclude an organic cause, e.g. an ovarian or uterine tumour. Arrange a pelvic ultrasound scan if appropriate.
- Check the serum FSH if the menopause is suspected.

Management

Treatment

- Advise the woman to keep a menstrual diary.
- If there is an IUCD in situ, consider its removal.

Prescribing

- Antifibrinolytics, e.g. tranexamic acid 1–1.5 g tds or qds at the start of heavy bleeding for 3–4 days.
- Mefenamic acid 250–500 mg tds: this should be taken during the worst few days of the period (it is used mainly for pain, and can be used in conjunction with tranexamic acid).

- COC: pills with a high progestogen content are more effective.
- To control torrential bleeding: prescribe norethisterone up to 10 mg tds. The bleeding should stop within 48 hours. The dose can then be reduced to 5 mg bd for 12 days. The patient will experience a bleed on stopping treatment.
- The IUS should be considered, particularly for women also requiring contraception (see p. 16).

Referral

If there is no response to treatment or if symptoms warrant it, consider referral for transcervical resection of the endometrium (TCRE), endometrial laser ablation (ELA) or hysterectomy.

Menorrhagia: referral criteria

Refer all women for gynaecological assessment if:
- the onset of menorrhagia is sudden
- there is a suggestion of an organic cause (e.g. an ovarian or uterine tumour, endometriosis, pelvic inflammatory disease).

AMENORRHOEA

A woman with absent periods is usually concerned about abnormal body function and future fertility, or about possible pregnancy.

Primary amenorrhoea. (i.e. when the menarche has not started by the age of 16 years):

- Causes: familial, structural (e.g. imperforate hymen), genetic (e.g. Turner's) and endocrine.
- Examine the external genitalia, and look for the development of secondary sexual characteristics.
- Check weight to exclude anorexia nervosa.
- Refer to a gynaecologist.

Secondary amenorrhoea. The usual cause is recent rapid weight loss, emotional upset or post-hormonal contraception, i.e. hypothalamic. (A common scenario is a young student starting college, having left home.) Always exclude pregnancy. The cause is otherwise nearly always hormonal.

Diagnosis

History. Ask about:

- date of the menarche
- LMP

- the normal cycle
- weight loss/eating disorder/stress
- drugs (e.g. the COC)
- galactorrhoea (this occurs in hyperprolactinaemia)
- menopausal symptoms (e.g. premature ovarian failure)
- hirsutism (this occurs in polycystic ovarian syndrome)
- general health (symptoms of, e.g. hypothyroidism, might be elicited).

Investigations

- Serum prolactin (raised in hyperprolactinaemia).
- Serum FSH/LH (raised in premature menopause).
- Serum testosterone (slightly raised, along with LH and sometimes prolactin, in polycystic ovarian syndrome).
- TFTs

Management

- If blood tests are normal, amenorrhoea can be assumed to be hypothalamic and the woman can be reassured that her periods will return.
- Secondary amenorrhoea due to anorexia nervosa should be referred appropriately.
- Contraception should be discussed, if appropriate. If the patient is trying to become pregnant, consider referral and/or treatment with clomiphene (see p. 60).
- If blood tests are abnormal, refer as appropriate.

PELVIC PAIN

Diagnosis

Try to exclude the following diagnoses on history and examination:

- Appendicitis.
- Ectopic pregnancy: consider this in all sexually active women with pelvic pain. If appropriate, do an immediate pregnancy test and arrange an urgent pelvic ultrasound (a negative pregnancy test does not always exclude an ectopic pregnancy). Arrange immediate referral if in doubt.
- A ruptured ovarian cyst.
- Acute pelvic inflammatory disease.
- Other pelvic pathology, e.g. endometriosis. (This last should always be considered when recurrent episodes of pelvic pain fail to respond to antibiotic treatment.)

Management of acute pelvic inflammatory disease (PID)

An HVS and endocervical swab (both in bacterial transport media) and an endocervical chlamydia swab (see p. 46) should be taken.

Treatment with antibiotics is usually given without a definite diagnosis, and should cover *Neisseria gonorrhoeae* and *Chlamydia* (the two major causes), and mixed aerobic and anaerobic infections. Treat with ofloxacin 400 mg bd and metronidazole 400 mg bd for 14 days.

IUCDs can be left in situ during treatment unless the infection is severe or persistent. Sexual contacts should be treated with doxycycline 100 mg od for 10 days. Always seriously consider referral to a GUM clinic. Admit the patient if symptoms are severe.

VAGINAL DISCHARGE

The most common causes of vaginal discharge in general practice are *Candida* and *Gardnerella* (bacterial vaginosis – BV). *Trichomonas* is a less common cause. *Chlamydia*, gonorrhoea and herpes simplex are rarely associated with vaginal discharge (see also STIs, p. 46).

- It is reasonable to treat first or occasional episodes of candida according to clinical findings, without doing swabs.
- An HVS in transport medium is needed for culture of *Candida*, BV, *Trichomonas* and most bacterial causes of pyogenic infection. An endocervical swab in transport medium is needed for gonococcal culture. An endocervical chlamydia swab is needed for chlamydia diagnosis. All three swabs should be taken in those with STI risk factors (see p. 2), although referral to a GUM clinic for investigation is preferable.
- Vaginal discharge is not, in itself, an indication for chlamydia testing (see p. 46).
- Non-infective causes of vaginal discharge include a cervical lesion or a foreign body.

CANDIDA

Candida is usually harboured by the woman, but can be sexually transmitted. The classic symptom is pruritus. The curdy white discharge may be minimal. It is often associated with dysuria and dyspareunia.

Management

Occasional symptoms. Treat with a topical imidazole, e.g. clotrimazole pessary 500 mg at night as a single dose. Clotrimazole 1% cream can be used in addition for vulval pruritus. Alternatively, treat with oral fluconazole 150 mg as a single dose. (All available OTC.)

Recurrent symptoms. (>3 per year):

- Advice, e.g. avoid nylon underwear and perfumed soaps.
- Exclude risk factors, e.g. antibiotics, diabetes, steroids.

- Treat the partner concurrently.
- Consider induction treatment as above, followed by a maintenance regimen for 3–6 months. Maintenance regimens include:
  - imidazole pessary (e.g. clotrimazole 500 mg) weekly
  - oral fluconazole 100 mg weekly
  - oral itraconazole 400 mg monthly, at expected time of symptoms.
- If *Candida* is caused by antibiotics, use prophylactic pessaries.
- If it is related to intercourse, insert a pessary after intercourse.

BACTERIAL VAGINOSIS (BV)

BV is not considered to be sexually transmitted. The thin, grey discharge is usually fishy-smelling.

Management

- Metronidazole 400 mg bd for 5 days.
- If symptoms are recurrent it may be worth treating the partner concurrently.

SEXUALLY TRANSMITTED INFECTIONS

In all STIs the partner should also be treated and sexual intercourse should be avoided until treatment is complete. Other recent sexual partners should be advised to seek medical advice.

Investigations should be performed to exclude the presence of any other STI. Referral to a GUM clinic is recommended for full investigation and for treatment of the patient and their sexual contacts (see p. 2 for considering possible STI risk).

TRICHOMONAS

Trichomonas is generally considered to be sexually transmitted and is often associated with other STIs. The discharge is usually frothy and yellow. Symptoms may include vaginal itching and soreness.

Management
Metronidazole 400 mg bd for 5 days.

CHLAMYDIA

See also p. 15 for opportunistic screening.

Chlamydia is a major cause of PID, tubal infertility and ectopic pregnancy. It is the commonest curable STI in the industrialised world. Most women with chlamydia are asymptomatic. An endocervical chlamydia swab should be taken.

Standard regimens for treatment of PID will cover chlamydia (see p. 44). Refer to a GUM clinic.

Management

- Doxycycline 100 mg bd for 7 days or azithromycin 1 g as a single dose. If pregnant or breast-feeding, erythromycin 500 mg qds for 7 days or 500 mg bd for 14 days.
- A test of cure investigation should be performed after treatment.

GONORRHOEA

Gonorrhoea is a major cause of PID. Patients should be referred to a GUM clinic. Remember chlamydia.

Management

- Treatment should be coordinated by the GUM clinic.
- Treat with e.g. single-dose ciprofloxacin 500 mg or ofloxacin 400 mg.

GENITAL WARTS

Genital warts are diagnosed by clinical appearance. They are caused by human papilloma virus (HPV).

Management

Treatment is usually coordinated by the GUM clinic

- Podophyllin paint is applied only to the warts. (Podophyllin should be avoided in pregnancy.) It should be left on for 4–6 hours, washed off, and reapplied every 3–7 days.
- Imiquimod cream is applied only to the warts, three times per week.
- Consider cryotherapy as an alternative treatment for external warts.
- Annual smears are recommended after a diagnosis of genital warts.

GENITAL HERPES

Genital herpes is usually diagnosed by symptoms and clinical appearance. Patients should know that one-third of genital herpes infections are acquired from a mouth lesion rather than via sexual contact, that the delay between contact and symptoms may be long, e.g. years, and that they are more likely than not never to have a further attack. A swab of suspicious lesions should be sent in viral transport medium.

Advice. Salt water baths and ice packs are helpful for painful lesions.

Management

- Analgesia, as appropriate.
- Treat with e.g. valaciclovir 500 mg bd for 5 days started as early as possible, but certainly within 7 days of the onset of symptoms.

Treatment of recurrent symptoms. Depending on the degree of severity, the following may be used: simple analgesia alone, aciclovir cream or oral valaciclovir (as above) within 48 hours of onset, or, if recurrences are severe or frequent, continuous low-dose oral aciclovir 200–400 mg bd may be prescribed, usually on consultant advice.

> A pregnant woman with a past history of genital herpes should have viral swabs taken in late pregnancy, as neonatal herpes can occur even when the mother has no overt signs of herpes.

HIV AND AIDS

See p. 201.

URETHRAL SYNDROME

In the urethral syndrome, symptoms of cystitis are present without a demonstrable UTI (i.e. an MSU shows $<10^5$ organisms per millilitre, or is sterile). Symptoms are usually mild and self-limiting, but may be recurrent. Patients are often anxious, and need reassurance.

Management

- The advice is similar to that for self-management of UTIs (see p. 65):
  - avoid scented soaps, bubble baths, etc.
  - alkalinise the urine with, e.g. sodium bicarbonate or potassium citrate mixture.
- It is worth considering treatment with an antibiotic, e.g. trimethoprim 200 mg bd for 3 days.
- Exclude intermittent infections by arranging MSUs, as appropriate.
- If the symptoms persist and are severe, refer to a urologist.

HIRSUTISM

In the vast majority of cases hirsutism is constitutional, especially in southern European women. Most hirsute women have increased androgen metabolism, at the high end of the spectrum of normality.

Diagnosis

Consider the following:

- a drug-related cause (e.g. phenytoin, corticosteroids, androgenic COC)
- a generalised endocrine disorder (e.g. hypothyroidism, Cushing's disease, acromegaly)
- inappropriate androgen production (raised serum testosterone and reduced SHBG) and polycystic ovarian syndrome (see below).

Management

Referral. Consider referral to an endocrinologist or to a gynaecologist if:

- the above apply
- galactorrhoea is present
- the hirsutism is worsening rapidly.

Advice. If investigations are normal and there are no associated features:

- Advise on cosmetic treatments (e.g. shaving, bleaching, waxing, depilatory creams, electrolysis). Electrolysis can be obtained on the NHS in severe cases.
- Encourage weight loss, if appropriate (serum testosterone levels increase with increasing weight).

Prescribing

- COC (particularly Dianette).
- Consider eflornithine cream for unwanted facial hair in women in whom alternative drug treatment cannot be used.
- Consider referral for treatment with high-dose cyproterone acetate.

POLYCYSTIC OVARIAN SYNDROME

The features of this common syndrome are polycystic ovaries on ultrasound together with irregular or absent periods and signs of excess androgens. Twenty per cent of asymptomatic women are found to have polycystic ovaries on ultrasound without the features of the syndrome. POS is thought to be related to insulin resistance. The patient often presents in her late teens or early twenties with some or all of the following symptoms:

- obesity
- virilisation with acne and hirsutes
- irregular or absent periods
- infertility (ovulation is sporadic or absent).

Investigations. Blood results may show: raised LH, increased LH/FSH ratio, raised prolactin and raised testosterone. Ultrasound shows characteristic ovaries. Also check fasting blood sugar and serum cholesterol (POS patients have higher rates of ischaemic heart disease (IHD), hypertension and diabetes).

Management

Advice

- Lose weight.
- Encourage exercise, a healthy diet and advise against smoking.
- Discuss contraception, which is still necessary, if appropriate.
- Consider referral to a gynaecologist for assessment.

Prescribing

- Treat hirsutism, if appropriate (see p. 48).
- Treat acne, if appropriate (see p. 131).
- The COC (e.g. Dianette) regulates bleeding and prevents endometrial overstimulation.
- Clomiphene will induce ovulation (see infertility, p. 59).
- Metformin (unlicensed indication) improves insulin sensitivity, menstrual disturbance and ovulatory function. Seek specialist advice.

BREAST SCREENING

The government-funded National Breast Screening Programme offers routine 3-yearly mammography to all women aged 50–64, by invitation. Women aged 65 and over may receive 3-yearly mammography, but only on request.

The screening programme is reducing breast cancer mortality by 20–40%. No significant reduction in mortality has been shown in women under 50 years of age, following screening.

Mammography is not a tool for investigating established breast lumps.

BREAST AWARENESS

Most breast cancers are discovered by women themselves. Routine, formalised breast self-examination is no longer advocated, as it has not been shown to reduce breast cancer mortality and can cause considerable unnecessary anxiety. A more general breast awareness should be promoted. This encourages women to recognise what is normal, to know what changes to look out for, and to seek medical advice about these changes without delay.

BREAST CANCER

See breast lumps (p. 265).

Advice. Lifestyle measures known to reduce the risk of breast cancer include:

- breast-feeding
- stopping smoking and reducing alcohol, if appropriate
- exercise and avoiding obesity
- avoiding HRT and the COC.

The following women are at higher risk:

- Those with one first degree relative (parent/child/sibling) with breast cancer at age <40.
- Those with one first degree and one second degree relative (grandparent/aunt/uncle/niece/nephew) with breast cancer at age <50.

Those at higher risk may be offered annual mammography from 40–49, genetic counselling, testing and prophylactic surgery.

BREAST LUMPS

See p. 265.

THE MENOPAUSE/CLIMACTERIC

The menopause is the process of inevitable ovarian failure leading to oestrogen deficiency. The average age of onset is 50.

Diagnosis

History. The diagnosis is usually made on the history alone.
Ask about:

- bleeding pattern/LMP
- flushes and sweats
- genitourinary problems, e.g. vaginal dryness and urinary incontinence
- psychological symptoms, e.g. anxiety and depression
- risk factors for osteoporosis (see p. 243).

Investigations

- Consider a pregnancy test.
- Consider thyroid function tests.

Check serum FSH if the diagnosis is in doubt, e.g. in:

- hysterectomised women
- those already taking the COC or HRT (see below) and experiencing regular withdrawal bleeds
- those experiencing amenorrhoea secondary to the POP or IUS
- those with oligomenorrhoea or amenorrhoea and menopausal symptoms under the age of 45.

A serum FSH of >20 U/l is diagnostic of the menopause, but even a mildly raised level may be suggestive.

Management
Discuss:

- the patient's understanding of the menopause
- life changes and stresses
- the prevention of cardiovascular disease and osteoporosis (see p. 244)
- HRT (see below).

Hysterectomy with ovarian conservation is associated with early ovarian failure.

Bleeding usually becomes increasingly infrequent as the menopause approaches. However, any bleeding which occurs 1 year or more after the last period is considered to be postmenopausal (see p. 40) and should be referred for investigation to exclude malignancy.

> Irregular, very heavy or painful bleeding should not be considered to be part of the normal menopause, and should be referred for endometrial biopsy.

HORMONE REPLACEMENT THERAPY (HRT)

HRT is indicated for:

- menopausal symptoms (see above) – the benefits of short-term HRT outweigh the risks in the majority of women
- the prophylaxis of osteoporosis in women with an early menopause, i.e. <50 years (not as first-line treatment for the prevention of osteoporosis in women >50).

Contraindications

- Oestrogen-sensitive malignancies (breast or endometrium).
- Major thromboembolic disease (in view of minor adverse effects on clotting factors and platelet function).
- Severe kidney or liver disease.
- Gall bladder disease.
- Otosclerosis (may worsen on HRT).

First appointment

History. See diagnosis of the menopause.

Examination

- BP.
- Weight.
- Discuss breast awareness.
- Consider vaginal examination.
- Check smear status.
- Mammography should be arranged for women with a family history of breast cancer (see also p. 51).

Advice

- Offer general advice relating to the menopause (see p. 52) and osteoporosis (see p. 244).
- Discuss contraception if appropriate (see p. 18). HRT is not a form of contraception.
- HRT is associated with a small increased risk of breast carcinoma, within 1–2 years of starting treatment, and related to duration of use. The risk is highest with combined preparations, less with tibolone (see below), and even less with oestrogen-only preparations, e.g. for 1000 women aged 50–64, taking combined HRT for 5 years there would be six extra cases of breast cancer. Any excess risk disappears within about 5 years of stopping.
- HRT is, in addition, associated with a small increase in the rates of stroke and thromboembolic disease, and a small decrease in the rates of colorectal and endometrial cancer.
- HRT does not prevent cognitive decline or coronary heart disease.

Prescribing. (The lowest effective maintenance dose should be prescribed.)

- Continuous daily oestrogen should be prescribed for hysterectomised women, e.g. Premarin 0.625–1.25 mg daily.

Only hysterectomised women may be treated with unopposed oestrogens.

- Oestrogen/progestogen preparations should be prescribed for women with an intact uterus (unopposed oestrogens may cause hyperplasia of the endometrium and possible endometrial cancer). Continuous oestrogen with 12–13 days of progestogen at the end of each monthly cycle (cyclical HRT), producing a regular monthly bleed, is commonly prescribed in the perimenopause, e.g. Nuvelle or Prempak-C. Amenorrhoeic regimens (using continuous combined oestrogen and progestogen) may be used for women who are at least 1 year postmenopausal, e.g. Premique or Kliofem. Irregular bleeding is a common side-effect of these regimens during the early treatment stages. If it continues, endometrial abnormality should be excluded, and consideration given to cyclical HRT instead.
- Oestrogen can be given as a transdermal patch or subdermal implant.
- The low-dose COC alleviates perimenopausal symptoms. In fit non-smokers it can be prescribed up to the menopause.
- Tibolone combines weak oestrogenic, progestogenic and androgenic activity. It is useful for women who cannot take oestrogen, for osteoporosis prophylaxis and symptom control. It does not produce withdrawal bleeds, but spotting is a common side-effect.
- Vaginal oestrogen creams, e.g. oestriol 0.1%, are useful for women with atrophic vaginitis. The smallest effective amount should be used to minimise systemic effects. Modified-release vaginal tablets and an impregnated vaginal ring are also available.

Follow-up
Follow-up should be at 3 months and subsequently 6-monthly or annually.

History

- Ask about any abnormal bleeding. (The bleeding pattern is commonly abnormal in the first 2–3 months, but should be regular subsequently.)
- Some women with an intact uterus do not experience a progestogen withdrawal bleed. This is not a cause for concern. Exclude pregnancy.

Examination

- BP.
- Weight.
- Vaginal examination. (This is only necessary routinely in the presence of unscheduled bleeding.)
- Check the smear status.
- Check the mammogram status (see also p. 50).

Hormone replacement therapy

	Brand	Oestrogen	Progestogen	Formulation	Bleed	RX*
SYSTEMIC Sequential combined therapy	Climagest	Oestradiol (1 mg, 2 mg)	Norethisterone (1 mg)	Tabs	M	2
	Clinorette	Oestradiol (2 mg, 2 mg)	Norethisterone (1 mg)	Tabs	M	2
	Cyclo-prognova	Oestradiol (1 mg, 2 mg)	Levo/norgestrel (0.25 mg/0.5 mg)	Tabs	M	2
	Elleste Duet	Oestradiol (1 mg, 2 mg)	Norethisterone (1 mg)	Tabs	M	2
	Estracombi	Oestradiol (50 µg)	Norethisterone (0.25 mg)	Patches	M	2
	Evorel Sequi	Oestradiol (50 µg)	Norethisterone (170 µg)	Patches	M	2
	Femapak	Oestradiol (40 µg, 80 µg)	Dydrogesterone (10 mg)	Patches + Tabs	M	2
	Femoston	Oestradiol (1 mg, 2 mg)	Dydrogesterone (10 mg)	Tabs	M	2
	FemSeven Sequi	Oestradiol (50 µg)	Levonorgestrel (10 µg)	Patches	M	2
	FemTab Sequi	Oestradiol (2 mg)	Levonorgestrel (75 µg)	Tabs	M	2
	Novofem	Oestradiol (1 mg)	Norethisterone (1 mg)	Tabs	M	2
	Nuvelle	Oestradiol (2 mg)	Levonorgestrel (75 µg)	Tabs	M	2
	Premique Cycle	Conj. oestrogens (0.625 mg)	Medroxyprogesterone (10 mg)	Tabs	M	2
	Prempak-C	Conj. oestrogens (0.625 mg, 1.25 mg)	Norgestrel (150 µg)	Tabs	M	2
	Tridestra	Oestradiol (2 mg)	Medroxyprogesterone (20 mg)	Tabs	Q	2
	Trisequens	Oestradiol (2 mg, 2 mg, 1 mg)	Norethisterone (1 mg)	Tabs	M	2
Continuous combined therapy	Angeliq	Oestradiol (1 mg)	Drospirenone (2 mg)	Tabs	X	1
	Climesse	Oestradiol (2 mg)	Norethisterone (0.7 mg)	Tabs	X	1
	Elleste Duet Conti	Oestradiol (2 mg)	Norethisterone (1 mg)	Tabs	X	1
	Evorel Conti	Oestradiol (50 µg)	Norethisterone (170 µg)	Patches	X	1
	Femoston Conti	Oestradiol (1 mg)	Dydrogesterone (5 mg)	Tabs	X	1
	FemSeven Conti	Oestradiol (50 µg)	Levonorgestrel (7 µg)	Patches	X	1
	Indivina	Oestradiol (1 mg, 2 mg)	Medroxyprogesterone (2.5 mg, 5 mg)	Tabs	X	1

(continued overleaf)

Hormone replacement therapy (continued)

	Brand	Oestrogen	Progestogen	Formulation	Bleed	RX*
	Kliofem	Oestradiol (2 mg)	Norethisterone (1 mg)	Tabs	X	1
	Kliovance	Oestradiol (1 mg)	Norethisterone (0.5 mg)	Tabs	X	1
	Nuvelle Continuous	Oestradiol (2 mg)	Norethisterone (1 mg)	Tabs	X	1
	Premique Low Dose	Conj. oestrogens (0.3 mg)	Medroxyprogesterone (1.5 mg)	Tabs	X	1
	Premique	Conj. oestrogens (0.625 mg)	Medroxyprogesterone (5 mg)	Tabs	X	1
Gonadomimetic	Livial	Tibolone (2.5 mg)		Tabs	X	1
Unopposed oestrogen (if uterus is intact an adjunctive progestogen must be used)	Aerodiol	Oestradiol (150 µg)		Spray		1
	Bedol	Oestradiol (2 mg)		Tabs		1
	Climaval	Oestradiol (1 mg, 2 mg)		Tabs		1
	Elleste Solo	Oestradiol (1 mg, 2 mg)		Tabs		1
	Elleste Solo MX	Oestradiol (40 µg, 80 µg)		Patches		1
	Estraderm MX	Oestradiol (25, 50, 75, 100 µg)		Patches		1
	Estraderm TTS	Oestradiol (25, 50, 100 µg)		Patches		1
	Estradot	Oestradiol (25, 37.5, 50, 75, 100 µg)		Patches		1
	Evorel	Oestradiol (25, 50, 75, 100 µg)		Patches		1
	Fematrix	Oestradiol (40 µg, 80 µg)		Patches		1
	FemSeven	Oestradiol (50, 75, 100 µg)		Patches		1
	FemTab	Oestradiol (1 mg, 2 mg)		Tabs		1
	Harmogen	Oestrone (0.93 mg)		Tabs		1
	Hormonin	Oestriol/Oestradiol/Oestrone 1 strength		Tabs		1
	Premarin	Conj. oestrogens (0.625 mg, 1.25 mg)		Tabs		1
	Progynova	Oestradiol (1 mg, 2 mg)		Tabs		1

	Progynova TS	Oestradiol (50 µg, 100 µg)	Patches	1
	Sandrena	Oestradiol (0.5 mg, 1 mg)	Gel	1
	Zumenon	Oestradiol (1 mg, 2 mg)	Tabs	1
Adjunctive progestogen	Climanor	Medroxyprogesterone (5 mg)	Tabs	1
	Duphaston HRT	Dydrogesterone (10 mg)	Tabs	1
	Micronor HRT	Norethisterone (1 mg)	Tabs	1
	Mirena	Levonorgestrel (20 µg /24 hr)	IUS	1
LOCAL **Oestrogen only**	Estring	Oestradiol (7.5 µg)	Vaginal ring	1
	Ortho-Gynest Pessary	Oestriol (0.5 mg)	Pessary	1
	Ortho-Gynest Cream	Oestriol (0.01%)	Vaginal cream	1
	Ovestin	Oestriol (0.1%)	Vaginal cream	1
	Premarin	Conj. oestrogens (0.0625%)	Vaginal cream	1
	Vagifem	Oestradiol (25 µg)	Vaginal tabs	1

Reproduced from *Monthly Index for Medical Specialities* with permission from Haymarket Medical Ltd 2007; updated monthly (www.mims.co.uk)

Bleed: M, monthly; Q, quarterly; X, no bleed

*Combination packs incur multiple prescription charges

CERVICAL CANCER

Cervical cancer kills 1000 women in the UK per year.

Discussion points for primary prevention of cervical cancer

- Stopping or reducing smoking lessens the risk of cervical cancer.
- An increased number of sexual partners (for both men and women) increases the risk.
- Ninety-five per cent of cervical cancer is caused by HPV infection (HPV vaccine is available to girls before sexual activity starts).
- Barrier methods of contraception are probably protective.
- Patients should avoid intercourse with partners with genital warts, unless a condom is used.

National cervical screening guidelines

- Invitation for first screening at age 25.
- Women aged 25–50 should be screened every 3 years.
- Women aged 50–65 should be screened every 5 years.
- Screening is unnecessary for women who have never been sexually active.
- Women aged 65 or over who have had regular negative tests do not need further screening. Women aged 65 or over who have never been screened, or who have not been screened since age 50, should be encouraged to do so.
- Instructions for follow-up or colposcopy referral will be given on smear reports.

Negative smear reports sometimes reveal incidental findings which require action as follows.

Specific infections

- *Trichomonas*: treat (see p. 46).
- *Candida*: treat if symptomatic (see p. 45).
- *Actinomyces*-like organisms (ALOs): these may colonise the genital tract in the presence of an IUCD. If the woman is asymptomatic, discuss the possible risk of pelvic infection. Leave the IUCD in situ and arrange 6-monthly follow-ups, including bimanual examination. Alternatively, remove or exchange the device (this usually leads to disappearance of ALOs) and repeat the smear after 6 months. If the woman is symptomatic (i.e. pelvic pain, dyspareunia or discharge), remove the IUCD, send the threadless device for culture and take an endocervical swab. If ALOs are found, treat with high-dose penicillin (2–3 g per day) or erythromycin for at least 2 weeks. Arrange an alternative method of contraception.
- Herpes simplex: no action.

- Inflammatory changes: no action, or consider taking swabs (see PID, p. 44) and treat as appropriate.

Tip
Clinical suspicion of cervical pathology should prompt referral for colposcopy, even if a cervical smear is normal.

INFERTILITY

Tip
Infertility is common, affecting about 15% of couples. It is important to note that 25% of cases of infertility remain unexplained.

The main causes of infertility are:

- disorders of spermatogenesis
- ovulation disorders
- tubal/pelvic pathology
- others, e.g. endometriosis, sperm/mucus problems.

Diagnosis

History

- Confirm regular intercourse during the fertile period. The fertile period is from day 8 to day 17 in a normal 28-day cycle (see calendar method, p. 16).
- Ninety per cent of women of proven fertility will conceive within 12 months. Investigation is therefore not usually undertaken until the couple have been attempting to conceive for 12 months or more.
- The couple should ideally be seen together.

Investigations. Before referral, the GP can arrange for semen analysis and confirmation of ovulation.

Semen analysis

A fresh warm specimen, produced after 48 hours of abstinence, should be examined in the laboratory within 2 hours of production.
Normal values:

- volume >2 ml
- count >20 million/ml
- motility >50%
- normal morphology >50%.

Confirmation of ovulation. Ovulation is suggested by:

- regular periods
- premenstrual symptoms
- ovulation pain.

Ovulation can be confirmed by the following:

- Basal body temperature: this rises by 0.2–0.5°C after ovulation. Basal temperature thermometers can be prescribed on an FP10. Basal temperature charts can be obtained from the Family Planning Association, or direct from pharmacists.
- Mid-luteal phase serum progesterone of >30 nmol/l. The blood test should be taken about 8 days before the next period is due (usually day 19 to day 21).
- Urinary LH kits: these can be bought over the counter. They detect the LH surge in mid-cycle.

Management

Clomiphene may be given to women who have been shown not to be ovulating, while awaiting hospital assessment. Their partner must have a normal semen analysis. Prescribe clomiphene 50 mg daily for 5 days starting on day 2. Ovulation can be confirmed by a rise in day 19 to day 21 progesterone. In the absence of ovulation, a second course of 100 mg daily for 5 days can be given. Three courses constitute an adequate therapeutic trial.

TERMINATION OF PREGNANCY REQUEST

The 1967 Abortion Act (revised in 1991) allows the following grounds for termination of pregnancy:

1. risk to the life of the woman or risk of grave permanent physical or mental injury to the woman (no time limit)
2. risk of injury to the physical or mental health of the woman (only legal up to 24 weeks)
3. risk of injury to the physical or mental health of existing child(ren) (only legal up to 24 weeks)
4. substantial risk of the child being born with serious abnormalities (no time limit).

(Most TOPs are performed under point 2.)

Assessment

History. Ask about:

- circumstances of pregnancy and request for TOP
- LMP and calculate gestation (was the LMP normal?)

- usual cycle
- date of last smear
- past history of STI
- previous births, miscarriages or pregnancy terminations.

Investigations. Carry out a pregnancy test. (Confirmation of the pregnancy should not usually be a cause for delay in referral.)

Management

- Help the woman to make a decision about the future of her pregnancy.
- Give information about the different methods of TOP, if appropriate, and refer to a gynaecologist:
  - surgical treatment
  - medical treatment with RU486 (mifepristone) and prostaglandins (only suitable for use in pregnancies of less than 9 weeks' gestation).
- Discuss future contraceptive plans.
- Arrange follow-up 2 weeks after the termination.

CHAPTER 4

UROLOGY

Urinary tract infection (UTI)   64

Proteinuria   66

Urinary stones   66

Urinary incontinence   67

Prostatism   70

URINARY TRACT INFECTION (UTI)

The average GP with a list of 2000 patients will see 30–40 cases of UTI a year. UTIs are particularly common in sexually active women, older menopausal women and men with prostatic hypertrophy. They usually present with urinary frequency, dysuria and cloudy urine, and sometimes suprapubic pain or tenderness, haematuria, urinary incontinence, or acute retention of urine. Pyelonephritis may present with loin pain, fever, rigors and/or vomiting. Up to half of all non-pregnant women with symptoms of lower UTI have no detectable bacterial infection, and therefore drug treatment is often unnecessary.

Diagnosis

History. Ask about:

- the above symptoms
- previous history of UTI
- form of contraception.

Some other causes of UTI symptoms

- Atrophic vaginitis.
- Trauma from intercourse.
- Bladder outlet obstruction, e.g. prostatism.
- Soreness from e.g. deodorants.
- Genital infections, e.g. candida and chlamydia.
- Urethral syndrome (see p. 48).

Examination. Examination is usually unnecessary, but look for suprapubic or loin tenderness, if appropriate.

Investigations. Dipstick urine to test for protein, nitrite (a bacterial metabolite) and leucocytes. If positive, treat for UTI.

An MSU for MC&S is usually unnecessary but should be sent in the following patient groups:

1. pregnant women
2. children
3. men
4. catheterised patients
5. patients who have failed to respond to initial antibiotic treatment
6. patients with persistent symptoms.

The MSU, taken prior to starting antibiotics, must show a pure growth in excess of 10^5 organisms/ml and white cells in excess of $50/mm^3$ in order to confirm a significant infection.

Management

Advise the patient to drink copious fluids, especially alkaline liquids, e.g. sodium bicarbonate or potassium citrate solution (available OTC).

Proteinuria and haematuria have many causes other than UTI. Negative urine tests for leucocytes and nitrite can reliably indicate that a UTI is not present.

First-line treatment of UTIs

Females with simple UTI. Trimethoprim 200 mg bd or amoxicillin 250 mg tds for 3 days.

Children aged >12, men, and women with clinical evidence of renal involvement (e.g. fever, loin pain). Trimethoprim 200 mg bd or amoxicillin 250 mg tds for 7–10 days. (Check dosage for young children.)

Management of recurrent UTIs in women

- If recurrent symptoms are due to the same organism, ensure that treatment is with an antibiotic to which the pathogen has been shown to be sensitive, check compliance and continue the antibiotic for 5–7 days.
- Discuss, if appropriate:
  - increasing fluid intake
  - urinating more frequently
  - using a lubricant with intercourse
  - passing urine after intercourse
  - improving perineal hygiene
  - avoiding tight clothing
  - avoiding scented soaps, bubble bath, etc.
  - contraception (e.g. a diaphragm may encourage UTIs).
- Consider topical oestrogen for peri- and postmenopausal women.
- Further investigations: consider blood tests (e.g. C&Es, fasting BS), a plain abdominal X-ray (to look for radio-opaque stones), followed by an ultrasound scan of the urinary tract or an IVU to exclude renal cortical scars from previous infections, or evidence of obstruction.
- If these investigations are normal, consider giving prophylactic antibiotics. One-quarter of the usual 24-hour dose should be given at night and continued until the urine has been sterile for 1 year, e.g. trimethoprim 100 mg nocte. Before starting on this regimen, consider referral for urological assessment.
- Patients whose UTIs are clearly related to intercourse may take a single dose of antibiotic within 2 hours of intercourse (e.g. nitrofurantoin 50 mg).
- Consider prescribing a 'spare' course of antibiotics for the patient to start at the onset of symptoms.

UTIs in men. See management of UTIs in general (p. 65). Further investigations (see p. 65) should be arranged after a first confirmed UTI. Consider PSA if aged >40. In men with BPH, alpha blockers reduce the incidence of UTIs. Consider referring men with a confirmed UTI to a urologist.

Men with symptoms of a UTI but no infection may have prostatitis. They usually have discomfort behind the testicles. Prostatitis can be diagnosed by sending the first urine of the morning (the early part of the stream) for microscopy and confirming the presence of threads of white cells. Treat with e.g. trimethoprim 200 mg bd for 28 days, or longer if the symptoms have not completely settled.

UTIs in children. See p. 90.

Administration
Dipsticks for nitrite and leucocytes are not prescribable on FP10.

PROTEINURIA

A trace of proteinuria on dipstick, in the absence of microscopic haematuria, is nearly always benign.

Management

- Exclude fever or recent exercise.
- Dipstick urine for nitrite, leucocytes and blood.
- MSU for MC&S.
- Check BP.
- Bloods for C&Es and fasting blood sugar, if appropriate.
- 24-hour urine collection for total protein excretion (150 mg of protein/24 hours is the upper limit of normal), if appropriate.

Tip
A patient with persistent proteinuria (i.e. dipstick positive for protein recorded on three separate urine samples, including an early morning urine), with or without microscopic haematuria, should be referred to a nephrologist for consideration of renal imaging/biopsy.

URINARY STONES

Ureteric colic usually presents with very severe unilateral loin pain, often radiating to the groin or genitalia, and often accompanied by vomiting. The diagnosis is confirmed by the presence of microscopic haematuria. Patients with undiagnosed backache or vague loin pain may be harbouring a stone.

Diagnosis

Investigations. (These are only necessary with the first stone.)

Urgent. Dipstick urine for blood.

Less urgent. (i.e. may wait until the next working day.)

- MSU for MC&S.
- KUB X-ray (90% of urinary stones are radio-opaque) and ultrasound scan.
- An IVU will indicate the exact location of any stone, the function of both kidneys and the presence of any obstruction.
- Bloods
  - FBC and ESR
  - C&Es and urate
  - calcium, phosphate and alkaline phosphatase.
- Chemical analysis of the stone, if appropriate.

Management

Treatment

- Most patients improve spontaneously without intervention due to spontaneous passing of the stone.
- Give diclofenac 75 mg im (or 100 mg PR) or pethidine 100 mg im, together with prochlorperazine 12.5 mg im, if required, for vomiting.
- Less severe pain can be controlled with e.g. oral NSAIDs or oral pethidine.
- Sieve urine to catch stone(s) for analysis.
- Push fluids.

Referral. Patients with the following should always be admitted urgently:

- Ureteric colic that does not resolve within 24 hours.
- Possible stones where the GP does not have access to imaging procedures.
- Obstruction on IVU.
- Large calculi which cannot be passed spontaneously.
- Reduced renal function.
- Infection.

> **Tip**
> Patients with first-time stones who do not need urgent admission should be referred to the urology outpatient clinic.

URINARY INCONTINENCE

Incontinence is involuntary leakage of urine and is a common and disabling condition. It is estimated that as many as 60% of the elderly population and 40%

of women over the age of 20 suffer from some form of urinary incontinence. It can be significantly improved by appropriate intervention, but is underdiagnosed because a large percentage of sufferers do not consult their doctor. Stress incontinence and urge incontinence are responsible for over 90% of cases of incontinence. The two often coexist, but the most useful distinguishing factor is the absence of urgency in stress incontinence.

Diagnosis

History. It is important to take advantage of routine screening opportunities to identify sufferers. Ask about:

- stress incontinence:
  - leakage of urine with exercise, coughing or sneezing
- urge incontinence:
  - urinary frequency, day and night
  - hurrying to get to the toilet
  - not being able to get to the toilet in time
- overflow incontinence (bladder outflow obstruction):
  - difficulty passing urine (hesitancy)
  - dribbling after passing urine
  - poor stream
  - nocturia
  - a sensation of incomplete bladder-emptying
- passive incontinence:
  - passing urine without knowing it
  - accidents in bed at night.

General questions. Ask about:

- dysuria (suggestive of UTI, atrophic vaginitis or obstruction).
- liquid intake (alcohol and coffee are diuretics).
- drugs, e.g. diuretics, antidepressants.
- the use of pads or towels.
- past history, e.g. stroke, dementia, Parkinson's disease, multiple sclerosis, prolapsed disc, spinal injury, previous pelvic surgery, obstetric history, etc.

Examination (abdominal, PR and PV). Look for:

- constipation
- a palpable bladder (overflow incontinence)
- pelvic masses, e.g. fibroids
- other local 'lumps', e.g. a large inguinal hernia
- prolapse
- local infections, e.g. candida

- atrophic vaginitis
- enlarged prostate } in men
- tight foreskin.

Assess the pelvic floor muscles by asking the patient to pull up the pelvic floor while you are performing a pelvic examination.

Investigations

- Dipstick urine for blood, sugar, protein, nitrite and leucocytes.
- MSU for MC&S.
- Consider blood for C&Es and fasting BS.
- A urinary diary, documenting frequency and volume of urine passed, and drinks taken, can be helpful.

Management
Most patients can be treated satisfactorily by the GP.

Stress incontinence. (due to weakness of the urethral sphincter.)

- Encourage reduction of intra-abdominal pressure by:
  - reducing weight, if appropriate
  - stopping smoking, if appropriate
  - avoiding constipation
  - avoiding heavy lifting.
- Regular pelvic floor exercises (i.e. repetitive squeezing of the pelvic floor) improve tone and support. Tighten the front (bladder) and back (bowel) passages. Count to four slowly, then release slowly. Do this several times and repeat every hour or so, if possible. These exercises, which can be done at any time, and are not evident to others, should ideally be continued for life.
- Consider referral to a physiotherapist for instruction on pelvic floor exercises, treatment with graduated vaginal cones or electrical stimulation of the pelvic floor (faradism or interferential treatment).
- Consider referral for urodynamic investigations and/or surgery, e.g. transvaginal tape, colposuspension, if:
  - the exact diagnosis is in doubt
  - conservative methods have failed
  - symptoms recur following surgery.
- Treat atrophic vaginitis with local oestrogen cream or systemic HRT.

Urge incontinence. (due to detrusor instability)

- Bladder retraining involves encouraging the patient to void increasingly larger volumes of urine at less frequent intervals, thus relearning inhibition of abnormal detrusor muscle contractions.

- Drugs to stabilise the detrusor muscle can be used in addition to bladder retraining, e.g. oxybutynin 2.5–5 mg bd or tolterodine 1–2 mg bd (sustained release preparations reduce the anticholinergic side-effects). Once continence has been regained, many patients are able to sustain the improvement without medication.
- The patient may need psychological support.

Living with incontinence

- Refer to a district nurse for advice on appliances, e.g. incontinence pads.
- Consider involving local continence advisors.

PROSTATISM

Prostatism, or symptoms of outflow obstruction in men, is common, particularly in the elderly, and often not volunteered by the patient.

Diagnosis

History. Ask about:

- poor urinary stream
- hesitancy
- frequency
- nocturia
- terminal dribble
- bone pain, which raises the possibility of malignant bony secondaries.

Examination. Look for:

- the enlarged bladder of urinary retention, which can be painless in chronic retention.
- enlargement of the prostate gland, by performing a DRE. (As a general rule, the malignant prostate is hard, craggy, irregular and often enlarged, with the central sulcus obliterated.)

Investigations.

All cases

- MSU, to exclude a UTI as cause of frequency.
- Blood for C&Es, to exclude obstructive uropathy.
- Serum PSA. A level greater than 4.0 raises the possibility of malignancy, but there are many false-positive results.

In suspected malignancy

- PSA will often be raised if there is clinical suspicion of malignancy.
- X-ray of a painful, bony area, e.g. the pelvis or hips, is a sensitive way of detecting bony secondaries.

Management

- Frequency and nocturia may be helped by a selective alpha blocker, e.g. indoramin 20 mg bd (relaxes smooth muscle, producing an increase in urinary flow rate).
- Refer for urological opinion in suspected malignancy, obstructive uropathy or symptoms of prostatism, which are resistant to treatment.
- For the patient too infirm for surgery, incontinence aids may become necessary. Consider monitoring C&Es in such patients, to detect obstructive uropathy.
- Catheterisation becomes necessary in acute retention, deteriorating renal function and as an alternative in incontinence control.

Tip
Patients significantly troubled by symptoms of prostatism should be offered referral, as a routine case, for consideration for surgery. Cases of malignancy, suspected on clinical or biochemical grounds, should be offered an urgent referral for tissue diagnosis.

Prevention/screening
There is much debate at present about the merits of screening for prostatic cancer. The three methods available are:

- regular digital examination
- transrectal ultrasound scanning
- serum PSA.

Although all methods should, in theory, enable the earlier detection of prostate problems, none has been shown so far to reduce mortality from prostate cancer.

MEN'S HEALTH

Erectile dysfunction   74

Premature ejaculation   75

Peyronie's disease   75

Sexually transmitted
infections   76

Scrotal swellings   77

Testicular pain   78

Testicular cancer   80

Abdominal aortic aneurysm
screening   80

ERECTILE DYSFUNCTION

Estimated to affect approximately 1 in 10 men, erectile dysfunction is increasingly seen in general practice. It is defined as the inability to get or maintain an erection sufficient for the completion of sexual activity.

Diagnosis

History. Most men have a combination of physical and psychological causes. Ask about:

- general health and current well-being
- pre-existing illness such as diabetes, prostatism, atherosclerosis
- lifestyle – smoking, alcohol, drugs, stress
- relationship problems
- depression, performance anxiety.

Examination. This is not usually necessary unless specific concerns have been raised, e.g. pain on erection suggesting Peyronie's disease (see p. 75)

Investigation. It is worth sending baseline bloods: TFTs, fasting glucose, testosterone, C&Es, LFTs and γ-GT if alcoholism is suspected.

Management

- Lifestyle advice: advise the patient to try to avoid stress and anxiety, to reduce smoking and alcohol and to discuss any problems of sexual dissatisfaction with his partner.
- All treatments can be used for both psychogenic and organic causes.
- Phosphodiesterase type-5 inhibitors are usually effective irrespective of the cause, e.g. sildenafil, at a starting dose of 50 mg (25 mg in the elderly) approximately 1 hour before sexual activity. It should not be used in those receiving nitrates.

> **Tip**
> Most patients will need private prescriptions.

An NHS prescription can be issued to patients whose erectile dysfunction is felt to be caused by:

- diabetes
- pelvic surgery/trauma
- prostate cancer
- neurological disease
- severe emotional distress.

Remember to endorse these prescriptions 'SLS'.

- Refer for psychosexual counselling, if appropriate.
- Consider referral to a urologist, e.g. for vasoactive injections, penile prostheses or vacuum devices.

PREMATURE EJACULATION

This is very common, particularly in young men having their first sexual relationships.

Assessment

History. Ask whether the problem has been lifelong or of recent onset. Most men establish a pattern of ejaculating too soon for their liking, but recent anxiety, change of partner or of sexual position/practice may be the cause.

Ask if the man has discussed the problem with his partner. Many men are too embarrassed to do this but successful treatment is more likely if the partner is involved.

Examination. This is not usually necessary, unless there is a complaint of penile/testicular pain or swelling.

Management

The general principle of treatment is to encourage the man to learn how it feels when he is about to ejaculate and to stop the stimulation before reaching that point, resuming when the feeling has declined. It can usually be treated satisfactorily by the stop/start or the squeeze technique: when the man feels close to ejaculation he should stop and relax for 30 seconds, or the woman should squeeze his glans for 30 seconds. Stimulation can then continue and the process may be repeated. The man will eventually improve his control.

Prescription of one of the SSRI antidepressants may help some men. Not only does the antidepressant effect help if there is associated performance anxiety, but the SSRIs, like most antidepressants, have the side-effect of delaying or preventing ejaculation in some men.

Referral for psychosexual counselling is often appropriate.

PEYRONIE'S DISEASE

Peyronie's disease is rarely seen in general practice despite being present in over 80 000 adult men in the UK. All ages can be affected but it is most common around 50 years of age.

Assessment

History. Ask about:

- a fibrous plaque in the shaft of the penis
- pain on erection
- angulation of the penis on erection.

Because the problem is often painful it can lead to erectile dysfunction/impotence. Micturition is unaffected.

Examination. A fibrous, flat plaque is palpable beneath the skin of the shaft of the penis. It is usually 1–3 cm in diameter and on either the lateral or the ventral surface. The overlying skin is normal.

Tip
Some men are concerned that they may have cancer of the penis when they present with Peyronie's disease.

Management

There are surgical and non-surgical techniques for Peyronie's disease, including surgical excision, extracorporeal shock wave therapy, injections, tamoxifen, verapamil and vitamin E.

Referral to a urologist, preferably with a special interest in penile disorders, is advised.

Management of any associated erectile dysfunction should be guided by specialist advice, especially if erection is painful.

SEXUALLY TRANSMITTED INFECTIONS

Chlamydia is the commonest sexually transmitted infection (STI) in men and is often asymptomatic. Other STIs include gonorrhoea, syphilis, HIV/AIDS, genital warts, herpes simplex and thrush.

Men present to their GPs in two ways:

- with symptoms or suspicions of infection
- having been advised to be treated as the partner of an infected person.

Refer to a GUM clinic. Patients can self-refer to any clinic.

Assessment

History. The symptoms of chlamydia in men can include:

- pain on micturition
- urethral pain

- urethral discharge
- testicular pain
- joint pains (Reiter's syndrome).

Examination. Examination is usually normal, even in symptomatic men. Look for signs of other sexually transmitted infections:

- genital warts
- herpetic ulcers
- urethral discharge
- inguinal lymphadenopathy
- candidal balanitis.

Treatment

Treatment depends on the infection identified. Empirical treatment is advised in contacts of diagnosed infection without the need for confirmatory testing. For infection or contact with:

- chlamydia, give doxycycline 100 mg twice daily for 1 week, or azithromycin as a 1 g single dose.
- thrush, prescribe clotrimazole cream to be applied to the glans twice a day for 1 week.
- other diagnosed STIs, refer the patient to a GUM clinic for testing, treatment and contact tracing.

Contact tracing

This is an essential part of the population control of STIs. Most GP practices lack the resources for adequate contact tracing, which often involves patients who are not registered with the practice. If a patient is diagnosed by the practice with an STI, it is important to encourage the patient to inform their sexual partner(s) to seek treatment, either from their own GP or from a GUM clinic.

SCROTAL SWELLINGS

The most common causes of a swelling in the scrotum are an epididymal cyst, an inguinoscrotal hernia or a hydrocele.

A sebaceous cyst of the scrotal skin may be described as a scrotal swelling.

Testicular tumours are rare (see p. 80).

Diagnosis

History. Ask about pain in the scrotum. The following are painless:

- inguinoscrotal hernia
- hydrocele
- epididymal cyst.

Otherwise, see testicular pain, p. 78.

A history of trauma suggests either a secondary hydrocele or haematocele.

Examination

- Examine the patient standing.
- If palpation above the swelling is impossible, it is an inguinoscrotal hernia.
- If palpation above the swelling is possible and the swelling is above the testicle, it is either an epididymal cyst or a varicocele: an epididymal cyst will transilluminate; a varicocele feels like a bag of worms.
- A hydrocele is usually large and tense and transilluminates easily. The testicle cannot be palpated as it is within the hydrocele.
- A sebaceous cyst is superficial and confined to the scrotal skin.
- Testicular tumours cause enlargement of a testicle.

Investigations. If there is any doubt about the diagnosis, particularly with regard to excluding a possible tumour of the testis, request a scrotal ultrasound scan.

Management

- Sebaceous cyst: reassure.
- Hydrocele: small hydroceles require no further action as long as a normal testis is palpable. Larger hydroceles may be aspirated (see below) or referred to a urologist.
- All other scrotal swellings: refer.

Aspiration of a hydrocele. Only attempt if the GP has the confidence to perform the procedure correctly. Otherwise, refer.

- Avoid the testicle by locating it with transillumination.
- Clean the skin with an alcohol wipe.
- Insert a green needle on a 20-ml syringe and draw off as much fluid as possible.
- Always palpate the testicle afterwards to exclude a tumour of the testis as a cause of the hydrocele.
- Repeat the procedure as necessary. Frequent recurrences need surgical treatment.

TESTICULAR PAIN

The most common presentation of testicular pain in general practice is mild and transient, and a cause is often not found.

Diagnosis

History

 Severe pain in the testicle suggests torsion or acute epididymo-orchitis. Nausea and vomiting often occur in torsion. Torsion is extremely rare over the age of 25.

- A recent history of cystitis, prostatitis or prostatectomy suggests epididymo-orchitis, as does a history of STI or urethral discharge.
- Mumps may be complicated by orchitis.

Examination

- In torsion the genitalia are often too tender to examine.
- In epididymo-orchitis there may be red skin over the infection, and the most tender part is often felt to be above the testicle.
- In both torsion and epididymo-orchitis there may be scrotal swelling due to oedema or inflammation.
- Examination of the painful testicle is often normal, in which case mild epididymitis is probably the cause.
- Other possible causes of pain in the testicle include:
  - ureteric calculi
  - inguinoscrotal hernia
  - groin strain
  - malignancy
  - psychological.

Management

Admit all cases of severe pain as possible torsion.

In less severe cases, where the examination is normal, it is wise to wait and see what happens with time. Most cases resolve spontaneously without any treatment. Those that do not settle may be helped by prescribing an anti-inflammatory, such as ibuprofen 400 mg tds.

If there are signs suggesting epididymo-orchitis, such as erythema and fever, take an MSU (and urethral swab for gonococcus and chlamydia, if appropriate) and treat with a broad-spectrum antibiotic such as ciprofloxacin 500 mg bd for 5 days. Consider referral to the GUM clinic.

TESTICULAR CANCER

Testicular cancer is rare. The highest incidence is in the 20–40-year age group.

Assessment

History. The commonest symptom of testicular cancer is a swelling or lump in one testicle. It is usually painless but can cause an ache. Very rarely testicular cancer presents with symptoms of metastatic spread, such as breathlessness due to pulmonary secondaries.

Examination. Examination of the normal testicles usually reveals similarly sized, smooth, ovoid testes with the soft epididymi along the posterior surface.

The most common abnormality is an epididymal cyst, which feels like a firm swelling distinctly separate from the testicle and within the epididymis. These are usually between a few millimetres and 1 cm in size.

Swellings within the body of a testicle should be considered suspicious of testicular cancer.

Don't forget the hydrocele. This is a swelling that feels distinctly fluid-filled and envelops the testicle. They usually transilluminate well with a good pen torch in a dark room.

Management

- If examination is suspicious, an urgent referral to a urologist is advised.
- If the diagnosis is uncertain, refer for an ultrasound scan on an urgent basis.

Screening

No national screening programme exists for testicular cancer. Men should be encouraged to examine their testes monthly, after a warm bath, to learn what feels normal for them and to report any changes.

ABDOMINAL AORTIC ANEURYSM SCREENING

There is no NHS screening programme for aortic aneurysms at present. Screening is, however, available privately.

When to screen

Current evidence suggests that men should have a single ultrasound examination to measure the diameter of their abdominal aorta at 65 years of age. Men over 65 should be screened once, up to the age of 80.

Follow-up

Aneurysm diameter:

- >6 cm diameter: refer for surgery
- 4.5–5.9 cm: re-scan 3 monthly
- 3–4.4 cm: re-scan annually
- <3 cm: no further screening is necessary.

Men screened in this way have a 63% reduction in mortality from abdominal aortic aneurysm at 5 years.

CHAPTER 6

PAEDIATRICS

Examination of the neonate 84

6–8-week check 84

**Routine childhood
immunisations** 85

Neonatal jaundice 85

Infant feeding 85

Weaning 86

Babies with colic 86

Constipation 87

Nocturnal enuresis 88

**Urinary tract infection in
children** 90

Sleep problems 91

Nappy rash 91

Preschool check 92

Growth problems 92

Respiratory problems 93

Convulsions and seizures 97

Child protection 99

Sudden infant death 101

EXAMINATION OF THE NEONATE

Examination of the neonate should be completed and recorded at all deliveries within 5 days of the birth. One in 40 newborns will be found to have a congenital malformation. The aim is to assess the baby's general condition and respiratory function, and to identify any special management requirements in the first few days.

Routine examination should include:

- *Measurements*: check weight and head circumference.
- *General appearance*: look for dysmorphic features. Assess general muscle tone. Jaundice appearing within 24 hours requires urgent attention.
- *Head*: look for abnormalities in the cranial shape, allowing for moulding. An unusually full anterior fontanelle suggests hydrocephalus and an ultrasound should be arranged.
- *Eyes*: look for eye-size asymmetry. (Discrepancy suggests an infection, a developmental defect, or congenital glaucoma, which is an emergency.) Look for the red reflex to exclude a cataract.
- *Nose*: look for signs of obstruction.
- *Mouth*: check the palate for clefts.
- *Chest*: observe respiratory movements. Auscultate, if appropriate.
- *Heart*: heart murmurs are common at birth. Checking for murmurs at 8 weeks is more selective.
- *Abdomen*: look for distension or organomegaly. Exclude a single umbilical artery.
- *Groins*: check femoral pulses which may be absent in aortic coarctation. Look for hernias.
- *Genitalia*: check that the testes are in the scrotum. Exclude hypospadias and epispadias, and sexual ambiguity.
- *Anus*: exclude imperforate anus. The passing of meconium excludes this.
- *Spine*: exclude a scoliosis. Exclude any possible spinal cord abnormalities by looking for naevi, lumps, pits or hairy patches over the spine.
- *Hips*: exclude congenital dislocation.

6–8-WEEK CHECK

This check is completed by the GP and is combined with the first immunisations. It should include:

- *Discussion of parental concerns*: ask about vision, hearing and general development. Ask how the parents and siblings are adjusting to the birth of the baby.
- *General observation*: look for alertness, response to handling, dysmorphic features, etc.
- *Skin*: ask about and look for blemishes and abnormalities.

- *Growth*: plot weight, head circumference and, where necessary, length on a centile chart.
- *Eyes*: look for abnormal movements, squint or failure of fixation.
- *Heart*: check for murmurs.
- *Genitalia*: check that the testes are in the scrotum. Exclude hypospadias and epispadias, and sexual ambiguity.
- *Hips*: exclude congenital dislocation.

ROUTINE CHILDHOOD IMMUNISATIONS

See p. 334.

All newborn babies should receive vitamin K to prevent vitamin K deficiency bleeding (haemorrhagic disease of the newborn). Some areas recommend a single intramuscular vitamin K injection at birth. Other areas recommend oral vitamin K, two doses to be given in the first week of life (usually by the midwife). Babies who are being >50% breast-fed should receive a third oral dose at age 4 weeks (usually given by the health visitor).

NEONATAL JAUNDICE

- Jaundice within 24 hours of birth is always pathological.
- Serum bilirubin should be checked in babies with significant jaundice. Refer if the level lies above the limit for the baby's age. (Discuss with laboratory.)
- 'Physiological' jaundice appears after 48 hours and usually disappears by day 7–10 of life.
- Jaundice persisting or presenting after 10 days of age (14 days in immature babies) is abnormal and the baby should be referred for assessment. If the prolonged jaundice is associated with breast-feeding it should fade by 6 weeks of age.

INFANT FEEDING

BREAST-FEEDING

See p. 35.

Breast-feeding is the preferred method from birth until weaning and beyond.

BOTTLE-FEEDING

Bottle-fed babies, like breast-fed babies, should be fed on demand and allowed to find their own pattern. Bottles and teats should be sterilised until the baby is >6 months old. Formula milk, as opposed to cow's milk (which has relatively low iron and vitamin A, C, D and E content), should ideally be given until the baby is 1 year old. The baby requires about 150 ml per kg body weight per day. This is usually given as about six feeds/bottles per day. In the first week or so, the baby takes about 50–70 ml 7–8 times per day.

Changing milks because the baby has colic or seems unsettled is of little value. Soya milks are often misused. They have no advantage over other formulae but should be reserved for proven cow's milk intolerance.

Milk feeds after 6 months

- Formula milk should ideally be continued for the first year.
- Cow's milk can be introduced after 6 months.
- Low-fat milk should not be introduced before the age of 2.

WEANING

Weaning is the transition from an all-milk diet to a varied diet using solid foods. Advice should be sought from the health visitor.

- Solid foods are usually introduced by 6 months, but not before 3 months.
- Food should be offered by spoon in small quantities. If a food is rejected, it should be tried again after a while.
- Early foods should be low in salt and sugar.
- Plain rice cereals mixed with milk are usually given first, followed by stewed and puréed fruit or vegetables.
- As the baby starts to cut down milk consumption, small quantities of protein foods, e.g. meat or fish, can be added.
- By 9–12 months infants should be encouraged to have three regular meals per day, eating normal chopped family food. They will need about 0.5 litre (1 pint) of milk (breast, formula or cow's) per day, as well as additional fluids. Only give drinks after meals, to avoid reducing appetite. Water should be encouraged, and fruit juices should be diluted with water.
- Avoid an excessively high fibre intake, as high-fibre foods are bulky and have a relatively low nutrient and energy content.
- Supplementary vitamins (A, D and C), 5 drops daily from 6 months to 5 years, may be given to children with an inadequate diet.
- If, from the age of 6 months, a child uses fluoride toothpaste, fluoride supplements (even in areas where there is no added fluoride in the water supply) are now considered unnecessary.

BABIES WITH COLIC

When called to see a crying baby, important physical causes must be excluded. Consider volvulus, intussusception or acute infection (e.g. otitis media or UTI).

Colic tends to start after 2 weeks of age, and usually settles by 4 months of age. The infant is often well in the morning, but by the evening may be distraught, pale and drawing up its legs. The parents are often quite unable to comfort the baby. They need reassurance that the problem is self-limiting and that they are not at fault since there is no clear cause. Involve the health visitor and encourage the parents to get as much rest as possible. Changing milk formulae is rarely helpful. Breast-feeding technique may need attention. A consistent feeding and sleeping routine may help, as may increased carrying and treatment with e.g. dimethicone (Infacol) 0.5–1 ml before feeds. Be alert for a child at risk (see child protection, p. 99).

Tip
Crying for long periods of time, especially in the evening, is usually due to 'colic'.

CONSTIPATION

CONSTIPATION IN INFANTS

Constipation is more common in formula-fed than in breast-fed babies. It is only considered to be a problem if hard stools cause straining and discomfort. The passage of a normal soft stool once a week, for example, is not a problem. The cause is not always clear, but it may be due to inadequate fluid intake or to inadequately diluted formula feeds.

Management

- Consider the possibility of Hirschsprung's disease if there is delay in first passing meconium and subsequent constipation.
- Exclude an anal fissure.
- Encourage the parent to give abundant fluids. (Unsweetened fruit juice can be given to babies in addition to milk.)
- Abdominal massage can be helpful.
- Laxatives are very rarely required.

CONSTIPATION AND SOILING IN OLDER CHILDREN

Hard stools may cause faecal retention and chronic constipation. This can lead to soiling due to a distended rectum, which leads to relaxation of the internal sphincter. The external sphincter is then put under considerable strain and is unable to prevent leakage of faeces. Most children are clean by 2.5 years of age and soiling may be viewed as abnormal after 4 years of age.

Acute constipation often follows febrile illnesses.

Diagnosis

History. Ask about:

- the child's diet and fluid intake
- previous bowel habit
- present management and how the parents are coping.

Examination. Check:

- the abdomen for a loaded colon
- the anus for an anal fissure
- the rectum for the presence of faeces.

Management

The aim of treatment is to regain the child's confidence in being able to defaecate painlessly.

- An enema may be required to dislodge a faecal mass. However, this can be distressing for a child, and a course of an oral stimulant laxative, e.g. senna syrup (age >6 years, 5–10 ml in the morning), and a faecal softener, e.g. lactulose solution (age 5–10 years, 10 ml bd), may be prescribed.
- Encourage copious fluids and a high-fibre diet.
- Refractory cases may require a prolonged course of senna and/or lactulose in gradually reducing dosage in order to amplify the gastrocolic reflex. Consider referral to a paediatric gastroenterology clinic.
- The child should be encouraged to go to the toilet, in unhurried time, after each meal, in order to encourage the gastrocolic reflex.
- The child with intentional defaecation in unacceptable places (encopresis) should, if appropriate, be referred to a child psychiatrist.

NOCTURNAL ENURESIS

Bed-wetting in children is a common problem. Most children are dry at night by the age of 3, 90% are dry by the age of 5 and >95% by the age of 10. The cause of bed-wetting is usually unclear, but the problem nearly always resolves with time. About 1% of children will have an organic problem, e.g. a congenital abnormality of the urinary tract, a urinary tract infection or a neuropathic bladder.

Diagnosis

History. Ask about:

- Whether the child has ever been dry. (A period of dryness suggests that the problem is not organic unless the child has an acute UTI.)
- Whether the child wets during the day. (After the age of 4 this suggests a neuropathic bladder and the child should be referred.)

- Family history: children often follow a familial pattern.
- Any behavioural or emotional problems.
- Heavy sleeping.

Investigations

- Dipstick urine for glucose, nitrite, leucocytes and protein
- send an MSU for MC&S.

Management

Involve both the parent and the child, as well as the health visitor. Some areas have specific enuresis clinics.

> **Tip**
> Specific treatment is unnecessary under the age of 7 years. Ten per cent of 5-year-olds still wet the bed.

Advice

- Drinks should be avoided in the evening.
- Lifting the child to the lavatory when the parent goes to bed may be helpful.
- A star chart with stars given for dry beds encourages the child.
- A child who is <7 years of age might wear nappies or trainer pants at night if the above methods are unsuccessful.

Treatment

An enuresis alarm can be used if the above methods fail (obtainable via health visitors, school nurses or the local enuresis clinic). This is placed in the child's bed so that the alarm rings when the child wets. Most children become dry within 2–3 months. Stop using the alarm after about 28 consecutive dry nights. Relapse responds well to re-treatment.

Drug treatment is usually helpful in children who do not respond to conservative measures. Use e.g. desmopressin nasal spray (synthetic analogue of ADH) 20–40 μg at bedtime. Withdraw treatment for at least 1 week for reassessment after 3 months. Desmopressin can be used intermittently, e.g. when staying away from home.

Refer to a urologist if history, examination or investigations suggest an organic cause, or if response to treatment is poor.

> **Tip**
> A child with a neuropathic bladder has daytime as well as night-time wetting. Examine for absent ankle jerks and a sacral dimple or hairy naevus. Refer to a urologist.

URINARY TRACT INFECTION IN CHILDREN

See also UTI, p. 64.

Eight per cent of girls and 2% of boys will have a UTI in childhood. From 25 to 50% of children with UTIs have associated urinary tract abnormalities (mainly vesicoureteric reflux). Appropriate and prompt antibiotic treatment reduces the risk of renal damage, which can occur in children as a result of recurrent UTIs.

Older children tend to present, like adults, with urinary frequency, dysuria, haematuria and/or abdominal pain.

Consider a UTI in any child who is failing to thrive or who has symptoms of fever, vomiting, diarrhoea, irritability and/or enuresis.

Investigation. Dipstick urine to test for protein, nitrite and leucocytes.

Send MSU for MC&S before treatment with antibiotics. In younger children special collecting bags or pads can be used to obtain a urine specimen.

Management

Initial treatment of a suspected UTI is with antibiotics, e.g. trimethoprim or nitrofurantoin (see BNF for dose according to age) for 7 days, without waiting for the MSU result. Advise analgesia, if appropriate, and copious fluids.

Follow local guidelines if available:

> All children under 5 years of age with a first confirmed UTI should be referred to a paediatric urologist for further investigation (e.g. renal tract ultrasound, micturating cystourethrogram, DMSA scan, IVP). Arrange an ultrasound while awaiting specialist assessment.

- Children over 5 years of age should have a renal tract ultrasound, including postvoiding residual urine volume, and should be referred to a paediatric urologist if this is abnormal.
- Antibiotic prophylaxis should be given to under 3-year-olds, and to older children where there is likely to be delay before investigation, e.g. trimethoprim 1–2 mg/kg at night or nitrofurantoin 1 mg/kg at night. Longer term antibiotic prophylaxis may be necessary in children in whom an underlying renal tract abnormality is confirmed, in order to prevent further renal scarring, and should be considered for children with recurrent UTIs in whom investigations have been normal.
- Arrange a repeat MSU for MC&S 1 month after the UTI, to ensure resolution.

SLEEP PROBLEMS

Sleep problems are very common and are nearly always simply habitual. Parents may be concerned that the child will not go to sleep, wakes during the night, or wakes very early. They are likely to be exhausted, and will need reassurance. Try to involve *both* parents in consistent management. Always consider involving the health visitor.

Exclude specific problems, e.g. unhappiness, fear, bed-wetting, environmental noise or illness.

Management

Advice

- An initial sleep diary, recording details of the sleep disturbance, is extremely useful. It should include waking time in the morning, times and lengths of naps during the day, time that the child went to bed, time of settling in bed, and times and lengths of waking during the evening and night, as well as parent management.
- Instil a disciplined bedtime routine.
- If the child gets out of bed, put them straight back with a firm reminder that it is time to sleep. Unless this plan is adhered to every time without fail, the child will continue to wake in the knowledge that the parent will eventually give way.
- Avoid rewards for night-waking, e.g. drinks, taking the child to the parents' bed.
- Ensure a satisfactory environment, e.g. night light, adequate warmth.
- As far as possible, reward success and avoid chastisement.
- Consider the short-term use of hypnotics, in addition to the above, especially if parents are experiencing difficulty coping, e.g. promethazine 15–20 mg (2–5 years), 20–25 mg (5–10 years), at bedtime.

NAPPY RASH

Nappy rash is nearly always either due to contact with ammonia from urine or due to *Candida* (thrush).

Management

- Change nappies frequently to avoid prolonged contact with urine.
- Encourage periods without a nappy, i.e. exposure of buttocks to air.
- Wash the nappy area with water at each change.
- Apply a barrier cream at each nappy change, e.g. zinc and castor oil cream.
- Regular use of bath oils and moisturising creams prevents skin dryness.

Candida dermatitis usually presents as erythematous spots with satellite lesions, and often affects the flexures. (Ammoniacal dermatitis tends to spare the flexures.) Use an imidazole cream or nystatin cream ± a steroid cream, e.g. Timodine.

PRESCHOOL CHECK

This check is carried out by the GP when the child is 3.5 years old. The aim is to detect any potential special educational needs, as well as physical and emotional problems, and arrange for referral and assessment where necessary.

- Discuss parental concerns, asking specifically about vision, hearing, language and behaviour.
- Growth: plot height and weight on a centile chart.
- Examine heart and testes.
- Further examination is only necessary if indicated by parental concerns.
- Immunisations (see p. 334).

GROWTH PROBLEMS

Growth reflects general health and also the nutritional and emotional environment of a child. (For standard growth charts for girls and boys see appendices, pp. 349–352.)

Regular weight and head circumference measurements are useful to detect abnormalities and to reassure the parents that the baby is thriving.

FAILURE TO THRIVE

If the infant's growth pattern is causing concern:

- Measure and plot the infant's weight and head circumference at 2-weekly intervals and plot all previous measurements.
- Discuss milk intake, diet, nature and frequency of stools, and parental attitude and concerns.
- Perform a full examination.
- Check urine for protein, nitrite and leucocytes and send for culture.
- Discuss with the health visitor and other members of the primary healthcare team who may be involved.
- Refer if concern persists.

The most common reason for poor weight gain in breast-fed babies is insufficient milk intake. After attention to feeding technique, a trial of complementary bottle-feeding should be considered.

> **Tip**
> Serious abnormalities affecting growth, in addition to poor weight gain, are usually accompanied by other symptoms and signs. Most babies who gradually cross centiles downwards are normal and are simply adopting their true growth trajectory.

FAT BABIES

Babies whose weight lies above the 97th centile should only be a cause for concern in extreme cases. Infant obesity is not a good predictor of adult obesity.

HEAD GROWTH

Large head
The most common cause of head enlargement is a familial large head, where the head circumference may cross centiles upwards, but additional symptoms are absent. Hydrocephalus usually presents as a head measurement that is crossing centile lines upwards, together with signs of raised intracranial pressure (e.g. tense fontanelle, suture separation, irritability).

- Measure the parents' head circumferences.
- Examine the baby for signs of raised intracranial pressure.
- Refer if there is concern.

Small head
Refer if the head circumference is below the 3rd centile.

SHORT/TALL STATURE

Short stature is considered to be a height below the 3rd centile, tall stature is above the 97th centile (see pp. 349–352). Both are usually normal variants. If there is concern about a child's height:

- Plot the child's height and weight together with previous recordings.
- To assess the expected final adult height of the child, plot the mean parental centile at age 19 (adult) on the growth chart:
  - for a boy this is [father's height + (mother's height + 12.5 cm)]/2
  - for a girl this is [father's height + (mother's height − 12.5 cm)]/2.

A height 8.5 cm above the mean centile is the 97th centile; 8.5 cm below it is the 3rd centile.

    If the child's predicted final adult height is reasonably consistent with the mean parental centile, monitor the height. Refer if this is not the case, if centile lines are crossed or if the final height is extreme and the parents/child are unduly concerned.

RESPIRATORY PROBLEMS

CORYZA

There is rarely any need for antibiotic treatment. Consider paracetamol syrup to reduce irritability, and nasal decongestants if feeding is difficult, e.g. xylometazoline paediatric nasal drops, 2 drops per nostril tds (maximum duration of use 7 days).

COUGH

Bronchiolitis
Bronchiolitis usually presents as an irritable cough with tachypnoea after coryzal symptoms in infants and toddlers, mainly in winter months. There may be feeding difficulty and a low-grade fever. The most common cause is respiratory syncitial virus. Examination confirms widespread crepitations, especially on expiration. Advise paracetamol, fluids and provision of warm moist air, if appropriate. Confident supportive care of the child is important. Refer if there is significant feeding difficulty or if the child is ill or distressed. Antibiotics do not help.

Croup
Croup involves fever, rhinorrhoea and sore throat, together with the diagnostic features of inspiratory stridor and a barking cough. Calm, confident management is important. Ask the parents to place the child in a steamy room (e.g. boil the kettle without a lid), and the symptoms will often improve after 10–20 minutes. Nebulised steroids, e.g. budesonide 2 mg, can be helpful. Antibiotics do not help. Refer if there is intercostal recession or if the child is ill.

Whooping cough (pertussis)
See p. 188.

CHRONIC ASTHMA IN CHILDREN UP TO AGE 12
See also p. 170.

> **Tip**
> There is no evidence that early diagnosis or treatment affects the long-term prognosis of asthma in children under age 5.

Acute viral wheezy episodes in very young children are probably clinically distinct from atopic asthma.

> **Tip**
> The diagnosis of asthma in young children relies almost entirely on history.

History. Ask about:

- a persistent nocturnal cough (a very common presentation in young children)
- recurrent wheezing (most commonly induced by exercise, upper respiratory tract infections and allergens).

Investigations. Consider a chest X-ray if e.g. the child has recurrent chest infections or there is poor response to treatment.

Management of chronic asthma

- Avoid provoking factors, where appropriate. (Parents who smoke should be strongly advised against it.)
- Consider the best method of drug delivery:
  - age 0–2: MDI + spacer and face mask. Bronchodilator syrups, e.g. salbutamol syrup 100 μg/kg tds prn (unlicensed at this age), have more systemic side-effects and are less effective, but are sometimes used in mild cases or for diagnostic treatment trials
  - age 3–12: MDI + spacer. Breath-actuated devices, or, in older children, dry powder devices, can be helpful.

  Nebulisers are rarely needed. Spacer devices are cheaper and as effective.
- Involve parents in a self-management plan as far as possible.
- Regularly review compliance, inhaler technique and parental concerns, especially before stepping treatment up or down.

Drug therapy. Start the patient at the appropriate step according to symptoms (see pp. 96, 97):

- inhaled short-acting β₂ agonist, e.g. salbutamol 2 puffs tds
- inhaled steroid, e.g. beclometasone 100 μg bd.

  Consider inhaled steroids if:
  - using inhaled β₂ agonists more than three times per week
  - symptomatic in the day more than three times per week or at night more than once per week
  - there has been an exacerbation of asthma in the last 2 years.

  Consider stepping down dose of inhaled steroids by 25–50% each time at intervals of 3 months or more. Maintain on the lowest dose of inhaled steroid which controls symptoms:

- leukotriene receptor antagonist, e.g. montelukast 4 mg in the evening
- long-acting β₂ antagonist (LABA), e.g. salmeterol 50 μg bd
- SR theophylline, e.g. Slo-Phyllin 60 mg bd.

A 5-day course of soluble prednisolone (<1 year, 1–2 mg/kg/day; 1–5 years, 20 mg/day; older children, 30–40 mg/day) should be considered at any time to gain rapid control.

Management of acute asthma. See p. 174.

Administration
Quality and Outcomes Framework for Asthma (see p. 175).

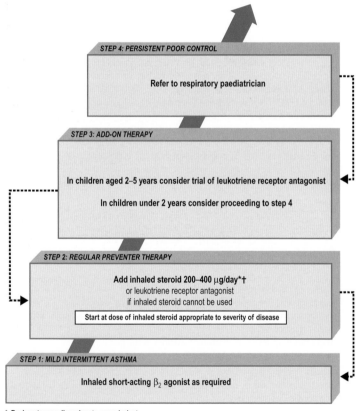

STEP 4: PERSISTENT POOR CONTROL

Refer to respiratory paediatrician

STEP 3: ADD-ON THERAPY

In children aged 2–5 years consider trial of leukotriene receptor antagonist

In children under 2 years consider proceeding to step 4

STEP 2: REGULAR PREVENTER THERAPY

Add inhaled steroid 200–400 μg/day*†
or leukotriene receptor antagonist
if inhaled steroid cannot be used

Start at dose of inhaled steroid appropriate to severity of disease

STEP 1: MILD INTERMITTENT ASTHMA

Inhaled short-acting β₂ agonist as required

* Beclometasone dipropionate or equivalent
† Higher nominal doses may be required if drug delivery is difficult

Summary of stepwise management of asthma in children aged <5 years, 2004. Reproduced with permission from the British Thoracic Society/Scottish Intercollegiate Guidelines Network Executive Committee.

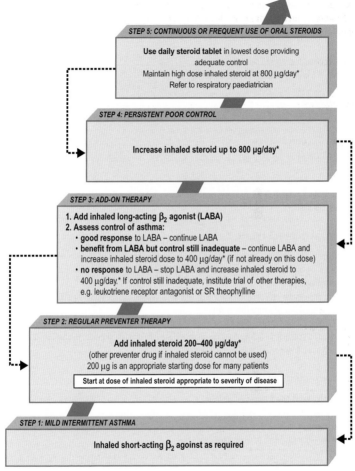

STEP 5: CONTINUOUS OR FREQUENT USE OF ORAL STEROIDS

Use daily steroid tablet in lowest dose providing adequate control
Maintain high dose inhaled steroid at 800 μg/day*
Refer to respiratory paediatrician

STEP 4: PERSISTENT POOR CONTROL

Increase inhaled steroid up to 800 μg/day*

STEP 3: ADD-ON THERAPY

1. **Add inhaled long-acting β_2 agonist (LABA)**
2. **Assess control of asthma:**
   - **good response** to LABA – continue LABA
   - **benefit from LABA but control still inadequate** – continue LABA and increase inhaled steroid dose to 400 μg/day* (if not already on this dose)
   - **no response** to LABA – stop LABA and increase inhaled steroid to 400 μg/day.* If control still inadequate, institute trial of other therapies, e.g. leukotriene receptor antagonist or SR theophylline

STEP 2: REGULAR PREVENTER THERAPY

Add inhaled steroid 200–400 μg/day*
(other preventer drug if inhaled steroid cannot be used)
200 μg is an appropriate starting dose for many patients

Start at dose of inhaled steroid appropriate to severity of disease

STEP 1: MILD INTERMITTENT ASTHMA

Inhaled short-acting β_2 agoinst as required

* Beclometasone dipropionate or equivalent

Summary of stepwise management of asthma in children aged 5–12 years, 2004. Reproduced with permission from the British Thoracic Society/Scottish Intercollegiate Guidelines Network Executive Committee.

CONVULSIONS AND SEIZURES

ABSENCE SEIZURES (PETIT MAL EPILEPSY)

During these episodes, the child suddenly ceases activity, and may stare blankly for a period of seconds. The child may seem to be day-dreaming, and the episodes may occur many times per day. Diagnosis relies on witness reports usually from family or school teachers.

Refer to a paediatric neurologist for investigation and management.

NON-FEBRILE CONVULSIONS

Diagnosis

History. Ask about:

- loss of consciousness
- shaking or jerking
- incontinence
- postictal state
- period of amnesia
- family history.

General management

- Admit all infants with a convulsion under the age of 6 months.
- Refer older children who have had a convulsion to a paediatric neurologist.
- Children with epilepsy should not cycle in traffic. They may swim in the presence of a responsible adult.
- The tendency to have seizures resolves during childhood in >60% of children. Anticonvulsant therapy can be stopped, on specialist advice, if the child has been free from seizures for 2 or 3 years.

Management of status epilepticus

- Ensure that the airway is patent.
- Give diazepam 0.3 mg/kg iv slowly, or rectally 2.5 mg (age <1), 5 mg (age 1–3), 10 mg (age >3).
- Admit the child if fitting continues.

FEBRILE CONVULSIONS

Febrile convulsions are very common, affecting about 4% of all children, usually in the second year of life.

Diagnosis

History. The child has usually been unwell with a high fever prior to developing a major motor seizure lasting a few minutes. There is often a family history of febrile convulsions.

Examination

- The child has a fever and often an upper respiratory tract infection.
- Look for signs of meningitis.
- Examine ears and throat, chest and abdomen.

Investigations. Send a urine sample for culture, if appropriate.

Management
Admit if:

1. meningitis is suspected
2. this is the first attack
3. the child is <18 months old
4. the fit lasts for more than 10 minutes
5. the child is clearly unwell
6. there are persistent neurological signs
7. more than one fit occurs during one febrile episode.

Tip
The child may be left at home if the fit lasts for <10 minutes and recovery is complete.

The risk of recurrence after one febrile convulsion is about 20%. This may be minimised by advising the parents to use tepid sponging and paracetamol whenever the child becomes febrile.

Paracetamol doses: age 3 months to 1 year, 60–120 mg, 4–6 hourly prn; age 1–5 years, 120–250 mg, 4–6 hourly prn; age 6–12 years, 250–500 mg, 4–6 hourly prn (maximum of four doses in 24 hours).

CHILD PROTECTION

Child abuse is often divided into four categories. Few cases in practice fall neatly into one category.

1. PHYSICAL ABUSE (OR NON-ACCIDENTAL INJURY)

Physical abuse should be suspected where the nature of the injury is not consistent with the account of how it occurred, or where there is reasonable suspicion that the injury was inflicted or knowingly not prevented. There is often delay in seeking medical attention. Suspicious injuries include:

- handslap marks
- facial and neck bruising

- bruising to soft body parts, e.g. buttocks, lower abdomen or thighs
- cigarette burns
- grip marks
- bite marks
- 'dipping' scalds
- torn frenulum.

Physical abuse includes Munchausen syndrome by proxy.

2. SEXUAL ABUSE

This includes direct and indirect (e.g. pornography and indecent exposure) sexual acts perpetrated on a child who is either too young to give consent, or is old enough to give consent but is in an exploitative relationship.

Examination is usually unhelpful, but there may be genital or anal injury, emotional disturbance or sexually inappropriate behaviour. The most common presentation is with a statement by the child or by another member of the family.

3. NEGLECT

This involves persistent neglect and failure to protect the child from exposure to danger or threats to health. It may involve persistent absence from school without reason or failure to seek appropriate medical care. It may present as failure to thrive, severe nappy rash, unkempt condition, developmental delay or behavioural and emotional disturbance.

4. EMOTIONAL ABUSE

This involves severe psychological mistreatment. The child is denied comfort, nurture, control and love. There may be persistent verbal denigration and humiliation in the absence of positive interest.

CHILD PROTECTION PROCEDURES

 The child's welfare is paramount. The duty of confidentiality is overridden by the duty to protect the child from abuse.

Children's best interests are served by being cared for within their own families wherever this is possible.

- Take a full history, and carefully record observations.
- Fully examine the child, except in cases of possible sexual abuse when examination should be carried out only by doctors with appropriate training.
- Expert anonymous consultative advice is always available in doubtful cases from e.g. child protection coordinators at Social Services.
- Discuss with other appropriate members of the primary healthcare team, particularly the health visitor.

If abuse is suspected:

- Refer as soon as possible to the Child Protection Investigation Team at Social Services. They will consider the need to remove the child to a place of safety.
- Refer immediately (see below) to the paediatric registrar/consultant for further medical examination.
- In the case of sexual abuse refer to an approved doctor.

The degree of urgency depends on the severity and type of abuse, the age of the child (younger children are more vulnerable) and continued exposure to risk.

- Involve the parents as far as is possible.
- Attend the case conference, or provide a written report. The child may be placed on the Child Protection Register for regular monitoring.
- The case may be taken to court where a supervision order or a care order may be issued.

SUDDEN INFANT DEATH

Sudden infant death syndrome (SIDS) is defined as the sudden, unexpected death of an infant or young child, for which post-mortem fails to show a cause. It occurs in 1 in 500 live births and there is a peak incidence between 2 and 3 months of age. It is rare after 6 months.

Management
The management of families suffering a sudden infant death has similarities with other cases of bereavement (see p. 327).

A phone call from parents whose baby has stopped breathing

- Call an ambulance if the parents have not done so.
- Tell the parents you will come immediately.
- Has resuscitation been attempted? Tell the parents how to attempt mouth-to-mouth resuscitation.
- Continue resuscitation until the ambulance arrives, unless the child is clearly dead (see below).

The 'near miss' (i.e. the apnoeic child has been resuscitated). Admit the child to hospital. The risk of further episodes or of sequelae, whether real or perceived, is lessened by hospital admission.

The dead baby.

Immediate action

- Confirm death (see p. 325).
- Comfort parents and siblings. Be prepared for severe grief reactions, including anger.
- Try to answer parents' questions, which often reflect their feelings of guilt.
- Inform the coroner/police, who will arrange for the baby to be taken to A&E or a mortuary. The police will usually take a statement from the parents.
- Encourage the parents to hold their dead baby.
- Suggest the parents call a close friend or family member to help. This also allows the GP to leave.

Later action

- Visit the family soon after the death.
- Listen to parents' and siblings' expressions of grief.

Common features of grief

These include guilt, anger, loss of confidence, fear of being alone and a sense of unfairness. Many parents have vivid dreams and hear the baby crying.

- Discuss suppression of lactation, if appropriate (see p. 36).
- Involve others in support, e.g.:
  - health visitor or midwife
  - Cot Death Helpline (Foundation for the Study of Infant Deaths) (see p. 357).
- Offer referral to a paediatrician for the parents to discuss the death.
- Offer continued support at home, in the surgery or over the telephone.

Parents' anxieties over the next pregnancy and baby following a sudden infant death.

- Common feelings are doubt, loss of confidence, and fear of loving the new baby too much.
- Reassure the parents that the risk of further SIDS is very low and involve others in supporting the family, e.g. health visitor and midwife, paediatrician and CONI (Care of Next Infant) (see p. 356).

- Apnoea monitors, room thermometers, weighing scales and charts are available from the Foundation for the Study of Infant Deaths (see p. 357).
- Offer same-day appointments for minor illnesses.

Primary prevention of sudden infant death

Advise all pregnant women and mothers of babies, to avoid:

- overwrapping the baby in the cot
- placing the baby face down to sleep
- smoking.

CHAPTER 7

ENDOCRINOLOGY

Diabetes 106
Thyroid disorders 111
Obesity 113

DIABETES

A GP with a list of 2000 patients might expect to have 50 patients with diabetes, 10–15 of whom will be receiving insulin at any one time. Diabetes occurs because of lack of insulin, or resistance to its action, and is diagnosed by raised blood sugars.

> **Tip**
> Active case-finding and organised screening of selected groups is the key to diagnosis.

Risk factors in diabetes

The following factors put people at increased risk of developing diabetes:

- >65 years old
- Asian or Afro-Caribbean origin
- obesity, particularly abdominal obesity
- a family history of diabetes or cardiovascular disease
- a history of gestational diabetes
- a history of having delivered a large baby (>4.5 kg) ⎫ in women.
- a history of unexplained foetal loss ⎭

Diagnosis

Patients are often asymptomatic and may be diagnosed during routine or opportunistic screening.

History. Patients with the following symptoms should be tested for diabetes:

- thirst, polyuria and weight loss
- recurrent infections, especially skin infections
- neuropathic symptoms, e.g. pain, numbness and paraesthesiae
- marked visual acuity changes
- unexplained symptoms, e.g. lassitude.

> **Tip**
> Diabetes is defined by WHO criteria, using venous samples, as:
>
> - a fasting blood glucose level of >7.0 mmol/l, or
> - a random plasma glucose level of >11.1 mmol/l.
>
> In asymptomatic patients the measurements should be duplicated on another day before the diagnosis is made.

Investigations Patients with a fasting plasma glucose between 6.1 and 7.0 mmol/l have impaired fasting glycaemia and need an oral glucose tolerance test.

The oral glucose tolerance test

- The patient should not have smoked and should have had a normal carbohydrate intake for the previous 3 days.
  - After an overnight fast, give 75 g of oral glucose (350 ml of Lucozade can be used).
  - Measure blood glucose 2 hours later.
- If ≥11.1 mmol/l, the patient is diabetic.
- If ≥7.8 and <11.1 mmol/l, the patient has impaired glucose tolerance.
- If <7.8, the patient has normal glucose tolerance.

Patients with impaired fasting glycaemia and impaired glucose tolerance should have annual follow-up with fasting blood glucose measurement.

Management

Referral. At the time of diagnosis, if the patient is ill, ketonuria is present or if the blood glucose is more than about 25 mmol/l, immediate referral should be arranged.

Admit all children and pregnant women.

Aims of diabetic care

- To keep the patient well and symptom-free.
- To keep the fasting blood glucose below 6.7 mmol/l, the maximum blood glucose below 10 mmol/l and the level 2 hours after a meal below 6.7 mmol/l. (It is generally believed that good diabetic control prevents the development of long-term complications.)
- To avoid fasting glycosuria.
- To maintain the HbA_{1c} below 7%.
- To minimise the risk of cardiovascular disease by vigorously treating hypertension (<130/80) and hypercholesterolaemia (reduce total cholesterol by 25% or to <4 mmol/l, whichever is the lower value) in conjunction with the diabetes. All diabetics should be prescribed aspirin 75 mg od if aged >50 and a statin, e.g. simvastatin 40 mg od if aged 40–80, or if younger and total serum cholesterol ≥5 mmol/l.
- To detect complications early, in order to reduce:
  - angina, MI and cerebrovascular disease
  - foot ulceration and limb amputation due to peripheral vascular disease and diabetic neuropathy
  - visual loss due to diabetic retinopathy
  - renal failure due to diabetic nephropathy.
- To offer effective education.

General management. Practice nurses and diabetes specialist nurses have a valuable role in sharing the management of the diabetic patient. Diabetes UK is the national association for diabetes (see p. 356) and offers excellent on-line advice to both patients and professionals.

Education

- Emphasise the importance of self-management.
- Advise against smoking.
- Self-monitoring:
  - All type 1 (insulin-dependent diabetes mellitus (IDDM)) patients should measure their blood glucose (and, ideally, their urine for ketonuria). Teach home glucose monitoring using a blood glucose test meter. Testing should ideally be carried out before each main meal and before bed.
  - Urine testing alone is satisfactory for older type 2 diabetics. The urine should be tested 2 hours after a meal. A series of three tests on one day per week is more useful than once-daily testing.
- Intercurrent illness:

> Diabetes therapy (insulin or tablets) should never be reduced or omitted during intercurrent illness. Insulin-dependent diabetics usually require more insulin during intercurrent illness.

  - Non-insulin-treated patients can occasionally become ketoacidotic during intercurrent illness and may require insulin therapy.
  - The frequency of self-monitoring should be increased.
  - Fluid intake should be increased.
  - Daily carbohydrate intake should be maintained, as liquid if necessary.
  - If the blood glucose is >13 mmol/l or the urine sugar is ≥2%, increase the insulin by 2–4 units per day until control is regained.
  - Admit if the patient is vomiting and unable to take liquid or carbohydrate, or is ketoacidotic or dehydrated.
- Give advice on foot care. Look out for problems, e.g. corns, ingrowing toenails, bunions, and refer to podiatry if appropriate.
- Discuss the warning signs of hypoglycaemia (unsteadiness, difficulty in concentration, headache and tremulousness).
- Diet:
  - Refer all newly diagnosed patients for dietary advice (practice nurse or dietician).
  - Overweight patients need advice on calorie reduction (according to desired BMI).

> **Tip**
> The main dietary message for diabetics is to eat 'healthily'. At least
> half of the energy intake should be made up of complex, fibre-rich
> carbohydrates. Intake of refined carbohydrate, fat, alcohol and salt should
> be low.

- Exercise: regular exercise should be strongly encouraged.
- Immunisations: offer influenza and pneumococcal vaccine to all diabetics.
- Driving: patients must notify the Driver and Vehicle Licensing Agency and their insurance company, unless their diabetes is controlled by diet alone.
- Free prescriptions: patients receiving treatment with either tablets or insulin are exempt from paying prescription charges.
- Occupation: hazardous jobs are no longer an option for patients with type 1 diabetes mellitus, e.g. police, armed forces.

Routine review. The patient should be checked at least 6-monthly (either by the GP, practice nurse or hospital diabetic clinic).
Look at:

- The patient's own records of blood or urine testing (self-monitoring).
- Fasting blood sugar HbA_{ic}.
- Weight/BMI (and discuss diet).
- Urine for protein. If present, send an MSU for MC&S, and check C&Es.

Refer to a nephrologist if there is persistent proteinuria or if the creatinine is raised >150 μmol/l. Tight hypertensive control is important. Proteinuria, rising BP and deteriorating renal function are indicators of nephropathy.
If proteinuria is absent, the urine should be checked for microalbuminuria (microalbuminuria precedes frank proteinuria, and antihypertensive treatment slows progression). If positive (≥20 mg/l), the patient should be started on an ACE inhibitor, even if normotensive, to delay the onset of nephropathy.
Check annually:

- BP. Aiming to reduce to below 130/80 ideally.
- Visual acuity.
- Fundi (dilate pupils with 1% tropicamide). Fundoscopy and fundal photography can be performed by accredited opticians throughout the UK.
- Bloods:
  - C&Es, to exclude renal failure
  - serum cholesterol, triglyceride and HDL, aiming to reduce total cholesterol by 25% or to <4.0 mmol/l, whichever is the lowest, by the use of statins.

- Feet:
  - pulses
  - reflexes
  - vibration and pinprick sensation
  - evidence of ulceration, etc. – treat infection, arrange Doppler, refer urgently to specialised foot care team and consider referral for angiography.

Therapeutic management of type 2 diabetes mellitus

> **Tip**
> The primary treatment of type 2 diabetes is diet, with the aim of reducing excess weight and avoiding refined sugar.

Tablets and insulin should not be used before an adequate trial of diet alone (2–3 months), unless the patient is very ill or has a very high blood glucose (>25 mmol/l).

Start with metformin 500 mg od (decreases gluconeogenesis and increases peripheral utilisation of glucose), provided renal and hepatic function are normal. Metformin is particularly useful for overweight patients, as it is less likely to cause weight gain than the sulphonylureas. Increase the dose monthly as appropriate, to a maximum of 1 g bd. Add a sulphonylurea (see below) if control remains inadequate, e.g. gliclazide 40–80 mg od (augments insulin secretion), adjusted according to response up to a maximum of 160 mg bd. Warn the patient of the hazard of hypoglycaemia.

Consider other antidiabetic agents:

- Glitazones, e.g. rosiglitazone (reduce peripheral insulin resistance). Use as second-line therapy and in patients who are unable to tolerate metformin and sulphonylurea in combination or in patients in whom either metformin or a sulphonylurea is contraindicated.
- Nateglinide and repaglinide stimulate insulin release. Both may be given in combination with metformin. The latter may be given as monotherapy.
- Acarbose is an inhibitor of intestinal alphaglucosidases. It may be used alone or as an adjunct to metformin or to sulphonylureas.

If control remains poor despite attention to diet and tablets, insulin therapy should be considered.

Therapeutic management of type 1 diabetes mellitus. Insulin doses are determined on an individual basis, by gradually increasing the dose but avoiding disabling hypoglycaemia. If the blood glucose is too high, increase the dose of insulin. If the blood glucose is too low, decrease it. Hypoglycaemia between 10 a.m. and lunchtime or between the evening meal and midnight is due to too much short-acting insulin in the morning or evening, respectively. Reduce the dose by 2–4 units.

Hypoglycaemia between 2 p.m. and the evening meal or during the night or before breakfast is due to too much long-acting insulin in the morning or evening, respectively. Reduce the dose by 4–6 units.

Hypoglycaemia. Treat with oral glucose.

If the patient is unconscious, treat with glucagon 1 mg im, sc or iv, or glucose gel (e.g. Hypostop). Both can be issued to responsible relatives for emergency use.

Administration

Quality and Outcomes Framework for Diabetes

- Record body mass index.
- Achieve an HbA_{1c} 7.5% or below.
- Record retinal screening.
- Record peripheral pulses.
- Test for neuropathy.
- Achieve a blood pressure of 145/85 or below.
- Test for microalbuminuria.
- Measure the creatinine.
- Treat microalbuminuria with an ACE inhibitor or A2 antagonist.
- Achieve a cholesterol of 5 mmol/l or below.
- Annual flu vaccination.
- Ask about depression.

THYROID DISORDERS

HYPOTHYROIDISM

Hypothyroidism is common, especially in elderly people in whom the presenting signs are often non-specific. The threshold for testing should therefore be low.

Diagnosis

- Serum thyroid stimulating hormone (TSH) is the best initial screening test, as a normal value virtually excludes hypo- and hyperthyroidism.
- If the TSH is high, measure free T4. If this is low, hypothyroidism is confirmed.
- In subclinical hypothyroidism the TSH is high but the free T4 is normal, and when to start T4 replacement is a matter of clinical judgement.
- Problems with interpreting thyroid function tests in the elderly usually result from non-thyroidal illness or drug treatment.

Management

Most cases of hypothyroidism, particularly in the elderly, can be managed by the GP. Refer those who are young or ill. Check for autoantibodies (their presence makes other autoimmune diseases more likely).

Treatment. Treat with oral levothyroxine. The initial dose is 50–100 µg daily (50 µg for those >50 years and 25 µg in the elderly and those with cardiac disease). Increase the dose by 25 or 50 µg at intervals of at least 4 weeks.

Check the TSH each month and stop increasing the thyroxine dose when the TSH is normal. The usual maintenance dose of thyroxine is 100–200 µg daily. Treatment is usually lifelong. If the TSH is suppressed in young people, the thyroxine dose should be lowered in order to avoid osteoporosis.

Follow-up. Once stable, TSH should be monitored annually.

Patients taking thyroxine replacement are exempt from prescription charges.

Administration

> **Quality and Outcomes Framework for Hypothyroidism**
> • Measure the TSH annually.

HYPERTHYROIDISM

Hyperthyroidism affects about 0.7% of the population.

Diagnosis
TFTs reveal a low TSH and a raised T4 or T3.

Management

> **Tip**
> Refer all patients to endocrinology. The aetiology must be determined and the commonest causes are Graves' disease (80% of cases), toxic multinodular goitre and toxic adenoma.

While awaiting assessment, use propranolol 40 mg tds for rapid relief of symptoms if necessary, in conjunction with carbimazole.

Start carbimazole 15–40 mg daily and maintain the dose until the patient becomes euthyroid, usually after 4–8 weeks. Then reduce the dose progressively to a maintenance of 5–15 mg daily. Assess every 6 months with TFTs. Carbimazole can rarely induce agranulocytosis, which may present as e.g. a sore throat. A white blood cell count should be performed if there is any clinical evidence of infection.

Carbimazole treatment is usually continued for 12–18 months in the hope of inducing lifelong remission. On stopping treatment, check TFTs. Follow-up beyond 1 year is not necessary, but patients should be warned about the possible recurrence of symptoms.

Treatment with radioactive iodine may be recommended. Thereafter, TFTs should be monitored long-term, as most patients become hypothyroid at some stage, even many years after treatment.

THYROID ENLARGEMENT

A thyroid swelling can involve the whole gland (goitre) or consist of an isolated nodule.

Check TFTs.

> All thyroid nodules should be referred to a thyroid surgeon, urgently, in order to exclude malignancy. A simple or multinodular goitre in a euthyroid patient need only be referred if it bothers the patient. This can be confirmed by arranging a thyroid ultrasound scan.

OBESITY

Obesity is defined in terms of body mass index (BMI) (see p. 152):

- 25–30, overweight (grade I)
- 30–40, moderate obesity (grade II)
- >40, severe obesity (grade III).

About 30% of the UK population have grade I obesity, 3% have grade II obesity and 0.3% have grade III obesity. Mortality rates double at a BMI of 35, and increase exponentially with increasing BMI. Obesity is often associated with psychosocial problems, and can exacerbate various medical problems, including:

- hypertension
- ischaemic heart disease
- diabetes mellitus
- respiratory problems
- arthritis
- gallstones
- varicose veins
- intertrigo.

Management

- In order to lose weight, energy output must exceed energy input.
- Discuss breaking the diet/weight-gain/diet cycle by encouraging normal eating patterns.
- Think in the long term. Set realistic goals and take things slowly.
- The patient might expect to lose 0.5–1.0 kg per week on a reduced-calorie diet of e.g. 1000 kcal per day.

- In general, avoid the use of drugs for treating obesity, as they tend to work only in the short term. However, consider:
  - Orlistat 120 mg tds at mealtimes if the BMI is >30 or if the BMI is >28 in the presence of other risk factors, e.g. type 2 diabetes, hypertension, hypercholesterolaemia. It must be prescribed in the context of support, monitoring and counselling (see BNF guidelines).
  - Sibutramine 10–15 mg daily. Similar guidance to orlistat license. BP must be checked regularly.
- Encourage regular exercise.
- Consider involving the practice nurse or hospital dietician. Outside agencies, e.g. Weight Watchers, can be very helpful.

CHAPTER 8

GASTROENTEROLOGY

Dyspepsia 116

Gastro-oesophageal reflux
disease (GORD) 118

Halitosis 118

Coeliac disease 119

Infective diarrhoea 120

Change in bowel habit 121

Diverticulitis 121

Inflammatory bowel
disease 122

Irritable bowel syndrome 122

Constipation 124

Rectal bleeding 125

Pruritus ani 126

Anal fissure 127

Jaundice 127

DYSPEPSIA

Dyspepsia covers a range of symptoms, including epigastric/oesophageal pain, fullness, early satiety, bloating and nausea. It accounts for 3–4% of GP consultations. The main causes are:

- non-ulcer or functional dyspepsia (60–70%)
- peptic ulcer disease (15–20%)
- gastro-oesophageal reflux disease (GORD) (15–20%)
- upper GI cancers (<2%) (less than 1 in 1 000 000 under-55 year olds with dyspepsia have cancer).

Diagnosis

History. Ask about:

- aspects of the epigastric pain, e.g. relationship to food, periodicity, waking at night
- associated features, e.g. nausea and vomiting, bloating, changes in appetite, dietary indiscretion, alcohol intake, weight loss.

Alarm symptoms
Patients with dyspepsia who fulfil these criteria require referral for urgent endoscopy:

- chronic gastrointestinal bleeding
- progressive unintentional weight loss
- dysphagia
- iron deficiency anaemia (excluding NSAIDs and menorrhagia)
- persistent vomiting
- epigastric mass
- suspicious barium meal.

Without alarm symptoms, patients of any age presenting with dyspepsia do not require an endoscopy. Exceptions to this are patients aged >55 who have persistent symptoms despite *H. pylori* eradication, if appropriate, *and* proton pump inhibitor therapy, continuing need for NSAIDs, previous gastric ulcer, gastric surgery or raised risk of gastric cancer.

Management

Advice

- Review medication (e.g. calcium antagonists, nitrates, theophyllines, bisphophonates, corticosteroids and NSAIDs).
- Stop smoking.
- Reduce coffee and alcohol intake.

- Lose weight, if appropriate.
- Consider stress factors.

Prescribing

For mild dyspepsia. Antacids/alginates: e.g. magnesium trisilicate 10 ml after meals and at bedtime or prn, or Gaviscon 10–20 ml after meals and at bedtime or prn.

For more significant symptoms

- Prescribe a proton pump inhibitor at full dose for 1 month (e.g. lansoprazole 30 mg od or omeprazole 40 mg od) *and* test for *H. pylori* and treat, if appropriate (see below).
- If symptoms persist, add an H_2 receptor antagonist (e.g. cimetidine 400 mg bd or ranitidine 150 mg bd) for 1 month *or* a prokinetic agent (e.g. metoclopramide or domperidone) for 1 month.
- Most patients who do not respond to these measures, and without alarm symptoms, have non-ulcer dyspepsia. Endoscopy does not alter management, but gastroenterology referral may be considered. In addition to *H. pylori* serology, investigations prior to referral should include FBC, LFTs and CRP, and consider endomysial antibody.

Ongoing treatment. When PPIs have provided symptom control, then the PPI may be continued at the lowest effective dose on a prn basis. Annual review is appropriate for patients requiring long-term management.

HELICOBACTER PYLORI

H. pylori is associated with >90% of DUs, >80% of GUs and >60% of gastric cancers. It is not associated with GORD. Long-term healing of DUs and GUs can be achieved rapidly by eradicating *H. pylori*. Reinfection is rare.

> **Tip**
> The presence of *H. pylori* should be confirmed before starting eradication treatment.

Tests for **H. pylori**

- Serology or faecal antigen testing are recommended for initial testing.
- Urea breath testing is recommended for those patients where it is necessary to confirm eradication of *H. pylori*, e.g. for recurrent dyspepsia after eradication therapy or treatment of complicated peptic ulcer. This is usually arranged via referral, although urea breath tests are prescribable on FP10.

H. pylori *eradication therapy regimens*

- Full dose PPI (e.g. lansoprazole 30 mg) bd + amoxicillin 1 g bd + clarithromycin 500 mg bd for 7 days *or*
- Full dose PPI (e.g. lansoprazole 30 mg) bd + metronidazole 400 mg bd + clarithromycin 250 mg bd for 7 days.

GASTRO-OESOPHAGEAL REFLUX DISEASE (GORD)

This is common. It usually presents as retrosternal pain, which is worse on lying flat, together with an acidic taste in the mouth. It is usually secondary to a hiatus hernia.

Management

Advice

- As for dyspepsia (see p. 116).
- Elevate the head of the bed.
- Avoid eating late in the evening.
- Avoid large meals.
- Lose any excess weight.
- Avoid foods which aggravate symptoms, e.g. fatty foods, alcohol, coffee, citrus fruits.

Prescribing. (Prescribe according to severity.)

- Antacids (as for dyspepsia).
- Prescribe a full dose PPI (e.g. lansoprazole 30 mg) daily for 1–2 months, followed, if necessary, by a double dose PPI for 1 month.
- If symptoms persist, add an H_2 receptor antagonist (e.g. ranitidine 150 mg bd) or a prokinetic (e.g. metoclopramide or domperidone) to the PPI for 1 month.
- When symptom control is achieved, then the PPI may be continued at the lowest effective dose on a prn basis.

Referral. Non-responders should be referred for a gastroenterological opinion. Patients with alarm symptoms should be referred for urgent endoscopy.

HALITOSIS

When persistent, this is a distressing complaint and is usually due to poor oral hygiene or dental or gum sepsis.

Diagnosis

History. Ask about:

- chronic sinusitis, tonsillitis, respiratory infections and mouth-breathing in children (adenoids)

- smoking and drugs, e.g. alcohol, nitrates, disulfiram
- dry mouth due to e.g. drugs, Sjögren's syndrome
- mood disorders which can present as halitosis.

Investigations. These are rarely necessary, but it may be appropriate to exclude nasopharyngeal malignancy, upper GI tract pathology or metabolic disorders.

Management

- Refer to a dentist for oral assessment.
- Advise on oral hygiene.
- Use a mouth rinse, e.g. 0.2% aqueous chlorhexidine gluconate.

Antibiotic treatment is rarely necessary, but consider treatment with e.g. metronidazole or amoxicillin for 2 weeks to eradicate bacterial overgrowth

COELIAC DISEASE

The prevalence of coeliac disease in adults is 1 in 300. Diagnosis requires a high index of suspicion. It is often wrongly diagnosed as irritable bowel syndrome. In children it commonly presents as growth retardation or delayed puberty. In adults the common presentations are anaemia, chronic fatigue and variable abdominal symptoms (discomfort, bloating, excess wind, aphthous mouth ulcers, altered bowel habit).

It should be considered especially if the patient also has:

- a family history of coeliac disease
- diabetes
- an autoimmune disease
- osteoporosis
- infertility
- an undefined neurological disorder.

Coeliac disease doubles the risk of GI tumours.

Diagnosis

Investigations

- Take blood for endomysial antibodies (positive predictive value $\Delta 95\%$), FBC, B_{12}, folate, Fe, albumin, calcium and IgA antibodies (patients with IgA deficiency have a false-negative endomysial antibody result). Antigliadin antibodies are also useful. Refer to a gastroenterologist if results are positive.
- The definitive test is a distal duodenal biopsy.

Bone density scans are recommended at diagnosis, at the menopause for women, at age 55 for men, or if a fragility fracture occurs at any age (coeliac disease increases the risk of osteoporosis).

Management

Refer to a dietician

A strict lifelong gluten-free diet (resolves symptoms and eliminates the extra risk of osteoporosis and malignancy).

Prescription charge exemption. Patients receiving gluten-free products on prescription are exempt from prescription charges.

INFECTIVE DIARRHOEA

Acute diarrhoea is usually due to food poisoning or a viral infection. Most patients recover spontaneously. Always consider alternative diagnoses, e.g. inflammatory bowel disease, drugs or ischaemic colitis.

Diagnosis

History. Ask about:

- ingestion of suspicious foods
- any contacts with diarrhoea
- occupation (food-handlers will require specific advice)
- recent travel abroad
- blood in the stools.

Investigations. Send stool specimen for investigation if:

- diarrhoea is particularly severe
- diarrhoea has been present for >7 days
- there is blood in the stool
- there is a recent history of foreign travel
- the patient works with food.

Management

Advice

- Fluid intake should be copious.
- Food should not be withheld.
- Rehydration solutions may be helpful, especially in children (e.g. Dioralyte).
- On the whole antidiarrhoeal agents should be avoided, especially in children and the elderly.
- If necessary, diarrhoea in adults can be treated with e.g. loperamide two capsules stat. then one capsule after each loose stool.

Prescribing. Indications for antibiotics are few, as they usually fail to influence the course of the illness and they can prolong and increase the frequency of the carrier state. Ciprofloxacin 500 mg bd for 5 days is occasionally used for prophylaxis against traveller's diarrhoea, but routine use is not recommended. Antibiotics are, however, indicated for:

- *Salmonella*, if severe (ciprofloxacin 500 mg bd for 5 days or trimethoprim 200 mg bd for 5 days).
- *Campylobacter* (erythromycin 500 mg qds for 5 days).
- *Giardiasis* (metronidazole 2 g daily for 3 days). Prompt response to antibiotic treatment is, in fact, a more reliable diagnostic test than stool examination in giardiasis, which is suspected with a >2-week incubation period, watery stools and excessive flatus without fever.
- *Shigella* (ciprofloxacin 500 mg bd for 5 days or trimethoprim 200 mg bd for 5 days).

Referral. Refer if:

- there is dehydration
- there is toxaemia, abdominal pain or abdominal distension
- the diagnosis is unclear.

Administration
Notify, if appropriate (see appendix, p. 347).

CHANGE IN BOWEL HABIT

- Remember to perform a rectal examination.
- Check for anaemia and perform faecal occult bloods.
- Refer if the cause is unclear.

Suspect colonic carcinoma when a patient presents with unexplained, persistent change of bowel habit, either constipation or diarrhoea.

DIVERTICULITIS

Ninety-five per cent of diverticula are in the sigmoid colon.
Acute diverticulitis usually presents with:

- lower abdominal pain (usually left iliac fossa)
- altered bowel habit
- fever.

There may also be:

- nausea and vomiting
- dysuria and urgency (if the affected area lies close to the bladder)
- rectal bleeding.

Chronic diverticulitis (diverticular disease) presents with abdominal pain (usually left iliac fossa) and altered bowel habit. Symptoms are often improved by defaecation.

Management

Acute diverticulitis

- Mild symptoms: prescribe co-amoxiclav 250 mg tds or metronidazole 400 mg bd and cefaclor for 7–10 days. Symptoms should improve within 2–3 days.
- Admit if there is:
  - high fever
  - significant peritoneal signs
  - inability to tolerate fluids.
- Exclude, if appropriate, other causes of rectal bleeding, abdominal pain or altered bowel habit, particularly carcinoma of the larger bowel.

Diverticular disease. Investigate for change in bowel habit. Once diagnosis has been confirmed, treat with high-fibre diet and consider antispasmodics, e.g. mebeverine 135 mg tds prn.

INFLAMMATORY BOWEL DISEASE

Diagnosis, treatment and management of exacerbations fall to the specialist. The GP's role is in the management of established disease only.

The inflammation of Crohn's disease affects any part of the GI tract, frequently in discontinuity (skip lesions). Ulcerative colitis is a chronic disease of the colon which always affects the rectum and extends proximally. Drug therapies include oral prednisolone, rectal corticosteroids, aminosalicylates (e.g. mesalazine), azathioprine and methotrexate. Antibiotics may be used in Crohn's disease for small intestinal overgrowth, perianal sepsis and abscesses associated with fistulae. Patients with Crohn's disease are more likely to require surgery at some stage.

IRRITABLE BOWEL SYNDROME

Irritable bowel syndrome (IBS) is a functional disorder which may involve any part of the GI tract. It is characterised by abdominal pain (colonic or dyspeptic) and disordered bowel habit (diarrhoea and constipation occurring alone or in combination). The patient is likely to be young and female, and there is often a variety of non-bowel complaints, e.g. general malaise, headache and backache. Many patients associate an exacerbation of symptoms with stress.

Diagnosis

History

Common symptoms in irritable bowel syndrome

The diagnosis is usually based on history alone. Five symptoms cluster together significantly more frequently than others:

- distension
- relief of pain by defaecation
- looser stools with the onset of pain
- the passage of mucus
- the sensation of incomplete evacuation.

Examination. This is normal other than occasional colonic tenderness.

Investigations. Hb, ESR and FOBs should all be normal.

Management

Advice

- Improvement with appropriate treatment helps to confirm the diagnosis.
- Discuss the nature of the illness and its relation to stress (relaxation techniques, psychotherapy, etc.).
- Discuss diet:
  - avoid foods which may exacerbate the symptoms (this varies between individuals)
  - encourage a high-fibre diet (see p. 124) and plenty of fluids
  - consider referral to a dietician for e.g. an exclusion diet.

Prescribing

- For constipation: laxatives, e.g. ispaghula husk one sachet in water bd after meals.
- For pain:
  - antispasmodics, e.g. mebeverine 135 mg tds 20 minutes before meals, or peppermint oil 1–2 capsules tds before meals
  - anticholinergic agents, e.g. amitriptyline 25–75 mg nocte.
- For dysmotility symptoms (e.g. bloating, nausea): metoclopramide 10 mg tds prn or domperidone 10–20 mg 4–8-hourly.
- For diarrhoea: e.g. codeine phosphate 30 mg 3–4 times daily.

Referral in irritable bowel syndrome

Patients should be referred if:

- they are aged >40, with recent onset of symptoms
- there are other significant symptoms, e.g. weight loss, blood loss, nocturnal symptoms
- the diagnosis is in doubt.

CONSTIPATION

Constipation is the passage of hard stools less frequently than the patient's own normal pattern. Ensure that the patient has no misconceptions about normal bowel habits and that the constipation requires treatment. Laxatives should generally be avoided, but if they are used, prolonged treatment is seldom necessary.

In children, a high-fibre/high-fluid diet is often sufficient treatment (see p. 88).

CHRONIC CONSTIPATION

Diagnosis

History. A good history is not always easy to obtain, as faecal build up is often very gradual.

Examination. Perform an abdominal and a rectal examination.

Management

Advice

- Encourage exercise.
- Encourage a high fluid intake.
- Allow sufficient time for defaecation, e.g. after meals (especially after breakfast, when colonic activity is at its highest).
- Encourage a high-fibre diet, e.g. fruit, vegetables, wholemeal bread, pasta, wheat bran, cereals, pulses.

Prescribing

- Stimulants, e.g. senna 2–8 tablets nocte, according to response, are useful for 'getting things going' on an intermittent basis.
- Bulk-forming agents, e.g. ispaghula husk, are rarely necessary if the diet is high in fibre. They are useful for patients with colostomies, ileostomies, haemorrhoids, anal fissure, IBS, etc.
- Osmotic agents, e.g. lactulose 15 ml bd or Movicol 1–3 sachets daily, retain fluid in the bowel, and are commonly used.
- Stool softeners, e.g. liquid paraffin and magnesium hydroxide emulsion 20 ml prn, may be used.

Referral. Refer for exclusion of a more serious underlying pathology if the history suggests it, e.g. constipation developing suddenly in a middle-aged person for no clear reason (see p. 121).

ACUTE CONSTIPATION

The basic advice remains the same as above.

- Try to anticipate the problem, e.g. postoperative, bed-bound, perianal pain, opiates.
- Use senna in sufficient dosage: 6–8 tablets nocte.
- Patients may require disimpaction, especially if they are in pain:
  - insert a glycerol or a sodium phosphate suppository, or
  - arrange (usually via the district nurse) for an enema or manual evacuation.
- Enemas:
  - mild: arachis oil enema (to soften impacted faeces) or sodium citrate microenema
  - more powerful: sodium phosphate enema.

RECTAL BLEEDING

FRESH BLOOD

Fresh blood is usually the result of pathology between the anal margin and the lower sigmoid colon, e.g. haemorrhoids, anal fissure, diverticulitis, anorectal carcinoma.

- If the bleeding is minor in a patient aged <40 where the cause is clearly benign, e.g. haemorrhoids, it is reasonable to monitor symptoms over a period of time, and advise on avoiding constipation, etc.
- Remember to perform a rectal examination.
- Check Hb, if appropriate.

> All patients aged >40, with new symptoms or where the bleeding is significant, or where there are associated symptoms, e.g. weight loss, change in bowel habit, should be referred for proctoscopy/sigmoidoscopy/barium enema, etc.

See also haemorrhoids (p. 268).

MELAENA OR ALTERED BLOOD

This suggests bleeding from the upper GI tract. Melaena is usually secondary to stomach pathology.

- Current symptoms: admit immediately.
- If the symptoms have settled: arrange urgent endoscopy.
- Stop NSAIDs.

OCCULT BLEEDING

This is suggested by anaemia with positive faecal occult bloods.

- Refer routinely.
- Stop NSAIDs.
- Treat with oral iron if iron deficiency anaemia is confirmed.

PRURITUS ANI

A clear cause for pruritus ani is not always found. Itch tends to occur if the anus is moist or soiled. In children, the usual diagnosis is threadworms, especially if the history is short.

Diagnosis

History. Attempt to exclude threadworms by asking about the presence of worms in the stools.

Ask about any perianal rash.

Examination. Attempt to exclude the following:

- anorectal disease, e.g. haemorrhoids, fissures
- skin disease, e.g. psoriasis, contact dermatitis (including allergic reactions to products used to treat the pruritus)
- infection, e.g. fungal
- systemic disease, e.g. diabetes mellitus (fungal infection) and chronic liver disease.

Management

Threadworms. Pruritus is due to perianal egg deposition. Examination is usually unnecessary. It is reasonable to treat only the affected child as long as the rest of the family are scrupulously attentive to hygiene. Alternatively, the whole family can be treated.

- Wash perianal skin each morning.
- Wash hands and nails after each visit to the lavatory.
- Treat with mebendazole 100 mg sachet stat. and repeat 2 weeks later if reinfection occurs, or piperazine powder one sachet stat. and repeat after 2 weeks.

General. If no treatable cause is found:

- Consider treating empirically for threadworms.
- Advise careful perianal hygiene after defaecation with thorough drying.
- Avoid use of allergenic substances.
- Hydrocortisone ointment is useful, especially at night, or topical antifungal/ steroid mixtures.

ANAL FISSURE

See p. 268.

JAUNDICE

The common causes of jaundice in adults are: viral hepatitis (see p. 199), alcoholic hepatitis and biliary obstruction due to gallstones or malignancy.

Investigations

- Test the urine for urobilinogen (which indicates haemolysis) and for bilirubin (found in hepatitis and obstruction).
- Take blood for LFTs, hepatitis A, B and C serology, FBC and coagulation screen.
- If obstruction is a possibility, arrange an ultrasound of the liver, gall bladder and pancreas. If obstruction is confirmed, refer.

CHAPTER 9

DERMATOLOGY

Benign superficial lumps   130
Skin malignancies   130
Acne   131
Hidradenitis suppurativa   133
Rosacea   133
Bacterial skin infections   133
Viral skin infections   134
Fungal skin infections   135
Generalised pruritus   137
Hair loss   138
Excessive sweating   138
Eczema   138
Psoriasis   140
Keratosis pilaris   141
Head lice   141
Scabies   142
Other skin infestations   142
Allergic rashes/urticaria   143
Venous ulcers   143
Arterial ulcers   144

BENIGN SUPERFICIAL LUMPS

Benign superficial lesions, including moles, seborrhoeic warts, skin tags and sebaceous cysts, can be removed easily in the surgery by one or other of the following: curettage, cautery, cryotherapy or excision.

SKIN MALIGNANCIES

MALIGNANT MELANOMA

A GP might expect to see one malignant melanoma every 5 years in a list size of 2000 patients. The only effective treatment for melanoma is excision. It is therefore essential that an early diagnosis is made, while the tumour is still thin. Melanomas are extremely fast growing, developing over only a few months.

Diagnosis

History. Ask about the following risk factors:

- A mole changing in shape or colour.
- Large numbers of normal naevi, particularly with a family history of malignant melanoma.
- A past history of primary malignant melanoma or severe sunburn.
- General skin type: people with blonde/red hair colour and poorly tanning skin are at greater risk.

Examination

> **Tip**
> Major features strongly suggestive of malignancy
> - Change in size or new lesion.
> - Irregular shape.
> - Irregular colour.

Also look for other suspicious features, e.g.:

- inflammation
- crusting or bleeding
- changes in sensation.

Management

All suspicious moles should be referred immediately for wide excision.

Patients with clearly benign lesions should be reassured, and prevention should be discussed; excise the lesion if appropriate.

Long-term prevention. High-risk patients should be advised to examine themselves regularly and to know the signs of malignancy. They should protect themselves from the sun, avoid sunbeds and use sunscreens that protect against UVA and UVB with a sun protection factor of >15, e.g. Uvistat 20. Sunscreens can be prescribed on FP10 only for patients with photodermatoses who require high protection (SPF >15). Prescriptions should be marked with 'ACBS' (Advisory Committee on Borderline Substances).

Low-risk patients should also be advised to protect themselves from the sun and to use sunscreens with an SPF of at least 10.

SOLAR KERATOSES

These are more common on sun-damaged skin and in the elderly. They look like dry, cracked plaques. They have very low malignant potential, and can be treated with cryotherapy or fluorouracil cream bd for 2–4 weeks.

BASAL CELL CARCINOMA (RODENT ULCER) AND SQUAMOUS CELL CARCINOMA

These are commonly related to sun exposure. They both have raised irregular edges and may be ulcerated. The BCC may have a pearly border. These should be referred early for excision, radiotherapy or cryotherapy.

ACNE

More then half of British teenagers develop acne severe enough to warrant therapy. Acne can cause great emotional distress, and is usually easily treatable. It is exacerbated by hot, sweaty conditions, and any cosmetics used should be light and non-greasy. Sensitivity and understanding are important. Most sufferers will have already self-treated with OTC preparations.

Diagnosis

History. Ask about past and present OTC and prescribed treatments.

Examination. Look for comedones, erythematous papules and pustules on the face, chest or back. There may be pitted scars.

Management

> **Tip**
> Most patients need to be reassured that their acne is very largely unrelated to the nature of their diet.

Mild acne. These topical preparations should be applied to the whole affected area after washing the skin, and are likely to cause some degree of skin irritation initially.

Inflammatory lesions

- Benzoyl peroxide (1–10%). Start treatment with lower strength preparations.
- Topical antibiotics (clindamycin, erythromycin or tetracycline).
- Azelaic acid.

Non-inflammatory lesions (comedones)

- Topical retinoids (e.g. adapalene, tretinoin).
- Topical retinoids may be used in addition to benzoyl peroxide or topical antibiotics. If used together, apply each once a day at different times.

Moderate acne

Oral antibiotics. These may be used in addition to topical treatments. Improvement may take up to 6 weeks and maximum improvement occurs at 3–4 months. It is worth trying an alternative oral antibiotic if the response to the first is inadequate after 3–4 months. Treatment may continue for several years, if necessary.

- Oxytetracycline 500 mg bd for 3 months, then reduced to 250 mg bd.
- Erythromycin 500 mg bd for 3 months, then reduced to 250 mg bd. (Both antibiotics can be increased to 1–2 g per day, if necessary.)
- Minocycline and doxycycline are only taken once a day. They are significantly more expensive. They are less affected by food.

The combined oral contraceptive in acne

The COC can be started in a patient who has been taking long-term antibiotics for acne without the need for extra contraceptive precautions. If the patient is already on the COC when first starting antibiotics for acne, or when switching to a different antibiotic, additional contraception should be used for the first 2 weeks to allow antibiotic resistance to develop among the bowel flora which are responsible for recycling oestrogens.

Hormonal treatment

- Dianette: this contains cyproterone acetate, an antiandrogen. It is the most effective oral contraceptive for acne, and if used for contraception, a prescription charge can be avoided by writing 'for contraception' on the prescription. It can be used with or without oral antibiotics and/or topical treatments.
- COC: other COCs that tend to improve acne are those with a relatively non-androgenic progestogen, e.g. Marvelon, Cilest, Femodene, Minulet and Yasmin.

Severe acne. (Also acne that fails to respond to the above treatment.) Refer for oral isotretinoin. This is expensive, teratogenic and has a high side-effect profile. All females of child-bearing age should be using effective contraception (usually Dianette) and should have LFTs and fasting lipids checked before their dermatology appointment.

HIDRADENITIS SUPPURATIVA

This causes chronic papules and pustules, with scarring, in the axillae and/or groins. It can be treated with long-term oxytetracycline 500 mg bd. Some patients require plastic surgery.

ROSACEA

 Topical steroids aggravate rosacea.

This is characterised by chronic, shiny facial erythema, especially over the cheeks and central forehead. It is exacerbated by heat, sun exposure, spicy food and alcohol. There may be papules and pustules. It occurs most commonly in middle-aged women. It can be treated with long-term oxytetracycline 500 mg bd, reducing, if possible, to a maintenance dose of 250 mg daily. Treatment may be continuous or intermittent. Metronidazole gel applied twice daily is an alternative treatment, and may be used, if necessary with oral antibiotics.

BACTERIAL SKIN INFECTIONS

CELLULITIS/ERYSIPELAS (STREPTOCOCCAL)

These two conditions may coexist. Erysipelas is a superficial infection, causing sharply demarcated tender erythematous areas. Cellulitis causes deeper infection, involving the subcutaneous tissues. Treatment is with oral penicillin (*and*, in the case of cellulitis, flucloxacillin, in case of staphylococcal involvement) or erythromycin alone if penicillin-allergic for 7–10 days. Advise bed rest. Occasionally, admission may be required for treatment with intravenous antibiotics.

BOILS (STAPHYLOCOCCAL)

See p. 198.

FOLLICULITIS (STAPHYLOCOCCAL)

This is sometimes seen in patients treated with topical steroid ointments for eczema, and as a result of shaving or skin friction. It should be treated with mild antiseptics, e.g. povidone-iodine, or, if severe, with oral flucloxacillin.

IMPETIGO

Impetigo is a common infectious condition of the skin, caused by *Staphylococcus*.

Diagnosis

History. Impetigo starts as a slough, which hardens to form a yellow crust. It is usually painless and occurs anywhere on the body, but is most common on the face.

It often complicates other skin problems that involve a breach of the skin surface, e.g. cracked lips, cold sores, eczema or grazes.

Cold sores can be indistinguishable from impetigo.

Management

- Fusidic acid cream tds rubbed on the crusts will help to soften them and prevent the further multiplication of bacteria.
- For widespread or stubborn lesions, use flucloxacillin 250 mg qds for 5 days.
- Erythromycin is effective in patients allergic to penicillin.

> **Tip**
> Inform the patient that impetigo is contagious and an individual towel and flannel should be used. It is not necessary to avoid school once treatment has started.

ERYTHRASMA

This usually presents as a brown, slightly scaly area in the armpits or groins. It is asymptomatic and is produced by a *Corynebacterium*. It can be treated with topical imidazoles, e.g. miconazole, or topical fusidic acid, or with a 2-week course of oral erythromycin.

VIRAL SKIN INFECTIONS

WARTS

Diagnosis

Look for firm papules with a rough hyperkeratotic surface. Plantar warts (verrucae) may look like callosities (hyperkeratosis) and often have a dark centre. They can cause pain on walking.

Management

> **Tip**
> Warts and verrucae usually resolve spontaneously, the patient's immune response overcoming the infection. Treatment is only necessary if the patient is troubled by the wart.

Treat with the daily application of a wart paint or gel containing salicylic acid (e.g. Salactol), having softened the wart in hot water for a few minutes and removed any dead tissue with an emery board or pumice stone. The paint should not touch surrounding healthy tissue. The treatment may need to be continued for 3 months.

Cryotherapy with liquid nitrogen can be used for warts resistant to wart paints. It is quite painful and therefore best avoided in small children. Warn the patient that a blister may occur after treatment. Multiple warts normally require more than one application, and the optimum interval between treatments is 3–4 weeks. Occasionally, resistant warts require treatment with curettage and cautery.

Planar warts should be left to resolve spontaneously, as they are difficult to treat effectively.

Children with verrucae should be allowed to use swimming pools, particularly if the verruca is covered with a plaster or a water-resistant gel (e.g. Salatac), or if a verruca sock (available OTC) is used.

For genital warts, see p. 47.

MOLLUSCUM CONTAGIOSUM

This consists of asymptomatic crops of firm, pink, pearly papules, some of which have a central depression. They resolve spontaneously usually after about 12 months, but occasionally they persist for up to 5 years. Resolution may be hastened by:

- squeezing each lesion in order to expel the central plug (parents of young children with molluscum can be advised to perform this)
- cryotherapy
- pricking the centre of each lesion with phenol on the end of a cocktail stick.

FUNGAL SKIN INFECTIONS

RINGWORM (TINEA)

This can involve feet (athlete's foot), body, groin, scalp and nails. It is usually indirectly acquired as a result of contact with fungal hyphae in keratin debris. Athlete's foot is frequently the source of groin ringworm.

Diagnosis

Examination. Tinea pedis usually starts with macerated, irritable skin between the toes and may spread to the soles and dorsum of the foot.

Tinea corporis is characterised by red, circular, slightly scaly lesions which clear centrally and spread from the perimeter.

Tinea cruris presents as a well-demarcated, red, slightly scaly groin rash, and is most common in young men.

Tinea unguium causes thickened, yellow friable nails, and most commonly affects one or a few nails only.

Investigation. Send off skin scrapings, subungual scrapings or plucked hair, as appropriate, for microscopy and culture. (Unfortunately, results are often negative despite the presence of tinea.)

Management

Skin. Keep the affected skin clean and dry. Treat with a topical imidazole cream, e.g. clotrimazole, econazole or miconazole (apply 2–3 times daily, continuing for 14 days after the lesions have healed). Resistant cases can be treated with e.g. oral terbinafine 250 mg daily for 2–6 weeks or itraconazole 200 mg bd for 7 days.

Nails. Most treatments need to be continued until the affected nails grow out (6 months for fingernails and 12–18 months for toenails).

Topical treatments

- Tioconazole nail solution: apply twice daily.
- Amorolfine nail lacquer: apply 1–2 times weekly.

Oral treatments

- Terbinafine 250 mg daily is expensive, but only needs to be continued for 6 weeks for fingernails and 3 months for toenails.
- 'Pulsed' treatment can be prescribed, e.g. itraconazole 200 mg bd for 7 days and subsequent courses repeated after 21-day interval (fingernails two courses, toenails three courses).

CANDIDA INFECTION

Buccal mucosa. This is common in babies. Treatment is with e.g. nystatin oral suspension 100,000 units qds after food or amphotericin lozenges 1 qds, both to be continued for 2 days after lesions have resolved.

Nappy rash. See p. 91.

Intertrigo/angular stomatitis/chronic paronychia. Keep the hands dry and use a topical imidazole cream.

PITYRIASIS VERSICOLOR

This is characterised by an area of scaly, confluent macules which are usually asymptomatic and on the trunk, upper arms or legs. Affected patches remain pale on tanned skin. Use a topical selenium sulphide, e.g. Selsun shampoo, on all affected areas. Leave on the skin for 10 minutes before washing off. Repeat every other night for 3 weeks. Persistence of hypopigmented areas does not signify treatment failure. Alternatively, use an imidazole cream each night for 2–4 weeks. Oral itraconazole 200 mg daily for 7 days is effective.

SEBORRHOEIC DERMATITIS

> **Tip**
> Seborrhoeic dermatitis is often confused with eczema.

This usually presents as red, scaly patches in the eyebrows or nasolabial folds. It is commonly associated with a scaly scalp (dandruff) and blepharitis. Use a topical antifungal, e.g. ketoconazole cream bd ('SLS' must be written on the prescription) or Canesten HC, continuing for a few days after the lesions have healed, and ketoconazole shampoo twice weekly for 2–4 weeks. Recurrence requiring repeat treatment is common.

PITYRIASIS ROSEA

This is an eruption of pink macules, mainly over the trunk, which are usually distributed in lines parallel to the ribs. No action is required, but a mild topical steroid will relieve irritation. The rash resolves spontaneously in 6–8 weeks.

GENERALISED PRURITUS

Where there is no obvious skin disease, all patients with persistent generalised pruritus should be investigated to exclude an underlying systemic disorder. Scabies is a common cause – burrows can be difficult to see (see p. 142).

Arrange FBC, ESR, LFTs, C&Es, fasting BS, TFTs, urine for protein and a CXR.

If no underlying cause is found:

- use an emollient regularly (see p. 139)
- consider use of a topical steroid cream and/or an oral antihistamine. Crotamiton cream can be helpful.

HAIR LOSS

Acute stress is often the trigger for diffuse hair loss. Thyroid disease, iron deficiency and drug side-effects should be excluded. There is no specific treatment other than treating any identifiable underlying cause.

Alopecia areata normally resolves within a few weeks, although episodes may recur. Exclude tinea and hairpulling or other trauma in patchy hair loss.

Androgenic alopecia may be arrested by the use of topical minoxidil, which is only available on private prescription or OTC.

EXCESSIVE SWEATING

GENERALISED

A cause is rarely identified, but consider menopausal flushing, hyperthyroidism or hyperpituitarism, and autonomic neuropathy.

LOCALISED TO THE AXILLAE, PALMS AND SOLES

- Apply 20% aluminium chloride hexahydrate roll-on antiperspirant (e.g. Driclor) to dry axillae, palms or soles each night, and reduce to 1–2 times weekly as improvement occurs.
- Smelly feet are usually due to bacterial superinfection of sweat. Treat with e.g. potassium permanganate soaks (1:10 000 aqueous solution) twice daily, until the smell has improved. (Potassium permanganate stains the skin.)
- Axillary odour can be treated with an antiseptic cream, e.g. chlorhexidine cream bd.
- Consider dermatological referral for iontophoresis, which may help palmar or plantar hyperhydrosis, or botulinum type A toxin injections (Botox). In intractable cases consider surgical referral for thoracoscopic sympathectomy (also treats severe facial blushing).

ECZEMA

Eczema affects 15% of children (clearing in 50% of them by the teenage years) and 2–10% of adults. Atopic eczema is not present at birth, but often appears within the first 2 years of life. It is associated with other atopic conditions (asthma and has fever).

'Eczema' is synonymous with 'dermatitis'. Treatment is basically the same, whether the eczema is exogenous (allergic and contact dermatitis) or endogenous (atopic).

Diagnosis

The main symptom is itching. The main signs are redness, papules, vesicles and hyperkeratosis, and there may be weeping and crusting.

Unlike fungal rashes, which have a well-demarcated edge, eczema is more diffuse.

Management

General. Sympathetic explanation is essential, especially to the parents of young children with atopic eczema. Assess possible irritants or trigger factors with a view to avoidance, if possible, e.g. contact with metals, detergent or woollen clothing, dietary factors, emotion, heat, cold. If appropriate, give details of local and national support groups (see p. 358). The skin should be kept clean and warm, and prolonged contact with water, detergent, etc. should be avoided. If the hands are affected, gloves should be worn at the sink etc.

Emollients. Emollients moisten dry, scaly skin, and are the mainstay of treatment. They can be used at any time on dry skin, but are particularly useful at bathtime, when different preparations can be used in combination:

- soap substitute, e.g. emulsifying ointment
- bath oil, e.g. Oilatum emollient
- emollient cream after bathing, e.g. aqueous cream.

Ointments are more effective than creams, but in view of their greasiness they are less user-friendly.

Topical steroids. Aim to use the weakest preparation sufficient to control the disease. Acute exacerbations should be treated with relatively potent steroids. The potency should be quickly reduced when control is gained. Try to avoid anything stronger than 1% hydrocortisone on the face or in infancy.

Steroid potency

- Mildly potent: e.g. hydrocortisone 0.5%, 1% (can be bought OTC for use on all parts of the body except the face) and 2.5%.
- Moderately potent: e.g. clobetasone butyrate 0.05% (Eumovate).
- Potent: e.g. betamethasone 0.1% (Betnovate).
- Very potent: e.g. clobetasol propionate 0.05% (Dermovate).

Other treatments. Secondary infection should be treated with topical antibiotic cream or ointment (e.g. fusidic acid) or oral antistaphylococcal antibiotics (e.g. flucloxacillin or erythromycin).

Severe eczema on the limbs can be treated with bandages (wet wrapping) which may be applied overnight on top of steroid ointment or emollients, e.g. zinc paste and ichthammol bandage, zinc paste and coal tar bandage or simple elasticated tubular bandage. A community paediatric/eczema nurse may be available to instruct parents on their use.

A sedative antihistamine at night may help itching in exacerbations e.g. alimemazine 2.5–5 mg tds for children over 2 years old.

The role of diet in atopic eczema is contentious. Cow's milk is the most commonly implicated food, and should be avoided for the first 6 months of life. Exclusion diets help a small number of children, and should only be undertaken with expert advice from a dietician.

Referral. Consider referral if:

- eczema is resistant or aggravated by conventional therapy
- eczema is severe, for consideration of phototherapy or immunosuppression (e.g. tacrolimus). Consider a short course of oral steroids while awaiting an urgent appointment (e.g. prednisolone 20–30 mg od for 5 days)
- infection is a problem (bacterial or herpes simplex)
- there is a need to use long-term potent topical steroids
- wet wrapping/paste bandaging techniques need to be taught
- patch testing is indicated to investigate contact dermatitis
- there are occupational factors.

PSORIASIS

In total, 1.5% of the population are affected by this chronic inflammatory skin disease during their lifetime. It most commonly presents as multiple, large, well-demarcated, red plaques with thick silvery scales in a symmetrical distribution, often involving elbows, knees and scalp. Nails may be pitted. There is no cure and it is usually lifelong, with exacerbations and remissions. The patient should therefore be given detailed information on self-management. The Psoriasis Association can be helpful (see p. 358).

Psoriasis is often exacerbated by trauma, stress or infections.

STABLE PLAQUES

Management

- Emollients (see p. 139). These help to control the scaling and irritation, and their use should be encouraged in addition to other treatments.
- Vitamin D preparations, e.g. calcipotriol (Dovonex) ointment or cream bd.
- Topical steroids, e.g. Eumovate or Betnovate RD ointment bd (see p. 139). Useful in stable disease and when plaques are few in number.
- Proprietary tar preparations, e.g. Alphosyl and Exorex, and mild steroid/tar combinations, e.g. Alphosyl HC.
- Proprietary dithranol preparations, e.g. Dithrocream. Preparations should be applied daily to plaques and washed off after 30 minutes. Old clothes should be worn during application. Start with a low concentration (0.1%) and

gradually build up to the maximum concentration which produces
a therapeutic effect without irritation (up to 2%).
- PUVA, oral retinoids, methotrexate, ciclosporin, etc. If psoriasis is extensive or
unresponsive to the above treatments, refer for these.

SCALP PSORIASIS

In contrast to the scalp changes of seborrhoeic dermatitis, the scalp lesions in
psoriasis are easily felt.

Daily shampooing with coal tar shampoo, e.g. Polytar, is helpful, but by itself
is unlikely to control thick plaques. Calcipotriol (Dovonex) scalp solution used
twice daily, or topical steroid lotions (e.g. Betnovate scalp application) used on a
daily basis or less frequently, may be prescribed in addition.

Mixtures of tar and salicylic acid, although messy, are particularly effective
for severe scaling, e.g. Cocois scalp ointment, which should be applied to the
scalp once weekly, or more often if necessary, and shampooed off after 2 hours
or left on overnight. Mixtures of steroid and salicylic acid, e.g. Diprosalic scalp
application, are also helpful.

GUTTATE PSORIASIS

These symmetrical plaques on the trunk and/or limbs are round, unlike the oval
lesions of pityriasis rosea. They usually clear completely in a few months, but
classic psoriasis may develop subsequently.

Perform a throat swab, as guttate psoriasis usually follows a streptococcal
throat infection.

Use a mild tar-based cream, e.g. Alphosyl or Alphosyl HC, and consider
referral for UVB phototherapy.

KERATOSIS PILARIS

This is a very common disorder where the hair follicles are plugged with
keratin, causing rough skin. The commonest sites are the posterior upper arm
and the lateral cheeks, and it usually presents in young women as a cosmetic
nuisance.

Treat with mild keratolytics, e.g. salicylic acid 2–4% in soft white paraffin, or
advise cosmetic exfoliation. Emollients are helpful.

HEAD LICE

Head lice are common, and a particular problem in young schoolchildren and
their families. They present as an itchy scalp.

Management

Nit combs

Daily use of nit combs, ideally on wet, conditioned hair, is now advocated in preference to insecticides (particularly if the lice are few in number, or have shown resistance to insecticides), in order to eliminate new lice and therefore to break the cycle. Nit combs can remove lice at all stages of development. They will not remove empty egg-cases, which persist on the hair for some time.

Insecticides clear the lice at all stages except the very young eggs. The treatments should therefore be repeated after an interval of 7–10 days.

Lotions should be used in preference to shampoos, which are relatively ineffective. Use e.g. permethrin cream rinse. Rub into damp hair and rinse after 10 minutes.

Resistance to insecticides is becoming increasingly common. If a course of treatment fails to cure, a different insecticide should be used for the next course. Insecticides can be bought OTC. Essential oils, e.g. tea tree oil, may be used, mixed with shampoo prior to nit-combing, to help clearance. All members of a household should be treated. Parents should notify the school so that all members of the class can be treated.

SCABIES

The scabies mite spreads by skin to skin contact, e.g. holding hands with an infected person or sleeping in the same bed. It can take up to 6 weeks to develop symptoms after being infected. All household members and intimate contacts should be treated, to avoid reinfection. Commonly there are just a few mites on the skin, creating burrows, but the allergy to them causes generalised itch and mild rash.

- Treat with malathion lotion or permethrin cream (available OTC).
- Apply over the whole body from the neck down. Wash off after the recommended time (8–24 hours). Reapply treatment to hands every time they are washed within the treatment period. Reapply the same treatment 7 days after the first application.
- The itch takes 2–3 weeks after treatment to subside. (This can be treated with e.g. crotamiton cream ± hydrocortisone cream.)
- Wash all worn clothes and bedding.

OTHER SKIN INFESTATIONS

CRAB LICE

These are capable of living in all hair except scalp hair, which is too dense for them. The most common site is pubic hair. They are transmitted by close physical contact, usually sexual. Infection of children is not evidence of sexual abuse. Use aqueous preparations of e.g. malathion over the whole body. Instructions for use are as for head lice.

FLEA BITES

These usually present as multiple lesions around the ankles and calves. Often, only one member of the family is affected.

Use hydrocortisone ointment or calamine lotion on spots to relieve the itching (both can be bought OTC). Deflea pets, and spray insecticide on soft furnishings and carpets. Professional exterminators, via the Environmental Health Department, are sometimes needed.

BED BUGS

These are suggested by very large lesions on the face or hands, particularly when new lesions are found each morning. Bed bugs live behind wallpaper and skirting boards, not in beds. The Environmental Health Department should be called to treat the house.

ANIMAL MITES

These are suggested by itchy papules, principally on the abdomen, thighs and arms (i.e. the main sites of contact with an animal sitting on the sufferer's lap). Treat the animal.

ALLERGIC RASHES/URTICARIA

It is often difficult to establish a cause; any potential cause should, if possible, be avoided. It is possible to become hypersensitive to an allergen after many years of uneventful exposure to it. Urticaria may be due to a viral infection.

Management

- Oral antihistamine, e.g. loratadine 10 mg od.
- Topical steroids help to relieve pruritus.
- If the urticaria is severe, consider a short course of oral steroid (e.g. prednisolone 30 mg od for 3–5 days in adults). See p. 348 for anaphylaxis.
- If the urticaria is recurrent and there is no clear cause, refer for allergy testing.

VENOUS ULCERS

These are the commonest type of leg ulcer and are associated with underlying venous disease. They commonly occur above the medial or lateral malleoli. Confirm aetiology by Doppler. The mainstay of treatment is to limit oedema by good compression bandaging. Nurses are very much the experts in this field.

Management

General measures

- Encourage weight reduction in those at risk. (This is usually extremely difficult to achieve.)
- Encourage mobility (and ankle flexing while lying and sitting). The leg should be raised above the level of the hip when sitting.
- Consider systemic causes. Check Hb and urine for sugar.
- Physiotherapy may be beneficial, e.g. exercises, gentle massage and local ultrasound.
- Consider the use of diuretics and analgesics.

Dressing and bandaging

- Clean the ulcer with saline or warmed tap water.
- Moisturise surrounding skin with e.g. 50% liquid paraffin and 50% soft white paraffin. If significant eczema is present, consider steroid ointments and/or a medicated paste bandage (allergy to these is not uncommon).
- Dressings should be changed only once or twice a week, or as necessary. The choice of dressing depends on the nature of the ulcer, patient comfort, presence of infection, etc. A non-adherent dressing may be all that is necessary if compression is being used.
- Compression must be avoided if there is any evidence of arterial insufficiency.
- When an ulcer has healed, a graduated compression stocking should be prescribed.

Infected ulcers

- Take a swab.
- Prescribe oral antibiotics, e.g. flucloxacillin, or, if foul-smelling, metronidazole.
- Treat cellulitis with oral penicillin and flucloxacillin, or erythromycin.

Slow-healing ulcers. Consider:

- dermatology (ulcer clinic) referral
- varicose vein surgery. In younger patients this may prevent recurrences (see p. 270).

ARTERIAL ULCERS

These tend to occur over the shin or around pressure points.

- Confirm aetiology by Doppler (usually assessed by nurse).
- Consider referral to vascular surgery if ankle:brachial systolic pressure index (ABI) ≤ 0.8.
- Use light bandaging only. Compression bandages should be avoided.
- Treat pain and infection, if appropriate.
- Arterial ulcers usually take longer to heal than venous ulcers.

CHAPTER 10

CARDIOLOGY

Primary prevention of coronary heart disease 146

Hypertension 149

Cholesterol 151

Intermittent claudication 153

Chest pain 154

Angina 156

Acute myocardial infarction (MI) 158

Postmyocardial infarction 160

Heart failure 161

Raynaud's phenomenon 163

Funny turns 163

Palpitations 165

PRIMARY PREVENTION OF CORONARY HEART DISEASE

Primary prevention relates to individuals who have not developed symptomatic cardiovascular disease (CVD) or other major atherosclerotic disease, such as stroke/TIA or peripheral vascular disease.

In order to calculate a patient's CVD risk the following information is required:

- Gender.
- Age.
- Smoking status.
- Total cholesterol.
- HDL cholesterol.
- Blood pressure.

The presence or abTof diabetes mellitus is now obsolete when calculating primary coronary/stroke risk. Patients with diabetes should be considered suitable for secondary prevention measures (see Tip Box below).

Apply this information to the graphs on pp. 147–148 to calculate the 10-year risk of developing CVD. Alternatively, use the computer CHD/CVD risk calculator in the clinical system holding the patient's medical record.

> **Tip**
> Patients >50 years old with a 10-year CVD risk >20% should take aspirin 75 mg od unless contraindicated. Patients <80 years old with a 10-year CVD risk >20% and a serum total cholesterol >3.5 mmol/l should, in addition, be prescribed a statin.

General lifestyle advice for prevention of CVD

- Stop smoking (see p. 313).
- Dietary advice:
  - aim for ideal weight (see obesity, p. 113)
  - reduce dietary fats (see cholesterol, p. 151)
  - consume five portions of fruit or vegetables per day.
- Encourage exercise: recommend at least 20 minutes of brisk exercise three times per week.
- Encourage stress reduction (see anxiety, p. 294).
- Avoid excessive alcohol intake (>14 units per week for women and >21 units for men).

Risk factors for CVD

- Male.
- Age >50 years.
- South Asian/Afro-Caribbean race.
- Smoking.

JOINT BRITISH SOCIETIES' CVD RISK-PREDICTION CHARTS

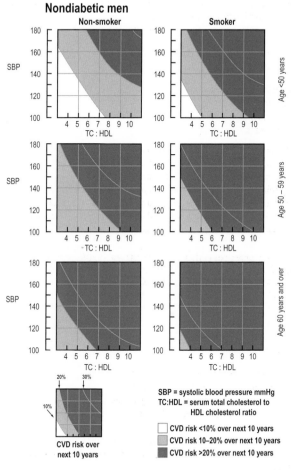

Nondiabetic men

SBP = systolic blood pressure mmHg
TC:HDL = serum total cholesterol to HDL cholesterol ratio

☐ CVD risk <10% over next 10 years
▨ CVD risk 10–20% over next 10 years
▦ CVD risk >20% over next 10 years

(continued overleaf)

JOINT BRITISH SOCIETIES' CVD RISK-PREDICTION CHARTS (*continued*)

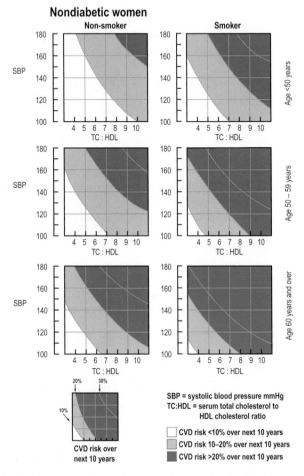

Nondiabetic women

SBP = systolic blood pressure mmHg
TC:HDL = serum total cholesterol to HDL cholesterol ratio

☐ CVD risk <10% over next 10 years
☐ CVD risk 10–20% over next 10 years
■ CVD risk >20% over next 10 years

Reproduced with permission from Professor P. Durrington, University of Manchester. Heart 2005; 91(Suppl V): VI–V52, copyright University of Manchester. These graphs underestimate the CVD risk in patients with a strong family history of premature CVD, and also those of Afro–Caribbean or South Asian origin.

Risk factors for CVD *(continued)*

- Obesity.
- Hypertension.
- Diabetes.
- Hyperlipidaemia.
- Other atheromatous disease (CVA/TIA, peripheral vascular disease).
- Family history of premature atheromatous disease.

HYPERTENSION

Hypertension affects approximately 15% of the population. It is asymptomatic unless extremely high. It can be managed almost entirely in general practice. The following advice is based on the British Hypertension Society's Guidelines 2004.

Diagnosis

The new hypertensive. On finding a raised blood pressure for the first time in a patient, the path described below can be followed.

- <139/89: no treatment, no follow-up (<130/80 in diabetics).
- >160/100: treat if consistently above this level on four or more consecutive readings over 2 weeks.

Tip
Ask the practice nurse to repeat the readings.

- Between 140/90 and 160/99: repeat BP reading four times over 3–6 weeks.

Diastolic BP of >120 and rising on subsequent examinations suggests malignant hypertension. Urgent referral or hospital admission is necessary.

After the fourth BP reading

- If any diastolic BP is <90 and the systolic is <140, no treatment is indicated (<130/80 in diabetics).
- If the BP is persistently in the range 140–160/90–99:
  - treatment is indicated if the patient is at high risk of cardiovascular disease (>20% 10-year CVD risk, see p. 146), or if there is evidence of target organ damage, as suggested by:
    - left ventricular hypertrophy (CXR or ECG)
    - transient ischaemic attacks

- o previous stroke, angina or MI
- o renal impairment (raised creatinine, proteinuria/haematuria)
- o peripheral vascular disease
- o hypertensive retinopathy.
- – treatment is not indicated if there is no evidence of target organ disease, and the 10-year CVD risk is <20%. Check the BP and reassess the CHD risk annually.

Initial investigations

- Blood tests: C&Es, fasting lipid profile to include total cholesterol and HDL cholesterol, urate, fasting plasma glucose.
- Urine tests: protein.
- ECG: for left ventricular hypertrophy.
- Patients under 35 years old: 24-hour urinary metadrenaline for phaeochromocytoma.
- Examine for retinopathy, abdominal aortic aneurysm, renal bruit, absent foot pulses.

Management

Advice. All hypertensives should be given advice on non-pharmacological methods.

See general lifestyle advice (p. 146).

Prescribing

- In patients over 55 or Black, initiate treatment with a calcium-channel blocker, e.g. amlodipine 5–10 mg daily.
- In patients under 55 or non-Black, initiate treatment with an ACE inhibitor, e.g. perindopril 2–8 mg daily.
- If the above are contraindicated, use a diuretic, e.g. bendroflumethiazide 2.5 mg daily in the over-65s/Black population or a beta-blocker, e.g. atenolol 50–100 mg daily in the under-65/non-Black population.
- Start aspirin 75 mg od in patients over 50 years old with satisfactory blood pressure control, if there is target organ damage or diabetes or established cardiovascular disease, or if the 10-year CVD risk is >20%.
- Start a statin (e.g. simvastatin 40 mg) in patients under 80 years old when serum total cholesterol is >3.5 mmol/l and the 10-year CVD risk is >20%, or if there is established CVD.

Follow-up

- Frequency of follow-up should be 4-weekly initially, unless there is a need to achieve more urgent control (e.g. BP >200/120).

Tip
If there are unacceptable side-effects, change to an alternative drug.

- Aim for BP of <140/85 ideally, but <150/90 is acceptable (<130/80 in diabetics).
- If control is not achieved, add a second drug from another class.
- If control is still not achieved, either add a third drug or consider referral (see below).
- Once control is achieved, follow up with BP check every 6 months. Arrange annual urinalysis for protein, and check C&Es and fasting blood sugar. Recalculate CVD risk every year.

Reasons for referral

- Malignant hypertension.
- Secondary hypertension (raised creatinine or proteinuria).
- Refractory hypertension (difficult to treat with two or more drugs).
- Hypertension of sudden onset.
- Hypertension that is worsening despite treatment.
- Hypertension under age 35 years with multiple cardiovascular risk factors.
- Pregnancy.

Stopping antihypertensives. If BP is consistently <130/80 and there is no evidence of target organ disease, antihypertensives can be gradually withdrawn.

Regular monitoring is essential and should be long-term.

Administration

Quality and Outcomes Framework for Hypertension

- Check the blood pressure of patients on the hypertension register 6-monthly.
- Achieve a blood pressure of 150/90 or below.
- Record the smoking annually.
- Offer smoking cessation to hypertensive smokers annually.

CHOLESTEROL

High cholesterol is principally a risk factor for the development of cardiovascular disease. GPs should consider the level of their patients' cholesterol when monitoring overall coronary risk.

Diagnosis

Test serum cholesterol if:

- The patient is at high risk of CHD:
  - hypertensive
  - diabetic

- has established atheromatous disease (angina, MI, CABG, CVA, TIA, peripheral vascular disease)
  - combination of risk factors, including smoking, obesity, lack of exercise
  - family history of heart disease: first-degree relative suffering coronary death under age 50 for male relative, age 60 for female relative.
- Family history of hyperlipidaemia.
- Patient's request.

Interpreting results

- Measurements of both total cholesterol and HDL cholesterol should be made.
- Readings should be applied to the Joint British Societies Coronary Risk Prediction Chart to assess 10-year coronary risk (see pp. 147–148).
- Very high serum cholesterol (say, >10) suggests a familial hyperlipidaemia.
- Serum cholesterol is elevated in:
  - diabetes mellitus
  - nephrotic syndrome
  - hypothyroidism
  - pregnancy.

Management

Advice. Give dietary advice:

- to achieve ideal weight
- to reduce overall fat intake
- to reduce saturated fat intake.

Dietary measures

(Send the patient to the practice nurse for advice.)

- Explain the role of diet in heart disease and the need for change.
- Measure weight and height and calculate body mass index from the formula BMI = weight (kg) ÷ (height (m))^2. Aim for a BMI of <25 for men and <23 for women.
- Ask the patient to keep an accurate dietary diary for 1 week.
- Review the diary with the patient, identifying sources of saturated fat intake.
- Suggest low-fat alternatives, aiming to substitute polyunsaturated fats or carbohydrates for saturated fats.
- Encourage compliance. Offer a follow-up appointment.

- Give advice on other risk factors (see p. 146).
- In the absence of established cardiovascular disease, treat patients under 80 years old with a statin if the 10-year CVD risk is >20% (see p. 146).

> **Tip**
> Patients with a history of ischaemic heart disease, CVA/TIA, peripheral
> vascular disease or diabetics over 40 years should be started on a
> statin (e.g. simvastatin starting at 40 mg on) to achieve a total
> cholesterol <5.0 mmol/l or a 20–25% reduction, whichever is the
> lower value.

- Total cholesterol >10 mmol/l: refer to the lipid clinic.

Follow-up

- At 3-monthly intervals, initially.
- If the serum cholesterol level is reduced, reinforce dietary measures and
  concentrate on other risk factors for cardiovascular disease.
- Check LFTs at the first follow-up if a statin has been started.
- Titrate the dose of statin to achieve target cholesterol.
- Remember the coronary risk rises with age. Reassessment of risk level may
  indicate treatment at some point in the future. Plan to reassess the patient at a
  suitable interval.

INTERMITTENT CLAUDICATION

Intermittent claudication is often a sign of more widespread atheromatous
disease, which should be sought.

Diagnosis

History. Ask about pain in the legs on walking, which is relieved by rest.
The calves are usually affected. Risk factors:

- smoking
- hypertension
- diabetes
- established atheromatous disease.

Examination. This may be normal, but:

- look for cold feet, no hair on legs, dry or flaky skin
- check BP and peripheral pulses
- check the feet for corns, fungal infections, badly cut nails.

Investigations. As for general atheromatous disease, i.e.:

- cholesterol
- fasting blood glucose
- ECG. Also consider Doppler pressures if available.

Management

- Document the distance at which claudication begins.
- Involve a podiatrist.
- Consider aspirin and statins (see p. 146).

Advice

- See general lifestyle advice (p. 146).
- Ask patient to report early signs of damage to the feet, e.g. blisters.

Referral. If this general advice fails to help, refer to vascular surgical outpatients for consideration for angiography to assess the arterial supply to the legs.

CHEST PAIN

The causes of chest pain can range from minor musculoskeletal aches to life-threatening cardiac ischaemia. Surprisingly, both conditions are relatively common in general practice.

Diagnosis

History. In diagnosing chest pain a good history is essential, especially if the initial contact is over the telephone.

The first question to ask yourself is, 'Is it an emergency?', i.e.:

- myocardial infarction
- dissecting aneurysm
- pulmonary embolus.

Ask about:

- The nature of the pain: central, crushing tight pain radiating to arms or neck suggests MI; central, tearing pain radiating to the back suggests dissection. PE causes pleuritic pain and often shortness of breath.
- The patient's appearance: collapsed, pale or grey, breathless and sweaty all suggest serious pathology.
- Risk factors for MI and dissecting aneurysm: see risk factors for CVD (p. 146).

- Risk factors for PE:
  - recent DVT
  - surgery
  - trauma
  - combined pill
  - smoking
  - history of thrombosis
  - long-haul flight (economy-class syndrome).

> If the history suggests MI, aneurysm, PE or a very ill patient, admit the patient to hospital by ambulance on 999 without delay (see p. 158).

If the initial impression is of non-urgent pathology, a more leisurely history and examination can be performed.

The main differential diagnosis then includes:

- oesophagitis/reflux
- angina/MI
- costochondral/musculoskeletal pain
- chest infection/tracheitis.

A detailed account of the nature of the patient's pain, including site, character, onset, duration, aggravating and relieving factors, associated symptoms and recent past medical history will usually provide a diagnosis.

Examination

- General appearance.
- Pulse.
- BP.
- Temperature.
- Chest, heart and abdomen. Do not forget to press on the chest wall to elicit musculoskeletal pain (common).
- Listen for the friction rub of pericarditis (rare).
- Epigastric tenderness suggests gastritis/reflux.

Investigations

- ECG: this may show evidence of acute MI or ischaemia, but may also be normal in both these conditions.
- CXR: this is of little diagnostic value, but it may confirm a chest infection, fractured rib or rib metastases.

> If the patient is unwell or the history suggests an MI, immediate admission to hospital is essential.

> **Tip**
> The diagnosis often remains unclear at this stage. The confusion is usually between myocardial ischaemia and oesophagitis/reflux.

A therapeutic trial of either a PPI or a nitrate/beta-blocker is then justified, e.g.:

- omeprazole 20 mg od, or
- GTN sublingual prn or atenolol 100 mg od.

The choice is governed by the 'best guess' based on the history and examination so far.

Follow-up. If the diagnosis is still in doubt after 24–48 hours on a therapeutic trial, referral to the cardiology outpatient clinic for the purpose of reaching a diagnosis can be justified. The following pages outline the management of ischaemic chest pain once a clinical diagnosis has been reached.

ANGINA

Angina is pain due to myocardial ischaemia.

Diagnosis

History. Ask about:

- the nature of the pain: central, tight or constricting, radiating to the arms or neck
- aggravating factors: exertion, walking uphill or into the wind, cold weather, large meals
- relieving factors: rest, nitrates
- risk factors (see p. 146).

Examination. Expect this to be normal. Look for:

- heart failure (ankles, lung bases and JVP)
- arrhythmias/murmurs.

Investigations.

- FBC: anaemia may unmask angina.
- ECG: a baseline ECG may be helpful for future reference, but expect this to be normal.
- CXR: this is unhelpful unless heart failure is suspected.

Tip

At this stage the diagnosis should fall into one of four groups:

- uncertain diagnosis (see p. 154)
- stable angina
- unstable angina
- suspected MI (see p. 158).

STABLE ANGINA

This is angina that is predictable, i.e. the symptoms are brought on by similar amounts of exercise every time; they are relieved by rest; and there is no change in the frequency of the attacks.

Management

Advice. See general lifestyle advice (p. 146). Warn the patient to report any increase in chest pain immediately.

Prescribing

- Start with a trial of a moderately cardioselective beta-blocker, e.g. atenolol 50–100 mg od.
- A long-acting calcium-channel blocker can be added if symptoms persist, e.g. amlodipine 5–10 mg od.
- Sublingual nitrate tablets or spray should be made available to the patient for the temporary relief of angina, e.g. one or two GTN tablets prn. (Warn of headache.)
- Oral nitrates can be added if the patient requires a regular daily dose of the sublingual preparation, e.g. isosorbide mononitrate 10–20 mg tds.

 All patients with angina should take aspirin 75 mg daily, unless contraindicated, and a statin (see p. 153).

Referral. Refer for exercise ECG/angiography in all new cases of suspected angina via fast-track chest pain clinic (i.e. to be seen within 2 weeks).

Follow-up. Continue lifestyle advice and attention to other risk factors.

UNSTABLE ANGINA

This is angina that has grown worse/more frequent over the previous month or less. Particularly worrying are rest pain and nocturnal pain.

Management

> Discuss with the cardiology team with a view to an urgent outpatient appointment or admission.

Otherwise the management is as for stable angina.

Administration

Quality and Outcomes Framework for Coronary Heart Disease
- All new cases of angina to be confirmed by exercise test/specialist referral.
- Record smoking status annually.
- Offer smoking cessation advice to current smokers annually.
- Measure and achieve blood pressure 150/90 or below annually.
- Measure and achieve total cholesterol 5 mmol/l or below annually.
- Prescribe aspirin or clopidogrel or warfarin.
- Prescribe a beta-blocker.
- Give a flu jab annually.
- Screen for depression annually.

ACUTE MYOCARDIAL INFARCTION (MI)

This is a true general practice emergency, for which immediate action has been shown to reduce mortality. Among a GP's 2000 patients there will be two episodes of acute MI per year.

> Call 999 and request ambulance paramedics as soon as an acute MI is suspected, even if this is before the patient has been seen.

Diagnosis

History. Ask about:

- the nature of the pain, e.g. central, crushing, tight chest pain radiating to arms or neck

- associated features, e.g. nausea, breathlessness, sweatiness, palpitations
- risk factors (see p. 146).

Examination. The general appearance is usually of an anxious, slightly sweaty patient.

Check the blood pressure and pulse to assess for cardiac output and arrhythmias. Examine for signs of heart failure. The heart sounds are usually unchanged.

Investigations

- ECG: if an ECG machine (or a defibrillator with cardiac monitor) is available, it is worth connecting it up, but this must not delay the calling of the ambulance. If the diagnosis is in doubt, a normal ECG will not rule out an acute MI.
- Cardiographic monitoring is most useful in the acute situation for the detection and treatment of arrhythmias.

> **Tip**
> If the diagnosis is in doubt, see: chest pain, diagnosis (p. 154).

Immediate management of suspected MI

- Reassure the patient.
- Make sure the ambulance has been called.
- Site an intravenous cannula.
- Give pain relief intravenously, e.g. diamorphine 2.5–5 mg or morphine 5–10 mg (the dose being titrated against the patient's response) with an antiemetic (e.g. prochlorperazine 12.5 mg iv or metoclopramide 10 mg iv).
- For heart failure give furosemide 40 mg iv.
- For hypotension (systolic pressure <100 mmHg) with bradycardia (<50) give atropine 300 μg iv. Repeat at 5-minute intervals to a maximum dose of 1.2 mg.
- Give aspirin 300 mg, unless contraindicated.
- Await the arrival of the ambulance and be prepared for the risk of cardiac arrest. Check the BP and cardiac rhythm regularly.
- Telephone the hospital to inform the medical team of the patient's imminent arrival. If there is time before the ambulance departs, write a covering letter, listing the time of onset of symptoms, drugs given and cardiac history.

Late presentation of MI

- If less than 24 hours have elapsed, admit the patient.
- If more than 24 hours have elapsed since the onset of severe chest pain, it is not essential to admit the patient, as long as there are no remaining symptoms or signs.

- If the patient is kept at home, examine regularly for signs of heart failure. Confirm diagnosis by taking bloods for cardiac enzymes (troponin).

POSTMYOCARDIAL INFARCTION

The aim of primary care after an acute MI is to support the patient and family in rehabilitation and secondary prevention. Hospital outpatient care should include assessment of the need for coronary revascularisation and also cardiac rehabilitation.

Diagnosis

Examination. Look for:

- arrhythmias, hypotension, murmurs, signs of heart failure
- the psychological effects of MI, which include
  - depression
  - beta-blocker side-effects
  - fear of physical exertion
  - insecurity
  - pessimism.

> **Tip**
> Pay attention to risk factors (see also p. 146).

Management
(In conjunction with cardiac rehabilitation.)

Advice. The patient should aim to return to normal activities by 6 weeks. This includes driving and sex. Graduated increase in the level of exercise should be limited by pain or tiredness. Regular daily exercise should be encouraged.

Prescribing. Ensure that the patient is taking:

- aspirin 75–150 mg od (unless contraindicated)
- a beta-blocker (unless in heart block)
- a statin
- an ACE inhibitor.

Check the patient understands the importance of long-term compliance.

Administration

Quality and Outcomes Framework for Myocardial Infarction*

- Prescribe an ACE inhibitor
*In addition to the targets for CHD (see p. 158).

HEART FAILURE

Congestive cardiac failure is a clinical syndrome of shortness of breath, fatigue and fluid retention. It affects about 1–3% of the population.

Tip
Swelling of the ankles is a common general practice symptom. The commonest cause is dependent oedema due to venous insufficiency. Once heart failure has been excluded, treat with support stockings and elevate the legs. A mild diuretic such as bendroflumethiazide 2.5 mg od may be used if necessary.

Diagnosis
There are two aspects: diagnosing heart failure and diagnosing its cause.

History. Ask about:

- symptoms of heart failure: shortness of breath, orthopnoea, paroxysmal nocturnal dyspnoea, swollen ankles, fatigue
- possible causes of heart failure: past MI, past heart surgery, anaemia, thyrotoxicosis, arrhythmia, CHD, NSAIDs (fluid retention).

Examination. Look for:

- signs of heart failure: raised jugular venous pulse, basal crackles, swollen ankles
- possible causes of heart failure: high output: anaemia (pallor), thyrotoxicosis (exophthalmos); low output: arrhythmia (irregular pulse, tachycardia), hypertensive disease (raised BP), valvular heart disease, e.g. aortic stenosis, mitral regurgitation (murmur)
- signs of associated cardiovascular disease: carotid bruits, absence of peripheral pulses.

Investigations. Consider:

- Bloods: FBC: anaemia; TFTs: thyrotoxicosis; C&Es: prior to treatment; LFTs: can be disordered in heart failure.
- CXR: left ventricular hypertrophy/aneurysm, cardiomegaly.
- ECG: LVH, arrhythmia, tachycardia, MI.
- Echocardiogram (by referral) for all patients.

Management

Is the patient in acute left ventricular failure? If so, treat as an emergency:

- Give:
  - diamorphine 2.5–5 mg iv
  - furosemide 40 mg iv
  - GTN sublingual
  - O_2 when available.
- Sit the patient up to decrease pulmonary oedema.
- Consider admission.

Treat the underlying cause specifically, if possible.

Advice. See p. 146.

Prescribing

To control symptoms. Diuretic, e.g. furosemide 20–40 mg mane.

To improve prognosis

- ACE inhibitor, e.g. lisinopril 2.5–20 mg od.
- Beta-blocker, e.g. carvedilol 1.25 mg od.

Method of starting ACE inhibition

- Check C&Es.
- Omit diuretics on the morning of initiating therapy.
- Increase the dose by a factor of 2 every week, if tolerated. Check C&Es at 2 weeks and BP with every dose increase.
- Avoid potassium-sparing diuretics and potassium supplements.

Follow-up

- Regular review, probably 6-monthly, but depends on the severity and underlying cause.
- Continued lifestyle advice and encouragement.
- Consider stopping treatment if the underlying cause is corrected.

Administration

Quality and Outcomes Framework for Heart Failure
- All cases of heart failure to be confirmed by echocardiography.
- Prescribe an ACE inhibitor or angiotensin receptor blocker.

RAYNAUD'S PHENOMENON

Raynaud's phenomenon is characterised by cold, blue fingers after exposure to cold. It can be caused by vibration, e.g. driving, and can also affect the toes.

Management

- Reassure the patient it is not dangerous.
- Encourage the patient to stop smoking.
- Advise keeping the hands warm, using gloves if necessary.
- Nifedipine 10 mg tds can be used if the symptoms are severe. Increase to 20 mg tds if there is no response after 1 week.
- Surgery: sympathectomy may help severe disease.

> **Tip**
> Consider other connective tissue disorders, e.g. scleroderma, systemic sclerosis.

> **Tip**
> Treat any underlying disease which may be associated, e.g. peripheral vascular disease (see p. 153).

FUNNY TURNS

Syncope is characterised by transient loss of consciousness, with or without a fall. Simple vasovagal faints are the commonest cause of syncope in young patients. The phrase 'funny turn' is often used by patients and relations to describe a wide variety of symptoms, which include syncope (see dizziness, p. 274).

The causes can be divided as follows.

Non-pathological

- Faints
- cough/micturition syncope.

Cardiovascular

- Arrhythmia
- valvular
- postural hypotension
- vertebrobasilar insufficiency.

Neurological

- TIA/CVA
- epilepsy.

Other

- Hypoglycaemia.

Diagnosis

History. Ask about:

- Preceding symptoms:
  - palpitations (arrhythmia)
  - aura (epilepsy)
  - emotional stress (faint)
  - cough/micturition (syncope)
  - chest pain (ischaemia).
- Witnessed account:
  - tonic/clonic
  - tongue-biting
  - asymmetrical weakness
  - urinary incontinence (epilepsy)
  - postictal drowsiness.
- Drug history (for postural hypotension): diuretics, nitrates, tricyclics, antihypertensives, sedatives, hypnotics, neuroleptics.
- Family history of sudden death: cardiomyopathy.

Examination. Look for:

- Cardiovascular:
  - pulse (irregular)
  - BP (postural drop)
  - heart sounds (aortic stenosis)
  - carotids (bruits)
  - extend neck (causes faintness in vertebrobasilar insufficiency).
- Central nervous system:
  - postictal
  - residual CVA/TIA deficit.

Investigations

- FBC.
- C&Es (if on digoxin/diuretics).
- Blood glucose.
- ECG.

Management

Treatment. The following are treatable in general practice:

- Postural hypotension:
  - advise the patient to rise slowly
  - surgical stockings
  - change responsible drugs if possible.
- Some arrhythmias (see below).
- Vertebrobasilar insufficiency:
  - explain the symptoms
  - advise the patient to avoid sudden neck movements.
- TIAs:
  - Rx (as per p. 281)
  - identify cause (e.g. AF).
- Hypoglycaemia:
  - if known diabetic: glucose orally or iv (50 ml of 50% solution)
  - may need to adjust daily insulin dose.

Referral

- TIA: to Stroke Clinic preferably.
- Some arrhythmias (see below).
- Valvular heart disease.
- New or poorly controlled epilepsy.
- Unexplained loss of consciousness. (Refer to either a cardiologist or a neurologist.)

Recurrent syncope

- Is the diagnosis correct?
- Advise the patient to avoid dangerous situations.
- The patient should inform the Driver and Vehicle Licensing Agency.

PALPITATIONS

Palpitations are an awareness of the heart beating due to either a change of beat or a heightened awareness of the normal cardiac rate and rhythm.

> **Tip**
> There are various ways of subdividing arrhythmias, but the most useful in general practice is the distinction between normal and pathological.

Normal (common)

- Increased awareness of the normal heart beat.
- Tachycardia: anxiety feedback loop.
- Menopausal flushing.
- Ventricular ectopics.

Pathological

- Paroxysmal supraventricular tachycardia.
- Atrial fibrillation
  - constant
  - paroxysmal.
- Second- and third-degree heart block.
- Ventricular tachycardia.

Diagnosis

History. Ask about:

- Rate and rhythm. (Ask patient to tap on the desk.)
- When the palpitations occur.
- Associated symptoms:
  - faintness/dizziness
  - loss of consciousness (see p. 163)
  - anxiety
  - tingling of the fingers or perioral area (hyperventilation)
  - hot flushes/sweats
  - shortness of breath.
- Exacerbating factors.
- Drug history.
- Cardiovascular history.

Examination

- Anaemia.
- Pulse, BP.
- Thyrotoxic?
- Heart sounds.
- Apex–radial delay (atrial fibrillation).

During attack

- Pulse, BP.
- Signs of heart failure (see p. 161).
- ?MI (see p. 158).

Investigations

- Bloods:
  - FBC
  - C&Es
  - TFTs
  - digoxin level.
- ECG:
  - routine
  - during attack.
(A 24-hour ECG is usually by referral.)

Management

Treatment. The following are treatable in general practice.

Non-pathological arrhythmias. Reassure (backed up by ECG).

Constant atrial fibrillation. If ventricular rate is >100 per minute and there is no murmur, give digoxin 0.25 mg po, then 0.25 mg 12 hours later, and then 0.125 mg daily for 1 week if C&Es are normal. Then assess ventricular rate and adjust dose accordingly.

    Anticoagulate with warfarin, over the age of 50, unless there are contraindications, in which case give aspirin, 75 mg daily (see p. 330).

Paroxysmal atrial fibrillation. Anticoagulate if there are no contraindications; otherwise give aspirin. Digoxin is of no benefit.

Symptomatic supraventricular tachycardia. Advise the dive reflex (plunge the face into a sink of cold water)/Valsalva manoeuvre/carotid sinus massage. Stop stimulant intake (coffee, tea, chocolate, cola, etc.).

Emergency treatment of arrhythmias following acute myocardial infarction includes:

- ventricular tachycardia: lidocaine 100 mg iv
- sinus bradycardia: atropine 300 μg iv
- ventricular ectopics: no treatment
- ventricular fibrillation: DC shock
- asystole: 1:1000 adrenaline 1 ml iv and CPR.

Referral. Refer if there is:

- no diagnosis (if symptoms are worrying patient or doctor)
- atrial fibrillation of recent onset (for DC cardioversion)
- atrial flutter
- paroxysmal ventricular tachycardia
- heart block
- associated valvular heart disease
- thyrotoxicosis
- SVT not responding to above advice.

Administration

Quality and Outcomes Framework for Atrial Fibrillation:

- All new cases to be confirmed by ECG.
- Anticoagulate all cases of AF unless warfarin contraindicated.

CHAPTER 11

RESPIRATORY MEDICINE

Asthma   170

Upper respiratory tract infection (URTI)   176

Acute cough   176

Chronic cough   178

Chest infection   179

Pneumonia   180

Haemoptysis   181

Chronic obstructive pulmonary disease (COPD)   183

ASTHMA

Asthma is a common chronic disease affecting approximately 5% of adults and 15% of children (see p. 94). It is a disease characterised by increased responsiveness of the airways to a variety of stimuli. The clinical picture is one of wheezing, coughing or shortness of breath, often worse at night. The following is based on the 2005 update of the British Thoracic Society Guidelines for Asthma first published in *Thorax* in 2003.

CHRONIC ASTHMA

Diagnosis

History. The suspicion of asthma should be raised if there is a history of chronic recurrent cough or wheeze.

> **Tip**
> A diagnosis can be made after more than two episodes of wheeze or cough which respond symptomatically to adequate bronchodilator or prophylactic therapy.

Ask about:

- the duration of symptoms and current treatment
- present symptoms and their effect on lifestyle, e.g. sleep disturbance, time off work or school, effort intolerance
- family history
- atopy
- active and passive smoking
- occupation
- drugs.

Examination/peak flow data

- Examine the chest.
- Measure height (and weight for children).
- Measure the PEFR and calculate the predicted PEFR.
- Prescribe a peak flow meter (if it seems appropriate and the asthma is chronic), available on FP10, and teach the use of the peak flow meter and peak flow charts.

In any patient over 12 years old, reversible airways obstruction should ideally be demonstrated via peak flow measurements by:

1. a 15% improvement in PEFR 5 minutes after an inhaled bronchodilator, or

2. a 15% variability in PEFR on a diary kept over a 2-week period when there are no exacerbating factors such as an infection, or

3. a 15% improvement in PEFR during a trial of high-dose oral steroids.

Management

Advice

- Discuss the disease and the principles of treatment (especially the difference between relief bronchodilators and prophylactic anti-inflammatory treatment).
- Teach an appropriate inhaler technique.
- Discuss a self-management plan, where appropriate.
- Emphasise the need for regular review by the GP or nurse.

Management principles

- Avoid provoking factors, e.g.:
  - smoking (active or passive)
  - house dust mite (cover mattresses and pillows with plastic covers and minimise carpets, soft furnishings and soft toys, especially in the bedroom)
  - pets
  - drugs: avoid aspirin, NSAIDs and beta-blockers (including eye drops).
- Discuss stress as a common exacerbating factor.
- Encourage self-management (see p. 173).

Tip
Advocate the use of prophylactic treatment even with mild asthma (in patients who need a bronchodilator three times per week or more). The need for bronchodilators is therefore kept to a minimum.

- Select an appropriate inhaler device. (Aerosol inhalers are always more effective if used with a spacer device.) The use of dry powder, e.g. disks, capsules or breath-actuated inhalers may be useful for those who find simple aerosol inhalers difficult to use because of poor coordination.
- Assess inhaler technique regularly, especially if control is poor.
- Treatment should be step-wise (see below), and should be started on the step most appropriate to the severity of the asthma.
- Treatment should be stepped up and down as necessary, depending on the symptoms, the extent of bronchodilator use and the PEFR.
- The need for relieving bronchodilators should be kept to a minimum.
- Use short-term oral corticosteroids for severe asthmatic episodes to bring asthma under control.

Drug therapy (for older children and adults)

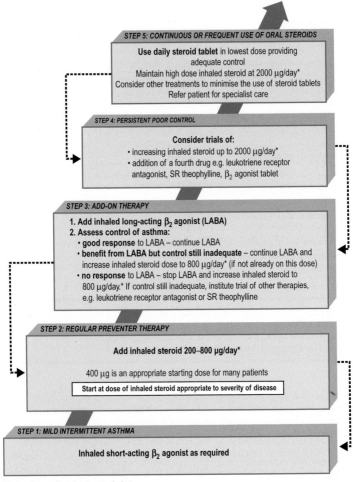

STEP 5: CONTINUOUS OR FREQUENT USE OF ORAL STEROIDS

Use daily steroid tablet in lowest dose providing
adequate control
Maintain high dose inhaled steroid at 2000 μg/day*
Consider other treatments to minimise the use of steroid tablets
Refer patient for specialist care

STEP 4: PERSISTENT POOR CONTROL

Consider trials of:
• increasing inhaled steroid up to 2000 μg/day*
• addition of a fourth drug e.g. leukotriene receptor
  antagonist, SR theophylline, β_2 agonist tablet

STEP 3: ADD-ON THERAPY

1. **Add inhaled long-acting β_2 agonist (LABA)**
2. **Assess control of asthma:**
   • **good response** to LABA – continue LABA
   • **benefit from LABA but control still inadequate** – continue LABA and
     increase inhaled steroid dose to 800 μg/day* (if not already on this dose)
   • **no response** to LABA – stop LABA and increase inhaled steroid to
     800 μg/day.* If control still inadequate, institute trial of other therapies,
     e.g. leukotriene receptor antagonist or SR theophylline

STEP 2: REGULAR PREVENTER THERAPY

Add inhaled steroid 200–800 μg/day*

400 μg is an appropriate starting dose for many patients

Start at dose of inhaled steroid appropriate to severity of disease

STEP 1: MILD INTERMITTENT ASTHMA

Inhaled short-acting β_2 agonist as required

*Beclometasone dipropionate or equivalent

Summary of stepwise management of asthma in adults, 2004. Reproduced with permission
from the British Thoracic Society/Scottish Intercollegiate Guidelines Network Executive
Committee.

Step one. Occasional symptoms: intermittent use of a short-acting bronchodilator to relieve symptoms, e.g. salbutamol 200 μg (two puffs of aerosol) prn.

Step two. More frequent symptoms, e.g. if bronchodilator treatment is required three times per week or more: regular use of inhaled anti-inflammatory agents, e.g. beclometasone 100–400 μg (1–4 puffs of beclometasone 100 aerosol inhalation) bd, plus short-acting bronchodilators as required.

Step three. Worsening symptoms or increasing requirement for bronchodilators: consider inhaled long-acting beta-agonists, e.g. salmeterol 50–100 μg (2–4 puffs of aerosol) bd.

Step four. Worsening symptoms or an increasing requirement for bronchodilators: as above, plus a sequential therapeutic trial of one or more of the following:

- Regular use of high-dose inhaled steroids, e.g. beclometasone 500–1000 μg bd plus short-acting bronchodilators as required. A spacer should always be used.
- Sustained-release theophylline, e.g. Slo-Phyllin 250–500 mg bd.
- Inhaled sodium cromoglycate or nedocromil, e.g. Intal aerosol inhalation 2 puffs qds.
- Long-acting beta-agonist tablets, e.g. Volmax 8 mg bd.
- High-dose inhaled bronchodilators, e.g. nebulised salbutamol. (Long-term use should be supervised by a chest consultant.)
- Leukotriene receptor antagonist, e.g. montelukast 10 mg tablet od.

Step five. If control is lost at any stage consider a short course of oral steroids, e.g. prednisolone 30–40 mg mane for 5 days, or until the peak flow has returned to at least 80% of the patient's best ever peak flow. Oral steroids can be stopped abruptly, even after courses of up to 3 weeks, but should not be stopped if the patient is on long-term oral steroids or if the patient's asthma is deteriorating subjectively or objectively.

Referral. Refer if:

- asthma remains poorly controlled or if the diagnosis is in doubt
- asthma is thought to involve occupational factors.

Self-management plan. Note the patient's predicted or best-ever PEFR, and calculate the 75% and 50% levels. These levels can be marked on a PEFR chart or on the peak flow meter itself. (Remember to recalculate the predicted or best-ever peak flow as the child grows.)

If the patient has an upper respiratory tract infection, is experiencing nocturnal wheezing or a persistent cough, or has a PEFR consistently between 50 and 75% of normal:

- Double the dose of the inhaled steroid for the number of days it takes to return to normal or until the PEFR returns to the previous baseline.

- Continue on this increased dose for at least the same number of days again. Then return to the maintenance treatment. Use a bronchodilator two puffs 4-hourly, or as appropriate.

If the patient is experiencing shortness of breath with normal activities, is increasing the use of bronchodilators or has a PEFR which is <50% of normal:

- Increase the dose of the inhaled steroids, as above.
- If arrangements have been made to use oral steroids at home:
  - See Step 5 (p. 173).
  - The patient should contact the GP within 24 hours.
- If oral steroids are not immediately available, the patient should contact the GP that day.

If experiencing difficulty with speaking, bronchodilators are ineffective or the PEFR is <30% of normal, the patient should contact the GP urgently, go directly to hospital or call 999.

ACUTE ASTHMA

Many asthma deaths are preventable. Factors include:

- underuse of corticosteroids
- failure of the patient or relatives to appreciate the severity of illness
- failure of the doctor to assess the severity of illness by clinical measurement.

Diagnosis

Examination

Signs of acute severe asthma. Seriously consider admission if more than one of the following features are present:

- inability to complete sentences
- a pulse rate of >110 beats per minute
- a respiratory rate of >25 breaths per minute
- a PEFR of <50% of the predicted or best-ever peak flow.

Signs of life-threatening asthma requiring urgent admission

- Silent chest
- cyanosis
- bradycardia or exhaustion
- oxygen saturation, measured with a pulse oximeter <92%.

Treat as below while awaiting an ambulance.

Management

Lower the threshold for admission if:

- an attack is late in the day
- the patient has had previous severe attacks
- the patient has had recent nocturnal symptoms
- social circumstances are unfavourable.

Treatment

- Treat with a nebulised bronchodilator, e.g. salbutamol 5 mg (2.5 mg in children), ideally via an oxygen-driven nebuliser. If a nebuliser is not available, use salbutamol inhaler via a spacer device, 6 puffs (given 1 at a time and inhaled separately), repeated at intervals of 10–20 minutes.
- Use oxygen 40–60%, if available.
- Give oral prednisolone 60 mg stat. For children aged <1 year, 1–2 mg/kg; aged 1–5 years, 20 mg stat; aged 5–12 years, 40 mg stat.
- Consider hydrocortisone 200 mg iv in adults.

If the response is good:

- Continue oral prednisolone 60 mg daily until recovery is full. For children aged <1 year, 1–2 mg/kg/day; aged 1–5 years, 20 mg/day; aged 5–12 years, 40 mg/day.
- Step up usual treatment including inhaled steroids.
- Arrange follow-up assessment the following day.
- Tell the patient to contact the GP again if the PEFR falls below 50% of its best.

Follow-up

- Assess the adequacy of maintenance treatment.
- Consider prescribing an emergency supply of oral prednisolone for the patient to keep at home.

ASTHMA IN CHILDREN

See p. 94.

Administration

Quality and Outcomes Framework for Asthma

- All new cases of asthma to be confirmed by peak flow >aged 8.
- Smoking status to be recorded after initial diagnosis >aged 14.
- Smoking status recorded annually.
- Smoking cessation offered to asthmatic smokers.
- Peak flow recorded annually.
- Asthma management assessed annually.

UPPER RESPIRATORY TRACT INFECTION (URTI)

Upper respiratory tract infections are responsible for about 30% of all GP consultations.

Diagnosis

History. Ask about:

- sore throat
- cough
- otalgia
- runny nose
- blocked nose
- dizziness
- aches and pains
- difficulty swallowing.

Establish the patient's expectations, e.g. antibiotics, sick note, reassurance.

Examination. It is usually sufficient to examine the throat, ears and cervical glands. If the patient has a cough, consider examining the chest.
    Look particularly for:

- quinsy (see p. 218)
- tonsillitis (see p. 218)
- otitis media (see p. 212)
- chest infection (see p. 179).

Management of uncomplicated URTI

- Reassure the patient that the condition is self-limiting and not serious.
- Discourage the use of antibiotics in general. It is often useful to discuss the body's natural immune response.
- Give advice on self-treatments such as paracetamol, soluble aspirin and fluids. Encourage a more self-sufficient approach to minor illness.

Administration

Sick notes are only needed after more than 6 days of continuous absence from work. Self-certificates, from the patient's employer, should be used for the first week.

ACUTE COUGH

The commonest presentation in general practice is of an acute URTI. There is a cough, sore throat, a blocked or runny nose or painful cervical glands. Earache or sinus pain may accompany these.

Other symptoms suggest an alternative diagnosis:

Diagnosis

History. Ask about:

- The character of the cough:
  - productive
  - dry (asthma, ACE inhibitors).
- Chest pain:
  - pleurisy of pneumonia
  - pulmonary embolus
  - pneumothorax.
- Haemoptysis:
  - pneumonia
  - tuberculosis
  - pulmonary embolus.
- Purulent sputum:
  - bronchitis
  - bronchiectasis
  - pneumonia.
- Breathlessness:
  - congestive cardiac failure
  - chronic obstructive pulmonary disease.
- Wheeze:
  - asthma
  - chest infection.
- Weight loss:
  - bronchial carcinoma.

Examination. Throat, ears, neck, pulse and chest. Pyrexia may be present in carcinoma and pulmonary embolism as well as infection.

Investigations

- CXR, if appropriate.
- ECG in e.g. pulmonary embolus and congestive cardiac failure.

Management

- Simple coughs due to URTI need no specific treatment but OTC cough mixtures, e.g. simple linctus, and steam inhalation can ease symptoms temporarily.
- Lower respiratory tract infections (LRTIs) need antibiotics. Amoxicillin and erythromycin are good first-line antibiotics, with co-amoxiclav or ciprofloxacin for second-line treatment in community-acquired infections.

Referral

- Ill patients with LRTIs should be admitted to hospital.
- Pulmonary embolus: admit the patient to hospital if this is suspected.
- Pneumothorax: admit the patient.
- Bronchial carcinoma: refer to a chest physician.
- Tuberculosis: refer to infectious diseases/chest clinic.
- Congestive cardiac failure (see p. 161).
- Asthma (see p. 170).
- COPD (see p. 183).

CHRONIC COUGH

Diagnosis

> **Tip**
> Any cough lasting more than 4 weeks falls into the category of chronic cough (see below).
>
> Consider the following:
>
> - asthma
> - carcinoma of the bronchus
> - gastro-oesophageal reflux disease
> - chronic bronchitis and bronchiectasis
> - tuberculosis
> - postnasal drip due to sinusitis.

History. Some features make one diagnosis more likely than another. For example, the child with a chronic, dry, nocturnal cough is likely to have asthma, whereas the lifelong heavy smoker aged 65 years with a chronic cough and weight loss is likely to have bronchial carcinoma.

Many adults, however, fall into the category of chronic cough with no obvious associated features.

Examination. Chest examination may give some clues, but is often normal in patients with a chronic cough.

Look also for:

- clubbing
- anaemia
- weight loss
- maxillary or frontal sinus tenderness
- cervical lymphadenopathy
- nasal obstruction.

Investigations. In suspected asthma, peak flow measurements before and after exercise and also pre- and post-inhalation of salbutamol may give the diagnosis (see p. 170).

A CXR is mandatory in patients aged over 40. Be prepared to repeat this after 6 weeks if the result is normal in patients who are losing weight.

Management

Management is of the underlying condition if this can be diagnosed. Often this is not possible, in which case a step-wise, empirical approach often produces results:

- Give 2 weeks of a broad-spectrum antibiotic, e.g. amoxicillin 500 mg tds.
- If there is no response, give 2 weeks of a PPI, e.g. lansoprazole 15 mg od.
- If this fails to cure the cough, try giving 2 weeks of inhaled beclometasone 400 μg bd.

If this regimen fails to relieve the symptoms, referral to a chest physician is justified.

Tip
The chronic cough of terminal chest disease can be relieved by pholcodine linctus or morphine.

CHEST INFECTION

Coughs and colds are the commonest presenting complaints in general practice in the winter and spring months.

Diagnosis

History. The commonest presentation is for an URTI to have 'gone onto the chest'.

Ask about:

- cough
- sputum production and colour
- chest pain
- haemoptysis
- breathlessness
- the facial pain of sinusitis
- history of chronic bronchitis or bronchiectasis
- smoking.

Examination. Look for:

- tonsillitis or the pharyngeal mucus of a postnasal drip in sinusitis (the temperature is usually normal)
- signs of pneumonia or bronchiectasis (focal crepitations over infected lobes).

Investigations. Consider CXR.

Management

- Is the patient unwell? If not, and there are no features in the history or examination to suggest anything other than a simple URTI with a cough, the patient can be reassured that there is nothing seriously wrong. Paracetamol 4-hourly can be advised. The condition should last no more than a week.
- Exacerbations of chronic bronchitis and infective episodes in bronchiectasis require antibiotics. The elderly commonly fall into this group. Oral amoxicillin 500 mg tds for 1 week is usually sufficient as a first-line choice, with erythromycin or tetracycline as alternatives. If this fails, co-amoxiclav 1 tds or ciprofloxacin 500 mg bd are good second-line choices.
- If pneumonia is suspected, see below.
- Steam inhalation or salbutamol via a metered-dose inhaler can help to loosen sputum.
- Consider asthma in patients with repeated episodes of cough or wheeze (see p. 170).

PNEUMONIA

Pneumonia presents either as a rapidly developing chest infection or as a consequence of a prior URTI.

Diagnosis

History. Ask about:

- cough, which is usually productive
- fever (not always present in the elderly or small children)
- breathlessness
- pleuritic chest pain
- haemoptysis
- vomiting or diarrhoea in children
- falls or confusion in the elderly.

Examination. Look for:

- tachycardia
- pyrexia (not always present in the elderly or small children)
- tachypnoea

- coarse crepitations, bronchial breathing and reduced air entry on auscultation of the affected lobe
- cyanosis
- grunting and intercostal recession, which may be found in small children. Some children may have no chest signs.

Investigations

- CXR if the diagnosis is uncertain.
- Sputum for microscopy and culture if obtainable.
- Dipstick urine for ketones if dehydration is suspected.

Management

 Ill patients should be admitted to hospital, as should all children and the immunocompromised, e.g. diabetics.

- Elderly patients may need admitting for social reasons, e.g. if they live alone.
- The otherwise fit, well-supported adult with no features of systemic toxicity can be started on oral amoxicillin 500 mg tds or erythromycin 500 mg qds.
- An NSAID, e.g. ibuprofen, can be useful for pleuritic pain.
- Patients dying of bronchopneumonia (e.g. nursing home residents) may need atropine or hyoscine im for excessive secretions (see p. 325).

Tip
Failure of the pyrexia to respond within 48 hours or the development of systemic features should prompt admission to hospital.

Pneumococcal vaccine
See p. 340.

HAEMOPTYSIS

The coughing up of blood may vary from slight streaking of phlegm to massive and fatal haemorrhage. A careful history usually allows distinction from haematemesis, although blood swallowed from the upper respiratory tract may be vomited back later.

Diagnosis

Consider the following possible causes:

- URTIs: tonsillitis, sinusitis.
- LRTIs: pneumonia, bronchitis, TB.
- Malignancy: bronchus, larynx, lung secondaries.
- Infarction: pulmonary embolus.

History

> **Tip**
> Most cases in general practice involve minor blood-speckling of mucus,
> produced from the upper respiratory tract due to excessively violent
> coughing.

Shortness of breath and pleuritic chest pain suggest a pulmonary embolus.
A productive cough suggests bronchitis or pneumonia. Chronic cough and
weight loss raise the suspicion of a bronchial carcinoma. Known or suspected
pulmonary metastases from e.g. a breast primary can present in general practice
as haemoptysis.

Examination

- The throat may reveal a possible source of bleeding if the tonsils are inflamed
  or the fauces injected.
- Chest examination may reveal pneumonia or bronchitis.
- Look for cervical and axillary lymphadenopathy in suspected carcinoma, and
  weigh the patient if malignancy is suspected.

Investigations

- ECG in pulmonary embolus shows S-waves in lead I and Q-waves and inverted
  T-waves in lead III.
- CXR to exclude e.g. TB, carcinoma and pneumonia.

Management

- Manage the underlying disease if a diagnosis is made.
- Haemoptysis can be very distressing. Diazepam orally or iv may be useful for
  acute distress (e.g. in terminal care).
- Refer for e.g. diagnostic bronchoscopy if the diagnosis is uncertain.

 Admit all cases of haemoptysis heavier than simple streaking of mucus,
unless the patient is expected to die, e.g. in palliative care at home.

CHRONIC OBSTRUCTIVE PULMONARY DISEASE (COPD)

COPD is very common in general practice, accounting for 30 000 deaths a year in the UK, and is the sixth leading cause of death worldwide. It is caused mainly by smoking. It is extremely unlikely to be present in patients under 50 or those who have never smoked. The following is based on the National Institute for Health and Clinical Excellence guidelines 2004.

Diagnosis

History. COPD should be considered in adults with persistent cough, sputum production or shortness of breath.
  Ask about:

- cough lasting more than 1 month, or recurrent cough
- sputum colour and volume
- shortness of breath, which is worse on exertion
- smoking (number of packs smoked and number of years as a smoker)
- any occupational exposure to dust or noxious fumes
- the effect of the respiratory problems on the patient's daily activities.

Grade breathlessness according to the MRC dyspnoea scale:

1. Only breathless with strenuous exercise.
2. Breathless when hurrying on the level or up a slight hill.
3. Walk slower than people of the same age due to breathlessness or have to stop for breath when walking on the level.
4. Stop for breath after walking 100 yards or after a few minutes on the level.
5. Too breathless to leave the house.

Examination

- Look at the chest. Hyperexpansion is common.
- Auscultate for wheeze (common) and signs of infection (also fairly common).
- Clubbing should be absent. Its presence suggests bronchiectasis or lung cancer.
- The heart should not be enlarged and the JVP should not be elevated, unless there is also coexisting heart failure.

Investigations

- CXR to help exclude e.g. malignancy and heart failure.
- Spirometry (in all cases). The characteristic feature of COPD is airway obstruction, defined as an FEV1:FVC ratio <70% and a measured FEV1 less than 80% of predicted (FEV1%).
- Reversibility testing: repeat spirometry 5 minutes after a 400 μg dose of inhaled salbutamol. An improvement in FEV1 of more than 500 ml, or normalisation of the FEV1, suggests asthma. Lesser improvements suggest bronchodilators will improve the COPD symptoms.

- PEFR. Variation in PEFR tends to be small in COPD. Serial home PEFR measurements may help to distinguish between COPD and asthma. A normal PEFR does not exclude COPD.

Referral. Consider referral to a chest physician if the patient is:

- under 40 years of age
- a non-smoker
- considerably disabled by dyspnoea
- diagnostically difficult.

Management

Take a step-wise approach to treatment, trialling the following drugs in order. Assess the response by asking the patient what effect there has been on objective measures such as exercise tolerance, and also by improvements in spirometry (FEV1%).

Mild COPD (either mild symptoms, or FEV1 no less than 50% predicted)

- Short-acting bronchodilator inhaler, e.g. salbutamol 100 μg, two puffs qds.
- Anticholinergic bronchodilator, e.g. ipratropium bromide inhaler 20 μg, two puffs qds or tiotropium 18 μg od (especially if there is excessive mucus).

Moderate to severe COPD (FEV1 <50% predicted, or disabling symptoms)

- Steroid inhaler, e.g. beclometasone dipropionate 200–250 μg, two puffs bd.
- Long-acting beta-agonist, e.g. salmeterol inhaler 25 μg, two puffs bd.

If symptom control is poor, consider referral to a chest specialist for e.g. possible home oxygen therapy.

Prevention

Smoking cessation. This is the only intervention proven to reduce the rate of deterioration in lung function in COPD patients.

- Assess the patient's motivation to quit.
- Offer referral to the practice's smoking cessation lead.
- Consider nicotine replacement therapy and bupropion hydrochloride.
- Hand out a leaflet on smoking cessation and arrange follow-up.

Immunisation. Offer all COPD patients an annual influenza vaccination and pneumococcal vaccination as a one-off (see p. 340).

Acute exacerbation of COPD

An acute exacerbation is a short-term worsening of symptoms, usually caused by infection.

- Increase bronchodilator use.
- Antibiotics, e.g. amoxicillin 500 mg tds for 1 week, followed by a second-line antibiotic if there has been no response, e.g. co-amoxiclav or ciprofloxacin.
- Oral steroids, especially if there has been a previous good response, or if the patient usually benefits from inhaled steroids. Give prednisolone 30 mg od for 6 days.
- Admit the patient to hospital if:
  - they are considerably disabled by dyspnoea
  - they fail to improve on the above treatment
  - they are unable to cope at home.

Administration

Quality and Outcomes Framework for COPD

- All cases of COPD to be confirmed by spirometry, including reversibility.
- Smoking status recorded annually.
- Smoking cessation advice to smokers annually.
- Reassessment by spirometry annually and FEV1 recorded.
- Inhaler technique checked annually.
- Influenza immunisation annually.

CHAPTER 12

INFECTIOUS DISEASES

Whooping cough   188

Meningitis   188

Scarlet fever   190

Glandular fever (infectious mononucleosis)   190

Hand, foot and mouth disease   192

Slapped cheek (fifth disease)   192

Chickenpox   193

Influenza   193

Pneumonia   194

Malaria   194

Conjunctivitis   196

Diarrhoea and vomiting   196

Impetigo   196

Cold sores   197

Shingles   197

Boils   198

Hepatitis   199

HIV/AIDS   201

Pyrexia of unknown origin (PUO)   202

Weil's disease   204

Lyme disease   205

Measles   205

Mumps   206

Rubella   207

WHOOPING COUGH

Whooping cough is now rare. After a catarrhal phase, it presents as an increasingly severe and paroxysmal cough. Send a nasopharyngeal swab for diagnosis. A differential white count shows a marked lymphocytosis. The treatment of pertussis is largely symptomatic. Erythromycin given for 10 days prevents spread of the illness. It should also be given to non-immunised child contacts (for pertussis vaccine, see p. 335). Admit if symptoms are severe (can cause apnoea in the very young).

> **Tip**
> Whooping cough is a notifiable disease.

MENINGITIS

There are 2000 cases per year of bacterial meningitis in the UK. Of these, 50% are due to *Neisseria meningitidis*. Viral meningitis is more common.

Diagnosis

History. Ask about:

- an acute illness of 24–48 hours' duration
- fever
- headache
- photophobia
- drowsiness
- vomiting
- neck stiffness
- rash (*N. meningitidis*).

Occasionally, meningitis may develop as a complication of a pre-existing pyrexial illness, such as otitis media, in which case the deterioration will be acute, although the total duration of the illness may be several days.

Examination. Look for:

- pyrexia
- cold peripheries
- pallor
- drowsiness

- vomiting
- pain on flexing the cervical spine
- pain on straight-leg raising
- decreased muscle tone in a baby
- irritability
- a petechial rash which does not blanch on pressure.

Tip
The early signs of meningitis are those of any pyrexial illness, e.g. pyrexia, irritability, vomiting and lethargy. Always be prepared to re-examine the patient if the condition deteriorates.

Always examine the patient for other causes of pyrexia, e.g. ears, throat, chest. Neck pain is more often due to the cervical lymphadenopathy of an upper respiratory tract infection.

Children without meningitis are able to kiss their knees.

Management

Any patient strongly suspected of having meningitis should be seen in hospital as soon as possible, even if there is a possible alternative explanation for the patient's condition, e.g. otitis media.

The vast majority of pyrexial patients will be found on history and examination to have no features of meningitis, and most will have an obvious alternative diagnosis. Treat as appropriate. Take the opportunity to advise the patient or the parents of the features of meningitis.

Close family and school contacts should receive rifampicin 5 mg/kg 12-hourly for 2 days.

For suspected meningitis give benzylpenicillin im/iv 600 mg under 2 years of age, 1.2 g over 2 years, immediately, before arranging urgent hospital admission. If allergic to penicillin, give cefotaxime im/iv 50 mg/kg under 12 years of age, 1 g over 12 years.

Tip
Meningitis is a notifiable disease. The hospital should notify the Environmental Health Department.

SCARLET FEVER

Scarlet fever has become less common over the last 50 years. It is caused by a β-haemolytic *Streptococcus*, group A.

The incubation period is 2–4 days.

Diagnosis

History. Ask about:

- sore throat
- rash
- flushed appearance
- headache
- vomiting.

Examination. Look for:

- tonsillitis with flecks of pus
- tender cervical lymphadenitis
- a furred tongue initially, which becomes red and smooth later
- a bright pink skin rash with tiny red spots (punctate erythema), which spares the circumoral region
- skin peeling, especially on the hands and toes, after a few days.

Investigations. Investigations are not indicated, although β-haemolytic *Streptococcus* can be isolated on a throat swab, and elevated ASO titres in blood are found. Usually, by the time the results are available in general practice, the illness is all but over.

Management

Prescribe penicillin V 250–500 mg qds orally for 10 days, or erythromycin if the patient is allergic to penicillin.

Tip
Small epidemics of scarlet fever are sometimes seen.

GLANDULAR FEVER (INFECTIOUS MONONUCLEOSIS)

Glandular fever is an acute viral infection, mainly affecting teenagers, and is a common general practice problem.

The incubation period is usually 7–10 days, occasionally longer.

It can occur either sporadically or in epidemics.

Diagnosis

History. Ask about:

- sore throat
- fever
- headaches
- tiredness
- malaise or anorexia.

These are usually of a short duration, but the condition may present after several weeks of a combination of the above, with prolonged, intermittent symptoms. Upper abdominal pain indicates hepatitis or splenic enlargement.

Examination. Look for:

- tonsillar enlargement with exudate, which can be difficult to distinguish from bacterial or viral tonsillitis
- petechial haemorrhages on the soft palate
- posterior cervical lymphadenopathy
- hepatosplenomegaly
- maculopapular rash.

Investigations.

- An FBC and film will show a neutrophil leucocytosis of $10–20 \times 10^9/l$.
- LFTs if jaundice is present.
- A Monospot/Paul Bunnell test will be positive in most cases of glandular fever, especially if taken at least 3 weeks after the start of the illness. False-negative results are common in the first week.

Management

- Advise rest, analgesia and fluids in the acute phase.
- Avoid alcohol.
- Be aware that amoxicillin may cause a rash in glandular fever.
- Avoid contact sports while the spleen is enlarged.
- Local anaesthetic throat lozenges may be helpful.
- Metronidazole 200 mg tds may help the oral lesions.
- Prednisolone 30 mg od for 1 week may help if the symptoms are prolonged or severe.
- If the continuing symptoms are dominated by depression, consider an antidepressant.
- If lymphadenopathy, fatigue and myalgia persist beyond 3 months, consider postviral fatigue syndrome (see p. 298).

HAND, FOOT AND MOUTH DISEASE

Hand, foot and mouth disease commonly occurs in epidemics. It affects mainly young children and the incubation period is 3–7 days. It is caused by a Coxsackie virus infection.

Diagnosis

History. Ask about mild fever and malaise, followed by red spots or vesicles in the mouth and on the lips and buttocks. Milky vesicles also appear on the hands and feet, and these may ulcerate.

Examination. Confirms the above. More widespread vesicular lesions suggest chickenpox.

Management

- Symptomatic relief is all that is necessary, using paracetamol and fluids. Benzydamine oral spray is useful for painful oral lesions.
- The illness lasts for 7–10 days.
- Other family members are often affected.

SLAPPED CHEEK (FIFTH DISEASE)

Fifth disease is an infectious upper respiratory illness of young children, which tends to occur in small epidemics.

Diagnosis

History. Ask about a mild illness characterised by erythema of the cheeks and accompanied by fever and irritability.

Examination

- Confirm the above.
- Exclude tonsillitis.

Management

There is no specific treatment. Paracetamol helps the fever and irritability. Associated with increased risk of miscarriage.

Tip
Red cheeks and mild fever may be due to teething in babies.

CHICKENPOX

Chickenpox is a common childhood illness in general practice, occurring usually in small epidemics.

The incubation period is 2–3 weeks.

After infection with chickenpox, the varicella-zoster virus remains dormant in dorsal root ganglia. Reactivation causes shingles (see p. 197).

Diagnosis

If the child is seen before the onset of the rash there may be a pyrexia and irritability. Otherwise the appearance of the rash is diagnostic.

Examination. The rash starts with one or two maculopapular spots which are rapidly joined by many others. Vesicles develop from these as new spots appear. The rash is very itchy and in children scratch marks can often be seen. The whole body can be affected including the palms, soles, oral mucosa and scalp. In the final stage of the rash, after 5–10 days, the spots scab over.

Complications. These are rare:

- chickenpox pneumonia (cough, wheeze and shortness of breath)
- encephalomyelitis (signs of meningism).

Management

- Paracetamol and calamine lotion are often all that are needed. Overheating tends to make the spots itch more. If impetigo develops in any of the spots, use fusidic acid ointment tds or oral flucloxacillin.
- In adults consider antiviral agent, e.g. aciclovir 800 mg five times daily for 7 days.

 Is the patient immunocompromised or pregnant? If so, varicella zoster immunoglobulin may be needed (see p. 343).

INFLUENZA

Influenza commonly occurs as a winter and spring epidemic.

The incubation period is 24–48 hours.

Diagnosis

History. Ask about:

- pyrexia
- headache
- coryza
- sore throat

- mild photophobia
- malaise and myalgia.

Examination. Look for:

- pyrexia
- blocked nose
- mild conjunctivitis
- red throat and cervical lymphadenopathy.

Exclude a chest infection, tonsillitis, otitis and meningitis.

> **Tip**
> Postinfluenza bronchopneumonia is more common in the elderly and infirm and is suspected at the onset of a productive cough, shortness of breath, pleuritic chest pain or prolongation of the fever. Treat with oral flucloxacillin 500 mg qds for 7 days.

Management

- Rest.
- Analgesic/antipyretic, e.g. aspirin or paracetamol.
- Good fluid intake.
- Reassure patient that they should make a full recovery in 5–6 days.
- Antivirals, e.g. oseltamivir or zanamivir, are recommended when influenza is circulating in the community and if an at-risk patient can start treatment within 48 hours of the onset of symptoms. At-risk patients are those eligible for immunisation against influenza.
- Oseltamivir is also recommended, within 48 hours of close contact, for postexposure prophylaxis in at-risk patients, >13 years, who are not effectively vaccinated or who live in residential care and if influenza is present in the establishment.
- For immunisation against influenza, see p. 340.

PNEUMONIA

See p. 180.

MALARIA

Malaria is becoming more prevalent in Britain with increased foreign travel. About 2000 cases occur every year in the UK, causing a dozen or so deaths.

Diagnosis

History. Ask about:

- Non-specific symptoms, similar to flu, including:
    - fever
    - malaise
    - headache
    - myalgia
    - sweating.
- A history of foreign travel. Visits to equatorial countries within the last year, including airport transfers, are relevant.

 Consider malaria in all patients with a fever after travel to an endemic area.

- The use of antimalarial prophylaxis (see below). A common problem arises when people assume they are immune to malaria, e.g. immigrants visiting relatives in malarious areas.

Examination. Examination is often unhelpful in suggesting or confirming the diagnosis. Findings may include fever, jaundice and hepatomegaly.

Investigations. Taking blood for a thick blood film for malarial parasites is essential in making the diagnosis. Send 5 ml of blood in a standard haematology tube and request a thick film for malaria. Mark the request urgent and ensure the results are available within 24 hours.

The result should identify the species of parasite.

If the result is negative, but the history strongly suggests the possibility of malaria, repeat the blood film at the height of the fever.

Management

Tip
If the diagnosis is confirmed or suspected, discuss the patient with the hospital medical team. An infectious diseases specialist is preferable, if available locally. Most cases are admitted, especially if the infection is due to *Plasmodium falciparum*.

Tip
Malaria is a notifiable disease.

Prevention

There are three important pieces of information to give to travellers about the prevention of malaria:

- Avoid being bitten, e.g. by using mosquito nets and insect repellents and wearing trousers and long-sleeved shirts in the evenings.
- Take antimalarial tablets as advised, making sure the course is completed (see below).
- Recognise the symptoms of malaria and seek medical help if suspicious: basically, report any febrile illness which occurs within 3 months of return from a malarious area.

Drug regimen. The choice of antimalarial depends on the area visited, and the advice changes from time to time depending on local resistance of the Anopheles mosquito to chloroquine. For up-to-date advice, refer to the travel guides published regularly in the free GP magazines or ask the patient either to telephone the Medical Advisory Service for Travellers Abroad (MASTA) (see p. 357) or obtain online advice at www.preventingmalaria.info.

 Whichever drugs are recommended, it is vitally important that they are started prior to travel and continued after leaving the malarious area.

Mefloquine should not be taken by patients with depression or other psychiatric disorders, any history of convulsions, or who are pregnant. The alternative antimalarials are less protective against malaria and the patient should reconsider the desirability of travelling to a malarious area.

CONJUNCTIVITIS

See p. 228.

DIARRHOEA AND VOMITING

See p. 120.

IMPETIGO

See p. 134.

COLD SORES

Dry, cracked lips are common, especially during winter, and these can be treated with Vaseline. True herpes simplex (HSV-1) lesions are less common.

Diagnosis

History. HSV-1 infection usually affects the lips, tongue, anterior buccal mucosa or nostrils. It is more common in children. It starts with painful ulcers or vesicles which form singly or in clusters and is often seen during another upper respiratory tract infection. The vesicles progress to crusts and often become secondarily infected, forming patches of impetigo (see p. 134).

Examination. Confirms the above. If the patient presents at the impetigo stage it can be difficult to determine whether or not the underlying lesion is herpetic.

Investigations. Herpes virus can be identified by electron microscopy of the vesicular fluid, but in practice this is rarely necessary.

Management

- Symptomatic treatment is often all that is necessary, with the use of analgesics, either orally or topically.
- Aciclovir is very effective in abating an attack of herpes, although its ability to eliminate the virus from the body is less certain.
- Aciclovir cream, 2 g, applied to the lesions five times a day, is usually sufficient if started at the first sign of an attack.
- For lesions inside the mouth, or if the vesicles are widespread in the mouth, valaciclovir tablets can be given 500 mg bd, or aciclovir suspension 200 mg (5 ml) five times daily over the age of 2 years, 100 mg (2.5 ml) five times daily under age 2 years.
- The total duration of treatment is 5 days.

SHINGLES

The rash of shingles is due to a reactivation of the chickenpox virus.

The incidence of shingles increases with age and is also more common in the immunocompromised.

It is mildly contagious, causing chickenpox, not shingles, in non-immune contacts. Shingles cannot be acquired by exposure to chickenpox.

Diagnosis

History. The patient experiences tingling, paraesthesia or burning pain in the distribution of a single dermatome (see p. 353). This is followed 24 hours later by the appearance of the rash, starting with erythema, then maculopapular and vesicular lesions and progressing to pustules, crusts and, finally, scars.

Shingles is always unilateral. It is most likely to occur on the trunk, but the face is often affected.

Complications

- Secondary bacterial infection of the vesicles is common, indicated by yellow slough or crusts.
- If the rash is in the trigeminal nerve root distribution, look for spread to the eye or nose.
- Postherpetic neuralgia, i.e. continued pain after the rash has gone, may complicate shingles, especially in the elderly.

Management

Prescribing

- Pain relief is often necessary, e.g. co-codamol, 1–2 tablets 4–6-hourly (max = 8 tabs/24 hours).
- Secondary bacterial infection can be treated with fusidic acid ointment tds or oral flucloxacillin 250 mg qds.
- Postherpetic neuralgia may be improved with amitriptyline 25–75 mg nocte or alternatively, gabapentin starting at 300 mg daily, increasing to a maximum of 1.8 g daily.
- Zoster-associated pain can be lessened by the use of an antiviral, e.g. oral aciclovir 800 mg 5 times daily for 7 days, in patients presenting within 72 hours of the onset of the rash.

Referral

- Arrange for the patient to be seen by an ophthalmologist if the rash involves the eye.
- Admit the patient under the medical or infectious diseases team if the rash becomes extensive.

BOILS

The boil, or furuncle, is a common skin infection, occurring even in people with adequate hygiene.

Diagnosis

History. A spot, almost anywhere on the body, becomes painful and inflamed. This progresses to a tense, swollen, erythematous lump. If left, the boil eventually points (forms a head) and either regresses or discharges its contents.

Boils often come in crops, one after another, and tend to be recurrent.

Examination. Look for:

- the above features
- lymphangitis from the boil to the regional lymph nodes
- lymphadenopathy.

Investigations

- A swab of the pus, if the boil is discharging, can guide antibiotic choice.
- For recurrent boils, take nasal swabs to check for *Staphylococcus aureus*, in case the patient is a carrier. Exclude diabetes.

Management

- Analgesia is often all that is required.
- Dress with magnesium sulphate paste under an absorbent dressing if the boil looks ready to discharge.
- Prescribe flucloxacillin 250 mg qds for 5 days if the surrounding skin is erythematous or if lymphangitis is present.
- If the boil is very tense and painful, relief may be gained by incising it through its pointing head with the tip of a scalpel blade, after spraying the boil with e.g. ethyl chloride. The boil can be gently squeezed to massage pus out and a dry dressing applied.
- If the patient is found to be a carrier of *Staphylococcus*, prescribe Naseptin cream, oral flucloxacillin and an antiseptic shower soap for 2 weeks.

HEPATITIS

Hepatitis A is the most common form of hepatitis seen in general practice in the UK. The incubation period is about 1 month. Infection spreads by the faecal–oral route, or by ingestion of infected food.

Hepatitis B is acquired parenterally, e.g. by blood transfusion, needlestick injury or sexually.

Prior to 1991, hepatitis C in the UK was usually caused by infected blood transfusion. Since the introduction of screening blood donors, the commonest cause of hepatitis C has been intravenous drug misuse. It is not easily spread through sexual contact.

Diagnosis

History. Patients may be asymptomatic, especially in hepatitis A. Infection with hepatitis B and C viruses is also usually asymptomatic, except in intravenous drug users, in whom 30% of hepatitis B infections are associated with jaundice.

> **Tip**
> By the age of 50 about 50% of the population in the UK is immune to hepatitis A.

Early symptoms of hepatitis

These can include:

- malaise
- nausea
- mild fever
- headache
- a distaste for cigarettes
- anorexia and diarrhoea
- upper abdominal pain
- pale stools and dark urine, which herald the onset of jaundice
- skin rashes and arthralgia, which can occur in hepatitis B.

Examination

- Jaundice is most evident in the sclerae.
- Lymphadenopathy and splenomegaly may be present.
- The liver is usually tender but not palpable.
- The urine tests positive for bilirubin, even in anicteric cases.

Investigations

- LFTs: show a raised AST and bilirubin.
- FBC: shows a lymphocytosis.
- Hepatitis viral screen: anti-HAV IgM shows a rising titre over 7–10 days in acute hepatitis A.
- Prothrombin time should remain normal. (A rising prothrombin time indicates hepatic failure.)
- Hepatitis B surface antigen is diagnostic of acute hepatitis B. Five to ten per cent of patients go on to develop chronic hepatitis. In these the surface antigen remains positive. If they are also e-antigen positive, they remain highly infectious.
- Antibodies to hepatitis C appear relatively late in the course of the disease. If clinical suspicion is high, test for hepatitis C virus RNA to establish the diagnosis.

Management

- No specific treatment is needed for hepatitis A or B.
- Bed rest is initially advisable, with simple analgesics for muscle or abdominal pains.

- The acute illness usually resolves in 3–6 weeks.
- A full, well-balanced diet and adequate fluid intake are recommended.
- Monitor for signs of fulminant hepatic failure (confusion, disordered LFTs).
- In hepatitis B and C warn the patient of possible spread to sexual contacts.
- Offer hepatitis B immunisation to family members and sexual contacts.
- Patients testing positive for hepatitis C should be referred for consideration for interferon alfa to reduce the risk of chronic infection.
- In acute hepatitis B check for hepatitis B surface antigen at 3 months. Only about 5–10% remain positive in the UK. All such patients should be referred for expert follow-up.
- For immunisation, see pp. 341–342.

> **Tip**
> General malaise for 2–3 months is common. Alcohol should be avoided for 6 months. Oral contraceptives can be resumed after clinical and biochemical recovery.

> **Tip**
> Viral hepatitis is a notifiable disease. Isolation is not necessary, but good personal hygiene is advisable to prevent the spread of infection. Children can return to school as soon as clinical recovery allows.

HIV/AIDS

Over 53 000 people in the UK are estimated to be HIV-positive, with about 6600 new cases per year. The main sources of transmission are sexual and through blood-to-blood contact. All persons who are sexually active should be advised on the prevention of HIV and AIDS. Safe- and low-risk sex should be promoted (see p. 2).

Increasing numbers of patients are requesting HIV testing in the wake of a growing public awareness of the disease and its risk factors. HIV testing is only performed with the patient's consent.

> **Tip**
> Not all GPs feel able to provide appropriate counselling. Genitourinary medicine clinics can.

The test must be performed at least 3 months after the at-risk exposure, as this is considered to be the time taken for seroconversion to occur.

Pre-test counselling

- Take a brief history to ascertain why the test is desired and the patient's likely risk. Risk factors include:
  - sexual contact
  - intravenous drug use
  - homosexual contact
  - needlestick injury
  - sex with men or women in high-risk countries, e.g. Thailand and sub-Saharan Africa
  - sex with prostitutes.
- Ask the patient to consider the implications of a positive result.
- Give advice on safe sex and needle use, if appropriate.

The follow-up appointment

- If the result is negative, the patient did not have antibodies to HIV at the time of the test. A further test is indicated if there has been possible exposure to the virus within the previous 3 months.
- Reiterate the advice on safe sex and needle use.
- Most HIV-positive people remain asymptomatic for many years. Patients have now survived over 20 years with HIV, and new drugs are being developed and used which delay the progression of the disease. There were fewer than 500 deaths from AIDS in the UK in 2003. (See: breaking bad news, p. 316.)
- Arrange further follow up in the GUM clinic.

HIV-positive patients

Patients with HIV-positive status should be followed up regularly in a GUM or specialist HIV clinic.

The GP should consider the HIV-positive patient to be immunocompromised, i.e. any pyrexial illness should be treated seriously. Patients with a low T4 count should be admitted.

Chest infections may be due to *Pneumocystis jiroveci* (formerly *P. carinii*). Tuberculosis is also not uncommon.

Close liaison with the patient's consultant is essential. There is a greater need to consider confidentiality as a sensitive issue in many cases of HIV disease.

PYREXIA OF UNKNOWN ORIGIN (PUO)

In theory, PUO is a pyrexia greater than 38°C, lasting more than 3 weeks, with no known cause after extensive investigation.

In general practice, thorough investigation is not possible. Many patients present with a temperature, and in some of these the cause will not be found with any great certainty. It is, however, rare in general practice for a genuine pyrexia to last more than 2 weeks.

History. Ask about:

- The method of recording the temperature. Patients may say they have a raised temperature when they actually mean they feel hot/sweaty/flushed. Advise the use of an aural thermometer if in doubt.
- Medication: drugs which can cause pyrexia include:
  - antibiotics
  - antituberculous drugs
  - anticonvulsants
  - propylthiouracil
  - procainamide.
- Other symptoms: rash, myalgia, weight loss, pain, cough.
- Contact with infectious disease.
- Past medical history: e.g. malignancies, HIV.
- Animal contact: parrots (psittacosis).
- Travel, especially to malarious areas.

Examination. Look for:

- clubbing, splinter haemorrhages, joint effusions, rashes
- ear, nose and throat infections
- cervical lymphadenopathy
- chest infection
- heart murmurs
- organomegaly.

Investigations

- FBC: infection, lymphoma, leukaemia.
- Glandular fever test.
- ESR: infections, malignancies, temporal arteritis.
- LFTs: malignancies, hepatitis.
- Urine: infection, renal cancers.
- Stool: tropical infection, *Clostridium difficile*.
- Viral titres and blood cultures.
- CXR: TB, sarcoid, lymphoma, psittacosis, metastases.

Management

> **Tip**
> Most persistent fevers can be diagnosed following a thorough history, examination and the above simple investigations. In the absence of a diagnosis, referral to an infectious diseases specialist is warranted if the pyrexia has lasted for more than 3 weeks.

> **Tip**
> The blind use of antibiotics is to be avoided in prolonged pyrexia. Refer for diagnosis first.

WEIL'S DISEASE

Weil's disease is the rare form of leptospirosis with jaundice that is usually caught from infected rat's urine and therefore affects mainly sewage workers, water board workers and people who swim in contaminated rivers.

History. Ask about:

- exposure to potentially contaminated water in the preceding 7–21 days
- abrupt onset of headache, severe muscular aches, chills and fever up to 39°C
- initial symptoms for 4–9 days followed by a recurrence of symptoms after a few days of relief
- jaundice (occurs on day 3–6 in Weil's disease).

Examination. Look for:

- conjunctival redness
- jaundice
- haemorrhages
- anaemia
- haematuria.

Investigations

- FBC: anaemia, neutrophil leucocytosis.
- LFTs: raised bilirubin.
- Serology: acute (days 2–4) and convalescent (week 3–4) for antibodies to leptospires.
- Blood cultures: for leptospires early in the disease, if suspected.

Management

> **Tip**
> In mild cases without jaundice it may be difficult to distinguish Weil's disease from a flu-like illness.

Jaundiced patients with a history of a biphasic febrile illness, headache, severe muscle pains and possible exposure to rat's urine should be admitted for investigation and intravenous antibiotic treatment of suspected Weil's disease.

The mortality in jaundiced patients is 10%.

LYME DISEASE

Lyme disease is a flu-like illness characterised by the rash of erythema migrans. It is caused by the spirochete, *Borrelia burgdorferi*, and is transmitted by tick bite, usually from deer ticks in areas such as the New Forest.

History. Ask about:

- a large, red, insect bite, usually on the thigh, trunk or axilla, often followed by smaller red marks around the initial area
- a severe headache
- myalgia, malaise, fatigue
- travel in an endemic area – New Forest, American North East
- history of tick bite.

Examination. Look for:

- a large, red, raised ring lesion with central clearing (the eschar)
- similar smaller surrounding lesions which come and go (migrans).

Later in the illness there may be signs of arthritis.

Investigations. Acute and convalescent antispirochetal antibodies confirm the diagnosis, but treatment can begin if the condition is suspected on clinical grounds.

Management

- Discuss the case with the infectious diseases department.
- Outpatient treatment is usually possible, with oral antibiotics such as amoxicillin 500 mg tds for 10–14 days or doxycycline 100 mg bd for 10–14 days.
- Most features of the disease respond well, especially if treated early.
- Complications include arthritis, Bell's palsy, heart block and lymphocytic meningitis. These are rare.

MEASLES

Measles is now uncommon in Britain due to the high uptake of the MMR vaccine and, previously, measles vaccines. Measles is more common towards the end of the year.

The incubation period is 2 weeks.

Diagnosis

History and examination. Upper respiratory features predominate initially, with conjunctivitis, rhinitis, otitis media and fever as well as Koplik's spots on the buccal mucosa (discrete, small, white spots).

This is followed 24–48 hours later by the appearance of the dusky pink macular rash, initially on the face and spreading peripherally.

Uncomplicated measles lasts 7–10 days.

Investigations. The diagnosis may be confirmed by a rising IgM titre between acute and convalescent sera.

Complications

- Bacterial otitis media.
- Bronchopneumonia.
- Purulent conjunctivitis.
- Giant cell pneumonitis (rare).
- Allergic encephalomyelitis (1:6000 cases).
- Subacute sclerosing panencephalitis (1:1 000 000 cases).

Management

- There is no specific treatment for uncomplicated measles.
- Secondary bacterial infections should respond to the appropriate antibiotic.
- Human normal immunoglobulin is advisable for immunocompromised patients.
- For childhood immunisation against measles, see p. 338.

> **Tip**
> Measles is a notifiable disease.

MUMPS

Mumps is becoming increasingly rare following the introduction of the MMR vaccine. It is most common in school-age children and young adults.

The incubation period is 18–21 days.

Diagnosis

History. Ask about fever and malaise for 1 or 2 days, followed by parotid gland swelling and pain.

Examination. The parotid gland swelling of mumps makes the angle of the jaw impalpable, helping to distinguish it from cervical or submandibular lymphadenopathy.

Investigation. Send saliva sample, during parotitis, for detection of virus.

Complications

- Orchitis affects 1 in 4 males who contract the disease after puberty.
- Abdominal pain, usually due to pancreatitis or oophoritis.
- Acute lymphocytic meningitis.

Management

- Most cases involve only a straightforward parotitis. There is no specific treatment for this other than pain and temperature control using paracetamol.
- Orchitis may respond to prednisolone 40 mg od in adults for 4 days.
- Abdominal pain may be managed conservatively at home with analgesia if the patient remains systemically well.
- In most cases the illness lasts for <15 days.
- For childhood immunisation against mumps, see p. 338.

> Mumps meningitis must be managed in hospital, even though the treatment is conservative, as a lumbar puncture is required to rule out the possibility of bacterial meningitis.

> **Tip**
> Mumps is a notifiable disease.

RUBELLA

Rubella is becoming increasingly rare with the widespread use of the MMR vaccine.

The incubation period is 2.5–3 weeks.

Diagnosis

History. Rubella is often a mild illness characterised by conjunctival suffusion and rhinitis, followed, after 24 hours, by a discrete, light pink maculopapular rash.

Examination. Examination confirms the features in the history. Also present are enlarged lymph nodes in the postauricular and suboccipital groups.

Investigations. Investigations are unnecessary except in pregnant women without proven immunity who are in contact with a suspicious rash. Send 10 ml of clotted blood to the virology laboratory for haemagglutination and IgM titres. Repeat serology may be requested after 10 days.

Differential diagnosis. The commonest confusion is with roseola infantum and non-specific viral rashes. Rubella is unusual without a certain amount of lymphadenopathy, which is often lacking in the non-specific illnesses.

Complications. Complications are very unusual. Joint pain is probably the most common.

Management

- Symptomatic treatment is usually all that is required. The rash should last no longer than 5 days.
- Refer for foetal assessment if blood tests suggest an acute infection in pregnancy.
- For immunisation, see p. 338.

> **Tip**
> Rubella is a notifiable disease.

CHAPTER 13

EAR, NOSE AND THROAT

Deafness 210

The discharging ear 211

Earache 212

Tinnitus 213

Hay fever 214

Epistaxis 215

Blocked nose 216

Sore throat 218

Cervical lymphadenopathy 219

Hoarseness 220

Gum disease 221

Snoring 221

DEAFNESS

Ear wax is the commonest cause of reduced hearing in general practice but it rarely causes deafness.

Diagnosis

History. Ask the patient:

- whether the deafness is unilateral or bilateral, and whether the deafness was of sudden or gradual onset
- if there are any associated symptoms, such as tinnitus or vertigo, which may suggest a labyrinthine disorder
- whether any drugs have been taken which may affect the acoustic nerve, such as streptomycin and gentamicin.

In the case of children, the parents' account of hearing loss or delayed speech development must be taken seriously.

Examination

- Test the hearing with a whispered voice in each ear in turn.
- Examine to exclude wax, otitis media and a perforated eardrum. (The canal needs to be completely blocked before wax can be held responsible for the hearing loss.)
- Decide whether the problem is conductive or sensorineural using Weber's and Rinne's tuning fork tests.

Weber's test. Place the foot of a vibrating tuning fork on the vertex of the patient's skull and ask in which ear the sound is loudest. An asymmetrical Weber's test indicates conductive deafness on the loud side or sensorineural deafness on the quiet side.

Rinne's test. Place the foot of a vibrating tuning fork on the patient's mastoid process. As soon as the sound fades away, hold the tines of the same tuning fork by the external auditory meatus. The normal ear should be able to hear the noise from the tines after the sound from the foot has faded. If bone conduction is louder than air conduction, a conductive loss is likely.

Management

Children with hearing loss and glue ear need considering for grommet insertion.

Referral

> **Tip**
> Unilateral sensorineural hearing loss, of recent onset, should be referred urgently in case of acoustic neuroma.

If the principal symptom is bilateral hearing loss and there is no external or middle ear problem to account for it, refer to ENT outpatients. In the elderly this is the commonest scenario and is due to the presbyacusis of old age. It can be helped by a hearing aid, which may be obtained by referral to the ENT outpatient department, or by direct referral to a hearing aid department, according to local policy.

Administration

Referral to a social worker for the deaf may be helpful, if this has not been done by the hospital.

THE DISCHARGING EAR

The commonest cause of discharging ear in general practice is otitis externa. It is usually unilateral.

Diagnosis

History. Ask about:

- any tendency to excessive ear wax
- earache
- the likelihood of a foreign body in the ear
- bleeding and deafness associated with the discharge.

Examination. Examine the ear, looking for:

- wax
- a foreign body
- otitis externa
- otitis media
- a furuncle
- perforated eardrum.

Investigations. Take a swab of the discharge and send it to bacteriology.

Management

Wax. See p. 213.

Foreign body. Remove any foreign body, if accessible; refer if not.

Otitis externa. See p. 213.

Otitis media. See p. 213.

Perforated eardrum. Perforations of the eardrum usually heal spontaneously within 4–6 weeks. It is reasonable to prescribe antibiotics e.g. amoxicillin 250–500 mg tds for 5–7 days at presentation. The perforated eardrum may require referral to ENT if healing has not occurred within 6 weeks. If the perforation is near the margin of the eardrum, as opposed to the centre, consider an earlier referral; cholesteatoma can present as a chronic discharging ear with a marginal perforation.

EARACHE

Earache can be very painful and makes children miserable. Parents of small children soon learn the importance of keeping a stock of paediatric paracetamol in the house.

Diagnosis

History. Ask about any symptoms of an upper respiratory tract infection. Patients with colds who develop earache will usually have either otitis media or eustachian tube dysfunction.

Other causes include:

- otitis externa
- trauma to the canal
- foreign body
- perforation of the drum as a result of otitis media (accompanied by the relief of pain).

Unusual causes to consider are:

- shingles
- temporomandibular joint dysfunction
- mastoiditis
- toothache.

Examination. If the eardrum is red, bulging or dull, middle ear infection is suspected. If the eardrum is normal, eustachian tube dysfunction is likely, i.e. increased pressure in the middle ear due to a blocked eustachian tube.

Look also for:

- a boil in the canal
- the vesicular rash of shingles
- inflammation behind the earlobe, suggesting mastoiditis.

Investigations. Take a swab of any discharge from the ear and send it to bacteriology.

Management

Otitis media. Treat with regular analgesia, e.g. paracetamol. Antibiotics, e.g. amoxicillin 125 mg tds under 3 years of age, 250 mg tds over 3 years, may be given if symptoms persist >48 hours.

Eustachian tube dysfunction. For eustachian tube dysfunction advise regular analgesia and warm drinks. (The action of swallowing helps.) The role of decongestants is more controversial.

Otitis externa. For otitis externa prescribe an antibiotic eardrop, such as Gentisone HC eardrops, with or without an oral antibiotic, such as amoxicillin. If there has been no response in 1 week, try an alternative eardrop, e.g. Otosporin or Locorten-Vioform, with or without oral erythromycin. Refer for aural toilet if there is no response.

Wax. Ear wax can be painful, but usually responds to the use of olive oil eardrops for 1–2 weeks. Syringing may be necessary if the wax persists.

Boil. A boil in the ear canal requires analgesics. Antibiotics or incision and drainage may be necessary if the pain is severe.

Shingles. See p. 197.

 If mastoiditis is suspected, refer the patient to ENT urgently.

Temporomandibular joint dysfunction. This also requires analgesics. Reassure the patient that the condition is self-limiting. Advise a dental opinion if the pain persists.

Toothache. This is best dealt with by prescribing analgesics and advising patients to contact their dentist. For dental abscesses prescribe penicillin V and metronidazole (see p. 221).

Perforated eardrum. See p. 212.

TINNITUS

Tinnitus is a ringing, buzzing, hissing or pulsating in the ears.

Diagnosis

History. Ask about associated symptoms, e.g.:

- hearing loss
- dizziness
- earache.

Is the tinnitus bilateral or unilateral and what is the duration of symptoms?

Examination

- Check the ears for otitis media, otitis externa and wax.
- Check BP.

Investigations. FBC to exclude anaemia.

Management

- Patients with tinnitus often present for the first time with fear of a sinister underlying disease, such as a brain tumour or high blood pressure. Reassure the patient if appropriate.
- Treat associated depression.
- The majority of cases resolve. Distraction techniques, such as increasing background noise, are often useful.
- Treat wax or otitis if present.
- If there is no response and the patient is still suffering, referral to ENT outpatients is indicated.
- 'Maskers' are available through ENT outpatients.
- Suggest the Tinnitus Association for educational support (see pp. 355–356).

> **Tip**
> In persistent, unilateral tinnitus of recent onset, refer to ENT to exclude acoustic neuroma.

> **Tip**
> In Ménière's disease and other longstanding causes of tinnitus, patients should be told that drug treatment is mainly ineffective and that, while the ringing will not go away, they will gradually become less aware of it.

HAY FEVER

In some areas hay fever is the commonest condition presenting to GPs in May and June.

Diagnosis

History. Hay fever is characterised by the variable combination of:

- seasonal rhinitis
- conjunctivitis
- occasionally, sore throat and wheeze.

Examination. Examination is usually unnecessary.

Management

Advise the patient to avoid situations in which exposure to pollen will be highest – being outside in the evening, driving with car windows open, sleeping with bedroom window open.

- Prescribe an oral antihistamine, e.g. loratadine 10 mg od or cetirizine 10 mg od. Most preparations are available OTC.
- Steroid nasal sprays are useful for the rhinitis of hay fever, e.g. beclometasone, two sprays bd per nostril.
- Mast cell stabilisers, e.g. sodium cromoglycate eyedrops, two drops qds, help to relieve allergic conjunctivitis.
- A bronchodilator inhaler, e.g. salbutamol, may be needed for wheezing.
- An intramuscular steroid injection may help in severe cases, e.g. Kenalog.

Tip
A step-wise approach to prescribing will reduce costs but a combination of types of treatment will often be necessary.

EPISTAXIS

Patients with nose bleeds present in general practice both acutely, with bleeding, and afterwards, for the prevention of recurrence.

Diagnosis

History. Ask how much blood has been lost, which nostril the blood comes from and whether the patient has any disorder of blood clotting.

Examination. Measure BP. Look up the nose to try and identify a bleeding point. Little's area, on the nasal septum just inside the nostril, often contains some large, delicate blood vessels.

Management

Nose bleeds are very common in young children and are often recurrent. No specific preventive treatment is necessary, as the tendency often remits spontaneously.

To stop acute bleeding

- Advise the patient or parent to squeeze the nose just below the bony part of the nasal bridge. The pressure needs applying continuously for 15 minutes, and it is best if this is timed with a watch. This stops most bleeds.
- If the bleeding does not stop within 15 minutes of continuous pressure and the bleeding is heavy, admit the patient. Alternatively, pack the nose with an adrenaline-soaked wick by pushing it gently towards the *back* of the nasal cavity with McGill forceps. A nasal balloon catheter may be used instead. Admit the patient if this does not control the bleeding.

To prevent further bleeding

- The recurrent bleeding nose is probably best cauterised. If a bleeding point can be identified in Little's area the blood vessel can be touched with the tip of a silver nitrate stick.
- Consider referral for nasal cautery if the bleeding point cannot be identified or controlled.

BLOCKED NOSE

Nasal obstruction can be either bilateral or unilateral, although distinguishing between the two is of little diagnostic use in general practice, except when a foreign body in the nose is suspected. A more useful distinction is between acute blockage (of a few days) and chronic blockage (of, say, more than 3 weeks).

ACUTE BLOCKAGE

Diagnosis

History. Ask about:

- symptoms of upper respiratory tract infection (URTI)
- the likelihood of a foreign body
- a blood clot following a nosebleed.

Consider also trauma (septal haematoma) and hay fever.

Examination. Using the largest auroscope, look up each nostril for:

- a foreign body, if suspected
- a septal haematoma, if there is a history of trauma
- the hyperaemia of Little's area associated with nose bleeds (see p. 215).

Management
If symptoms warrant treatment in an URTI, advise normal saline nose drops. Failing this, xylometazoline nose drops will help if used for a short while.

Hay fever. See p. 214.

Sinusitis. The blocked nose of acute sinusitis is associated with yellow, green or blood-streaked nasal discharge and facial tenderness. Treat with amoxicillin or doxycycline. For chronic sinusitis, treat initially with steroid sprays or decongestants, e.g. beclometasone two sprays bd per nostril. Otherwise, refer for sinus X-rays or CT and antral lavage if indicated.

CHRONIC BLOCKAGE

Diagnosis

History. Ask about:

- Nasal speech and the tendency to nasal discharge during URTIs. This may suggest:
  - adenoid hyperplasia
  - nasal polyps
  - septal mucosal hyperplasia.
- Sleep apnoea syndrome in adults, in which the sleep is interrupted by respiratory tract blockage at night, making daytime sleepiness a problem. This has been associated with chronic nasal blockage.
- Glue ear (in children) and snoring, which can also result from chronic nasal obstruction.

Examination. Examination is often normal in general practice. Look for nasal polyps. Measure the neck circumference in snoring as a collar size greater than 17 inches is positively associated with sleep apnoea syndrome.

Management
Nasal steroid sprays, e.g. beclometasone, may provide partial relief, as will treatment of acute infective exacerbations with antibiotics.

Referral. Referral for e.g. adenoidectomy should be considered for nasal speech, recurrent infections or glue ear in children, and for e.g. submucous resection or polypectomy, if appropriate, on failure of medical treatment in adults. For snoring/obstructive sleep apnoea advise weight loss and alcohol reduction if appropriate. Consider referral if symptoms are severe or daytime somnolence is significant (see p. 221).

SORE THROAT

Acute viral or streptococcal sore throats are a very common feature of general practice. Glandular fever, quinsy and the sore throat of postnasal drip in sinusitis are less common.

Diagnosis

History. Ask about:

- The duration of the symptoms: most acute viral and streptococcal sore throats get better spontaneously within 5–7 days.
- Symptoms of systemic illness: fever, sweating, myalgia and fatigue all suggest a more severe infection.
- The patient's expectations: some patients expect a prescription for antibiotics; others want reassurance or a medical certificate.

Examination

- Examine the throat with a good light.
- Look for the presence of pus on the tonsils, suggesting tonsillitis, and for the creamy white film of glandular fever.
- Palpate the cervical lymph nodes.

Investigations. Investigations are usually unnecessary and unhelpful in the majority of cases of sore throat. Throat swabs take at least 3 days to give a result, by which time most patients are better.

Blood-testing for glandular fever becomes more sensitive after the first 3 weeks, so repeat the test if a first early test is negative and the patient is no better 1–2 weeks later.

Management

Viral infections. Viral throat infections are best treated with analgesics. Antiseptic or analgesic mouthwashes may also help.

Bacterial infections. In streptococcal throat infections the duration of the illness can probably be shortened by 24 hours with the use of penicillin. (Unfortunately there is no quick way of distinguishing between viral and bacterial throat infections. The use of antibiotics is therefore difficult to justify.) If the patient is toxic, prescribe an antibiotic that is effective against streptococci, e.g. penicillin V, or erythromycin, 250 mg qds for 5 days.

Quinsy. Painful, marked swelling of a single tonsil suggests a quinsy, especially if a collection of pus can be seen to point from within the tonsil. Refer the patient to ENT casualty for incision and drainage.

Glandular fever. See p. 190.

Chronic sore throat. Consider physical causes of irritation of the throat, such as snoring, dust inhalation, gastro-oesophageal reflux.

Recurrent sore throat. Reinfection within families is a cause of recurrent throat infection, particularly with *Streptococcus pyogenes*. Send a throat swab and treat the family with penicillin or erythromycin if positive. Consider referral for tonsillectomy if more than five episodes of tonsillitis a year and/or significant snoring or apnoea.

 If a patient on carbimazole develops a sore throat, consider neutropenia. Check an FBC urgently.

Mouth ulcers. See p. 221.

CERVICAL LYMPHADENOPATHY

The isolated, enlarged lymph node in the neck is usually an associated finding with URTIs. Enlarged lymph nodes occasionally present alone, either with tenderness or without.

Diagnosis

History. Ask about symptoms relating to the following possible diagnoses:

- sore throat
- earache
- runny nose
- scalp laceration or infection
- other local infection
- pyrexial illness.

Examination. Examine the ears, nose and throat, and the scalp if necessary. Consider looking for other glands in the axillae and groins (and liver and spleen for thoroughness).

Management

- Often the cause is a non-specific viral illness and the gland returns to its normal state after a few weeks.
- Treat any underlying infection, as appropriate.

- If no infection can be found it is reasonable to wait and see for 3–4 weeks in the absence of other symptoms.
- If the gland remains enlarged, an FBC with differential white count, ESR and a glandular fever test will reveal most haematological malignancies and glandular fever. If the blood tests are negative, refer the patient to the ENT outpatient department for a biopsy to exclude tuberculosis or malignancy.

HOARSENESS

Hoarseness and loss of voice commonly present in general practice as acute problems in association with URTIs. Acute viral laryngitis is the usual cause, for which the treatment is symptomatic: analgesia for the sore throat and resting the voice.

Diagnosis
If the problem lasts more than a few weeks, consider the following diagnoses:

- overuse of the voice (e.g. singing)
- snoring
- oropharyngeal thrush (e.g. from steroid inhalers)
- hypothyroidism
- carcinoma of the larynx or lung (recurrent laryngeal nerve palsy)
- vocal cord disease.

Investigations. Baseline tests include:

- FBC
- TFTs
- CXR.

Management

- Manage any of the specific diseases above, if detected.
- Rest the voice if it is being overused.
- If inhalers cause thrush, advise the patient to rinse the mouth out after use. Nystatin oral suspension or amphotericin lozenges will help.
- Refer the patient to ENT if in doubt.

All patients with unexplained hoarseness for more than 3 weeks need referral to ENT to exclude carcinoma of the larynx.

GUM DISEASE

DENTAL ABSCESS

A dental abscess produces a painful tender swelling of the cheek adjacent to an infected tooth root. Often the carious tooth can be identified. It is worth excluding a parotid gland swelling by making sure the angle of the jaw is palpable.

Management

Prescribe analgesia, e.g. co-codamol, 1–2 tablets 4–6-hourly (max = 8 tabs/24 hours), and antibiotics, such as penicillin V 500 mg 6-hourly and metronidazole 800 mg 8-hourly.

Refer patients to their dentist.

GINGIVITIS

Gingivitis is inflammation of the gums, making them fragile and prone to bleeding on brushing. It occurs in the presence of dental caries, although not exclusively.

Management

Advise patients on general dental hygiene and suggest they see a dental hygienist. Chlorhexidine oral rinse 0.2% is useful in some cases.

MOUTH ULCERS

Painful acute ulceration is nearly always benign, but consider carcinoma of the oral cavity for ulcers that do not resolve over 4 weeks.

Management

- Mouth ulcers are usually aphthous, but can occasionally be viral. Most respond to symptomatic treatment with an analgesic oral gel.
- Prescribe nystatin oral suspension 1 ml qds if thrush is likely.
- Adcortyl in Orabase applied to the ulcers often speeds up the healing.
- Benzydamine spray is useful for ulcers of the tongue.

SNORING

Snoring affects everyone some of the time, and some people most of the time! Most requests for medical help come from partners whose sleep is affected by the patient's snoring.

In most cases of snoring the cause is unknown, or due to obesity.

History. Ask about:

- weight
- neck size
- alcohol intake
- nasal obstruction
- daytime somnolence.

Examination. Look for:

- nasal polyps
- septal deviation
- enlarged tonsils
- enlarged uvula.

Management

- Advise weight loss if the BMI is greater than 26 or if the collar size is >17 inches.
- Advise alcohol moderation in drinkers.
- Encourage patients to sleep on side and avoid excess pillows.
- Consider beclometasone nasal spray for nasal congestion.
- For nasal obstruction advise the use of AirFlow nasal plasters, or Nozovent. Both these are devices for holding the nostrils open at night, and are available from most pharmacies.

Referral. Refer to ENT for consideration for surgery, e.g. septal straightening, polypectomy, turbinate reduction, tonsillectomy or uvulopalatopharyngoplasty.

Refer to a sleep clinic or local chest physician if the patient complains of daytime somnolence. Sleep apnoea can be a complication of snoring, especially in patients with a collar size >17 inches. This condition is treatable with continuous positive pressure ventilation via a nasal mask at night.

CHAPTER 14

OPHTHALMOLOGY

The discharging eye 224
The dry eye 225
Eyelid problems 225
Squint 226
The acute red eye 227
The painful eye 230
Sudden visual loss 231
Progressive visual loss 233
Cataract 234
Chronic glaucoma 234
Floaters 235

THE DISCHARGING EYE

Eyes water as a result of either excessive tear production or inadequate tear drainage.

Excessive tear production

Common causes

- Wind
- dust
- ingrowing eyelash
- corneal or tarsal foreign body
- hay fever.

Impaired tear drainage

Common causes

- URTI
- ectropion
- entropion
- blocked tear duct.

Diagnosis

History. Ask about symptoms of URTI, allergy and possible trauma.

Examination

- Examine the cornea for foreign bodies.
- Inspect the eyelids for:
  - ectropion
  - entropion
  - ingrowing eyelash
  - the presence of an eyelash in the tear duct
  - signs of conjunctivitis.
- Evert the eyelid if the history suggests a foreign body in the eye.

Management

For a chronically sticky eye in a baby, show the parents how to massage the lacrimal duct with gentle pressure from the index finger over the medial palpebral fold twice daily. Only use antibiotic eyedrops if the eye is red. Regular swabbing with moistened cotton wool helps. Refer for duct probing under anaesthetic if there has been no improvement by 6 months of age.

Eyelashes in the tear duct can be easily removed with fine forceps.

Refer the patient with an ectropion, entropion or ingrowing eyelash for corrective surgery. Avoid antibiotic drops or ointment unless obvious conjunctivitis is present.

THE DRY EYE

Dry eye is a symptom that has many causes. The patient may mean gritty, sore, irritating or even painful eye (see p. 230).

Diagnosis

History. Ask about known conditions that may cause the eyes to be dry. The commonest are idiopathic and old age.

Conjunctivitis commonly causes the eye to feel dry. The symptoms also include itching, a sticky discharge and a bloodshot appearance.

Other rare causes are:

- Sjögren's syndrome (rheumatoid arthritis)
- sarcoidosis
- *Chlamydia trachomatis* infection
- exposure keratitis
- Stevens–Johnson syndrome
- pemphigoid.

Examination. Look for signs of infection, ectropion and entropion.

Investigations. A conjunctival swab may be indicated in conjunctivitis. Schirmer's test, in which a strip of special blotting paper is hung from the lower lid margin, may give an idea of the degree of dryness, but in practice is of little help in the management of the dry eye.

Management

- Give antibiotic eyedrops for suspected conjunctivitis.
- Hypromellose eyedrops prn are often the most useful treatment for the chronically dry eye.
- Manage any underlying disease as appropriate.
- Refer for eye surgery in cases of ectropion and entropion.

EYELID PROBLEMS

STYE

Styes are very common. They are infected eyelash roots and produce a red, painful swelling at the lid margin.

Management

Advise regular warm steaming. Consider antibiotic eyedrops, e.g. chloramphenicol or fusidic acid.

MEIBOMIAN CYST (CHALAZION)

This is less common than a stye and produces a red, uncomfortable eyelid swelling at a distance from the lid margin.

Management

For the acute infection advise regular warm steaming. The cyst usually bursts through the conjunctival surface of the eyelid after a few days.

   If the problem is recurrent or if the cyst remains, consider referral to an ophthalmologist for incision and curettage.

BLEPHARITIS

Blepharitis is chronic inflammation of the lid margins. It gives the eyes a sore, tired appearance, with red lid margins.

Management

- Advise the patient to avoid rubbing the eyes and pay attention to cleaning the lid margins carefully with warm water.
- Baby lotion or diluted baby shampoo wiped over the lid margins with a cotton wool bud often helps. Consider treating exacerbations with a topical antibiotic, e.g. Fucithalmic ointment.
- Treat any associated seborrhoeic dermatitis (see p. 137).

SQUINT

A squint is a misalignment of the visual axes of the two eyes. It is normal in very new babies, until they are old enough to focus on near objects.

Diagnosis

History

- When does the child have the squint (e.g. when tired)?
- Ask if there have been any developmental problems.

Examination. Attempt to confirm the squint, as prominent epicanthic folds often give the false impression of a squint.

The corneal light reflex. With the child looking at the light of a pen torch from a distance of about half a metre, the reflection of the light is symmetrical in each eye in the non-squinting child.

The cover test. Get the child to look at a small toy. Cover one eye while observing the other eye. If the uncovered eye moves to take up fixation on the toy, the child probably has a squint.

The red reflex. In babies check for the rare conditions retinoblastoma, retinitis pigmentosa and cataract using the red reflex. Observe the eyes through the ophthalmoscope from a distance of 20 cm. The normal eye has a uniformly red reflection in the middle of the pupil. Any abnormality of this reflex is suspicious.

Management

 If there is an abnormal red reflex, refer immediately.

- If the squint is confirmed, routine referral to the ophthalmology outpatient department is indicated.
- If a squint is not confirmed, refer if the history is convincing. The latent squint may appear only when the child is tired. Otherwise reassure the parents and offer to review the patient in 6 months.
- Reassure the parents that most squints can be corrected without surgery, e.g. by the use of patching or spectacles.

THE ACUTE RED EYE

There are many causes of red eye, even in general practice. The lists below give the principal distinguishing features.

- Most red eyes in general practice are not painful.
- The acute, painful, red eye usually needs urgent referral to ophthalmology.
- The very painful, red eye should be referred immediately.

Diagnosis

History

- Assess the level of pain.
- Ask about visual acuity. (Test if in doubt.)
- Is there any discharge?
- Is there any photophobia?
- Could there be a risk of a foreign body in the eye?

Differential diagnosis

Causes of the painless red eye

- Conjunctivitis.
- Subconjunctival haemorrhage.

Causes of the painful red eye

- Corneal abrasion.
- Herpes zoster infection.
- Arc eye/snow blindness.
- Corneal foreign body.
- Episcleritis and scleritis.
- Acute glaucoma.
- Acute iritis.
- Acute keratitis.

CONJUNCTIVITIS

Conjunctivitis is the most common eye condition seen by GPs. It is usually seen in the context of an upper respiratory tract infection or hay fever. It is mild and self-limiting.

Diagnosis

History. Irritation, grittiness, dryness, itching, stinging or soreness are common complaints in conjunctivitis. In most straightforward cases this is followed by the bloodshot eye, and discharging green/yellow sticky pus which glues the eyelids together overnight.

Any combination of the above symptoms may occur.

 If the eye is painful, consider an alternative diagnosis.

Examination. Look for:

- vasodilation of the conjunctiva
- cobblestone oedema of the conjunctiva under the eyelids
- purulent discharge.

Differential diagnosis

- See: the acute red eye (p. 227)
- the dry eye (p. 225)
- the painful eye (p. 230)
- the discharging eye (p. 224).

Management

- The eye should be kept clean. Hygiene advice is important. Treat with topical antibiotics, e.g. chloramphenicol drops qds, only if the symptoms have not improved after a few days.

- If there is no response, a swab of the discharge can be sent for microscopy, culture and sensitivities. At the same time, the treatment can be changed to fusidic acid eyedrops bd for a further week.
- In hay fever, the conjunctivitis is likely to be allergic, and treatment with antihistamine tablets, e.g. loratadine 10 mg od, or eyedrops, e.g. sodium cromoglycate qds, should be tried initially.
- If there is no response, consider referral.

> **Tip**
> Children with conjunctivitis do not need to be excluded from school or nursery.

SUBCONJUNCTIVAL HAEMORRHAGE

- Common.
- Completely painless.
- Normal acuity.
- No discharge or photophobia.
- No trauma.
- Usually only a part of the cornea is densely red.
- The pupil is normal.

Management
No treatment is usually required as spontaneous resolution occurs.

CORNEAL ABRASION

- Frequent.
- Mild to moderate pain.
- Acuity sometimes slightly reduced.
- Watering eye; no discharge.
- Little or no photophobia.
- Usually a history of mild trauma.
- Fluorescein stain is taken up by exposed keratin.

Management
Apply tetracaine drops, chloramphenicol ointment and an eyepad initially. Thereafter use antibiotic ointment tds.
   Review after 24 hours to check for healing.

HERPES ZOSTER INFECTION

- Not uncommon.
- Periorbital vesicular rash.
- Watering eye.
- Soreness.

Management
Refer urgently, to exclude a dendritic ulcer. Treat with oral aciclovir.

ARC EYE/SNOW BLINDNESS

- Uncommon in general practice.
- Moderate to severe pain.
- Slightly decreased acuity.
- Watering eye.
- Some photophobia.
- History of exposure to welding arc or snow.

Management
Anaesthetic eyedrops and an eyepad are usually sufficient, as spontaneous resolution occurs rapidly.

CORNEAL FOREIGN BODY

- Uncommon in general practice.
- Moderate pain.
- Slightly decreased acuity.
- Watering eye.
- Little or no photophobia.
- A history of something going into the eye.
- A foreign body is usually visible on the surface of the cornea or under the eyelids. (These may need everting.)

Management
Apply tetracaine drops. Remove the foreign body with a needlepoint under magnification. Consider the possibility of an intraocular foreign body.

Prescribe chloramphenicol ointment tds and apply a pad for 4 hours. Check for the presence of a rust ring after 24 hours.

Alternatively, refer to the eye casualty department.

THE PAINFUL EYE

A useful distinction to make in general practice is between the red painful eye and the normal-looking painful eye.

THE RED PAINFUL EYE

See p. 227.

THE NORMAL-LOOKING PAINFUL EYE

Possible causes of the normal looking painful eye:

- Commonly:
  - long-sightedness
  - migraine
  - sinusitis
  - stress headache.
- Rarely:
  - dental pain
  - retrobulbar neuritis
  - temporal arteritis
  - temporomandibular joint dysfunction.

SUDDEN VISUAL LOSS

 Sudden loss of vision is an ophthalmological emergency and requires immediate referral to hospital.

Causes

- Retinal artery embolus.
- Retinal vein thrombosis.
- Retinal detachment.
- Acute angle closure glaucoma.
- Giant cell arteritis.
- Retrobulbar neuritis.

Immediate management

Most of these conditions can be adequately dealt with by arranging immediate transfer of the patient to the eye casualty department.

If there is likely to be any delay, there are two conditions for which treatment started at home or in the surgery can save sight:

- giant cell (temporal) arteritis
- acute angle closure glaucoma.

GIANT CELL (TEMPORAL) ARTERITIS

Diagnosis

History. The patient is elderly and complains of a temporal headache and tenderness, accompanied by blurring or loss of vision in one eye.

Examination. Examination reveals a tender, hardened temporal artery and perhaps a mild fever. The eye looks normal.

Management

In the presence of such typical features take blood for ESR and give prednisolone 80 mg po. Arrange for the patient to go to hospital as soon as possible. A temporal artery biopsy can then be arranged to try and help confirm the diagnosis. See also p. 242.

ACUTE ANGLE CLOSURE GLAUCOMA

Diagnosis

History. The patient has a severely painful red eye, may be vomiting, and complains of having seen haloes around lights.

Examination. Examination reveals a cloudy cornea and a dilated pupil compared with the good eye.

Management

Instillation of 4% pilocarpine drops every minute for 5 minutes, then every 5 minutes will reduce the intraocular pressure. If available, an injection of 500 mg of acetazolamide iv will also help. Alternatively, a 250 mg acetazolamide tablet can be given if the patient is not vomiting. Arrange for the patient to go to hospital as soon as possible.

OTHER CAUSES

Cerebrovascular accident

The sudden onset of a homonymous hemianopia associated with a stroke is not unusual but can occasionally be the only neurological consequence of a posterior cerebral artery infarct. Referral is indicated for complete neurological assessment and rehabilitation (see p. 280).

Migraine

The visual changes accompanying a migraine attack are usually described as flashing lights, blurred vision or spots or zigzags, rather than loss of vision.

If visual loss is reported as a presenting complaint for the first time, even in the presence of a migrainous headache, it is wise to discuss the case with the duty ophthalmologist.

PROGRESSIVE VISUAL LOSS

Children and young adults with progressive visual loss should be referred to an ophthalmologist. The causes in this group include:

- refractive error
- amblyopia of disuse
- diabetic retinopathy
- inherited retinal degeneration (e.g. retinitis pigmentosa)
- posterior uveitis
- pituitary tumour.

Adults with gradual blurring of the vision can be encouraged to see an optician first. They are most likely to need only spectacles.

The commonest causes of progressive visual loss in the elderly

- Refractive error.
- Cataract.
- Senile macular degeneration.
- Chronic open-angle glaucoma.
- Hypertensive retinopathy.

Diagnosis

History. Ask about:

- pre-existing diseases that are known to affect the sight, e.g. diabetes, hypertension, thyroid disorder
- the extent to which the loss of vision affects the patient, e.g. driving, reading, general mobility
- the speed of onset of the visual loss.

Examination

- Measure the visual acuity (VA) with a Snellen chart and record the results. A VA of 6/36 means the patient can read at 6 m what the average person can read at 36 m, i.e. only the bigger letters. Normal vision is a VA of 6/6.
- Check BP.
- Screen for diabetes.
- Assess the visual fields with confrontation testing to exclude the peripheral visual field loss of chronic open-angle glaucoma.
- Examine for cataract (see p. 234).

Management

Referral to an ophthalmologist is indicated in most cases of visual loss. The timing of the referral depends on a number of factors, including the suspected cause and the patient's need to try and recover some of the lost vision (see cataract, below).

Registration of a patient as partially sighted or blind is the statutory duty of the consultant ophthalmologist, not the GP.

Advice. Benefits and aids for the partially sighted are many. Refer the patient to the social worker for the blind unless this has already been done.

Inform the patient of the existence of the Royal National Institute for the Blind (see p. 358) and any local clubs for the blind and partially sighted.

CATARACT

Cataract, or lens opacity, affects approximately 25% of the population in the 65–75-year age range.

Diagnosis

History. Ask about progressive decrease in VA, and glare.

Examination. Look at the eye through an ophthalmoscope from a distance of 20 cm. The normal homogeneous red reflex is obscured by dark lines across the pupil. Fundoscopy is often difficult due to the obstructed view.

Differential diagnosis. See progressive visual loss (p. 233).

Management

The mainstay of treatment for cataract is surgical, but the timing of the referral will depend on a number of factors. As soon as the VA has deteriorated enough to affect the usual daily routine, the patient should be referred for a surgical opinion.

In the meantime, advise patients not to drive if they fail to meet the standards required by the Driver and Vehicle Licensing Agency, i.e. to be able to read a number plate at 67 ft (20 m) with at least one eye.

CHRONIC GLAUCOMA

Chronic open-angle glaucoma is usually suspected by finding a raised intraocular pressure, cupping of the optic discs or peripheral visual field loss on charting. These changes are usually detected by the optician on routine eye testing.

Referral to the ophthalmology outpatient department is indicated.

Confirmed cases are followed up in outpatients. Treatment usually consists of eyedrops to either reduce intraocular pressure or facilitate anterior chamber drainage. Occasionally, surgery is indicated (iridocentesis).

Issues for the GP include:

- Family members are at increased risk of chronic glaucoma.
- Repeat prescribing of eyedrops.
- Beta-blocker eyedrops can have systemic effects in e.g. asthma.
- Management of progressive visual loss (see pp. 233–234).

FLOATERS

Floaters are small, black spots, seen by the patient to be floating in front of the eyes. They are very common and patients need reassuring that there is likely to be nothing wrong with their eyes.

The fortification spectra of migraine may be described as black spots, but these are usually followed by the headache and are temporary.

Management

Nothing need usually be done, other than to reassure the patient that the condition is benign and usually self-limiting.

> If the floaters are described as large, dark blobs which appear suddenly and are associated with flashing lights, the cause may be retinal detachment and the patient should be referred immediately.

Occasionally the patient may have a cataract (see p. 234).

RHEUMATOLOGY AND ORTHOPAEDICS

Joint pain   238

Gout   239

Neck pain   240

Osteoarthritis   241

Polymyalgia rheumatica and giant cell arteritis   242

Osteoporosis   243

Rheumatoid arthritis   244

Shoulder pain   246

Tennis elbow   248

Tenosynovitis   248

Carpal tunnel syndrome   249

Ganglion   250

Paronychia   250

Low back pain   251

Knee pain   252

Sprained ankle   254

Painful heel (plantar fasciitis)   255

Ingrowing toenail   256

JOINT PAIN

Many patients present with multiple aches and pains and some of these may be described as joint pains.

Diagnosis

History. Ask about:

- The duration of symptoms: a short-term illness requires a diagnosis.
  In long-term problems, first find out what the patient wants: symptom relief or reassurance.
- Associated features such as viral illness, depression or fatigue.
- Generalised or localised symptoms.
- Diurnal symptoms.
- Joint stiffness.

Examination. Look at:

- the affected area for inflammation, deformity or restricted movement
- nearby structures, such as the neck in shoulder pain
- whether it is a joint problem, periarticular or muscular
- tender spots, as in tennis elbow and fibrositis
- other areas as suggested by the history.

Causes of joint pain

It is worth having a checklist of causes of joint pain in mind when seeing these patients. The commonest are given first:

- unaccustomed use
- repeated overuse
- viral illness
- osteoarthritis (see p. 241).
- non-articular rheumatic pain, e.g. tennis elbow (see p. 248)
- gout (see p. 239)
- polymyalgia rheumatica (see p. 242)
- rheumatoid arthritis (see p. 244)
- other connective tissue disorders
- malignancy and myeloma.

Investigations. If the diagnosis remains unclear having taken a careful history and examined the relevant parts, bloods can be requested for FBC, ESR and CRP, rheumatoid factor and serum uric acid. See the patient after 2 weeks.

Insignificant causes will produce normal results (except, perhaps, for a slightly raised ESR in viral illnesses).

Persistent abnormality prompts management as in the relevant sections listed in the box on p. 238, or referral for further diagnostic tests.

GOUT

Gout presents most commonly in middle-aged men. It may affect any joint, but is usually seen in the big toe, ankle or knee.

Diagnosis

History. Ask about the spontaneous onset of severe pain in one joint, exacerbated by movement.

Examination. Look for:

- inflammation of the joint (red, hot and swollen)
- gouty nodules around ears, bursae or tendons, which suggest chronic gout.

Investigations

Serum uric acid. This is usually raised in gout, but is non-specific.

C&Es. In chronic gout it is necessary to exclude kidney damage.

Lipids. Hyperlipidaemia often coexists with gout.

Joint aspiration. The diagnosis of gout is usually obvious after the history and examination. If in doubt, aspirate fluid from the joint. Uric acid crystals in the synovial fluid are diagnostic.

Management

Advice. Give general advice about reducing the risk of gout:

- Reduce alcohol intake.
- Avoid being overweight.
- Avoid purine-rich foods (e.g. offal, oily fish, pulses).

Prescribing. A therapeutic trial of a strong NSAID (see below) may help to exclude other diseases, as the acute attack of gout should subside within a few days.

Stop any thiazide diuretics.

- For the acute attack, prescribe indometacin 50 mg tds or naproxen 500 mg bd.
- If the patient has a contraindication to NSAIDs, use colchicine 0.5–1 mg qds.

- For recurrent attacks prescribe allopurinol 100 mg daily. This can be increased, up to 600 mg daily, if attacks recur. Do not start allopurinol until after an attack has subsided.

Referral. Refer severe or resistant cases to a rheumatologist.

NECK PAIN

Neck pain is commonly a mild, self-limiting nuisance due possibly to muscle tension.

Diagnosis

History

- Ask about the duration of the symptoms. A short history of neck pain, usually on one side of the neck more than the other and with a twisting of the neck, suggests acute torticollis. This sort of acute pain, but without the twisting, is common in whiplash injuries.
- Ask about chronic pain and stiffness in the neck. These symptoms may be due to degeneration in the cervical intervertebral discs, suggestive of cervical spondylosis. Early morning stiffness may be a feature of osteoarthritis of the cervical spine. Severe acute cervical spine pain, usually accompanied by occipital headache, suggests meningism, especially in someone not accustomed to neck pain.
- Exclude radiculopathy and myelopathy by asking the patient about symptoms of pain or weakness in the arms or legs.

Examination. Look for:

- Tenderness in the neck muscles. If the head is held to one side and the patient cannot straighten the head, think of acute torticollis.
- A reduced range of movement of the cervical spine, which suggests cervical spondylosis or arthritis.
- Weakness and wasting in the arms or legs, which suggest a radiculopathy or myelopathy, are not uncommon in cervical spondylosis. Examine for this if there are suggestive symptoms.

Investigations. If the diagnosis is in doubt or if the patient is particularly requesting it, an X-ray of the cervical spine may be useful. Cervical spondylosis and arthritis usually show up after 6 months of disease.

Management

- Physiotherapy helps to improve the range of pain-free movement in both acute and chronic cases of neck pain.
- A collar often helps by temporarily resting the neck.

- Prescribe NSAIDs or simple analgesics for pain.
- Diazepam tablets 2–5 mg tds help relieve the muscle spasm of acute torticollis.
- Refer all cases with neurological complications.

OSTEOARTHRITIS

Osteoarthritis is the most common joint disease seen in general practice, its incidence increasing with age. It is a progressive, debilitating disease, mainly affecting the weight-bearing joints and hands.

Diagnosis

History. Ask about pain and early morning stiffness, usually in a knee, hip or ankle. Symptoms will have been present for some months and may have been exacerbated by recent injury or overuse.

Examination

- Look for a reduced range of movement or pain on movement of the affected joint or joints.
- Crepitus may be felt by laying a hand on the joint while moving it.
- The soft-tissue swelling of osteoarthritis produces a 'fattened' joint and fluid effusions are often absent.
- The patient may have a limp, use a stick or have difficulty getting on to the examination couch.

Investigations

- X-rays are unhelpful in the early stages of the disease, although 6 months of osteoarthritis will usually show characteristic X-ray changes.
- Blood tests exclude other causes of arthritis (see rheumatoid arthritis, p. 244).

Management

Advice

- Aim for ideal weight.
- Encourage mobility/activity.
- Social Services will advise the patient about allowances and benefits and a disabled parking permit.
- Educational leaflets and support groups are a useful source of information for patients.
- Be on the lookout for depression and carer stress.

Treatment

- For the relief of pain, start with simple paracetamol and increase if necessary to co-codamol or co-dydramol.

- Stiffness can be relieved by NSAIDs. A big evening dose is useful in early morning stiffness, e.g. ibuprofen S/R 800 mg, two tablets nocte.
- Beware of the risk of gastric irritation from NSAIDs in the elderly. Prescribe a proton-pump inhibitor such as omeprazole 10 mg daily.
- Consider glucosamine 1500 mg a day as an adjunct for pain relief (only available OTC).
- Physiotherapy is useful for maintaining joint mobility.
- Consider intra-articular injection of corticosteroid if only one or two joints are affected (e.g. for knee joint, methylprednisolone 40 mg).
- Walking aids such as sticks and frames can be obtained by referral to the local occupational therapy or physiotherapy department or from the day hospital.
- Occupational therapy can also help with activities of daily living and modification of the home.

Referral. Consider referral for joint replacements. The timing of referral depends on the effect of the disease on the patient's life in terms of immobility and pain. Generally, the patient who is being woken at night despite full doses of anti-inflammatories and non-addictive analgesics should be considered for surgery.

POLYMYALGIA RHEUMATICA AND GIANT CELL ARTERITIS

Polymyalgia rheumatica is a common condition in Caucasians, mainly affecting women over 55. It coexists with giant cell arteritis in about 30% of cases (see p. 232).

Diagnosis

History

Polymyalgia rheumatica. Ask about pain and stiffness around the shoulders or, occasionally, the hips, which is worse in the mornings.

Giant cell arteritis. Ask about temporal headache, visual loss or diplopia.

Both may present occasionally with fever, fatigue or weight loss.

Examination

Polymyalgia rheumatica. Look for mild tenderness on palpation of the shoulder muscles. Patients with PMR have difficulty in raising their hands above their heads. Examination of the shoulder joints and neck should be normal.

Giant cell arteritis. Look for a tender temporal artery on palpation.

> Giant cell arteritis is an ophthalmological emergency due to the risk of sudden blindness. If the diagnosis is suspected on the grounds of visual loss and/or temporal headache and tenderness in patients over the age of 55, the patient should be seen urgently by an ophthalmologist.

Investigations

- ESR: a result >50 is strongly supportive of the diagnosis of PMR. If a borderline raised ESR is obtained, repeat after 48 hours. Do not await the ESR result if there is a strong suspicion of giant cell arteritis.
- If the ESR is very high, exclude myeloma with serum electrophoresis (paraprotein band) and urine electrophoresis (Bence–Jones protein).
- TFTs: to exclude hypothyroidism.

Management

- For polymyalgia rheumatica: give prednisolone 10–20 mg daily.
- For giant cell arteritis: urgent referral if suspected, but the starting dose of steroids is 60–80 mg daily.
- For both: stay on the initial dose of prednisolone until the symptoms have come under control, then begin to reduce the daily dose of prednisolone by increments as long as there is no recurrence of symptoms or a significant rise in the ESR.
- Any recurrence of symptoms should prompt an increase in dose for 1 month.
- Most patients are maintained on less than 5 mg daily for the duration of the illness.

Tip
It is not unusual for these patients to require steroids for 2 years or longer, in order to maintain remission of symptoms.

- Beware the risk of osteoporosis in long-term steroid use. Use the minimum dose possible. Give osteoporosis prophylaxis (see p. 244) at the start of steroid treatment.

OSTEOPOROSIS

Osteoporosis is most common in postmenopausal women. It is characterised by a decreased bone density due to demineralisation and is responsible for 45 000 hip fractures a year in the UK.

Diagnosis

The condition itself is asymptomatic, but the following put patients at increased risk:

- postmenopause
- family history of osteoporosis
- smoking
- lack of exercise

- thin build
- steroids.

Examination. Patients present in the following ways:

- Fractured hip or wrist.
- Back pain which turns out on X-ray to be due to vertebral fracture.
- Loss of height or dowager's hump, both of which are due to vertebral collapse.

Investigations

- Bone densitometry can detect osteoporosis, but is not yet recommended for population screening.
- Blood tests should be normal in osteoporosis.

Management

- Treat the complications of osteoporosis, i.e. fractures.
- The deep bone pain of vertebral collapse usually responds to analgesia and bed rest in 2–4 weeks.
- For the prophylaxis and treatment of osteoporosis, including all patients with a history of low-impact hip fracture, bisphosphonates, e.g. alendronic acid or risedronate, are the drugs of first choice. For the prescribing regimen, see the BNF.

Prevention

- Stopping smoking reduces the risk of postmenopausal hip fracture by 25%.
- Regular weight-bearing exercise reduces the risk of postmenopausal hip fracture by up to 50%.
- Five years' use of oestrogen replacement therapy reduces the risk of postmenopausal hip fracture by 50–75% but the risk of osteoporosis is no longer considered to be a sole indication for initiating HRT (see hormone replacement therapy, p. 52).
- If a patient is on steroids, reassess the need.
- Maintain sufficient dietary calcium and vitamin D intake. Supplements are indicated in all elderly mobile patients in residential care and those at risk of falling or with a history of falls.

RHEUMATOID ARTHRITIS

The average GP list of 2000 will have 3–4 rheumatoid arthritis patients. It is three times more common in women. Patients are usually over 40, but may be younger.

Diagnosis

History. Ask about:

- Joint pain: symmetrical pain and morning stiffness are very common, especially in the small joints of the hands and feet. The distal interphalangeal joints are usually spared. Swelling of joints often occurs.
- Other symptoms, which include:
  - general malaise
  - weight loss
  - carpal tunnel syndrome
  - tenosynovitis.

Examination. Look for:

- Joints which are tender, hot, swollen and painful to move. The proximal interphalangeal, metacarpophalangeal and wrist joints are usually inflamed in the acute phase.
- Carpal tunnel syndrome (see p. 249), which is often associated with rheumatoid arthritis. Tender metatarsophalangeal joints may also be found.

Investigations. All suspected cases of rheumatoid arthritis should have ESR or CRP. If these are raised for the patient's age, organise the following:

- FBC.
- Rheumatoid factor: positive in 80% of rheumatoid arthritis patients, but 5% are false-positive results.
- Antinuclear antibody: should be negative to exclude SLE.
- Serum uric acid: should be normal to exclude gout.
- X-ray of the hands and feet: the characteristic appearances of rheumatoid arthritis appear after 6 months of disease.

> It is a mistake not to refer new cases of rheumatoid arthritis at an early stage, since disease-modifying drugs reduce erosive disease and resultant loss of function.

Management

Care of the acute case. Refer all patients in whom the diagnosis is suggested or confirmed by the above investigations. Resting acutely inflamed joints reduces pain. Passive movements help prevent deformity.

Drug treatment

- Simple analgesics may be equally effective, e.g. paracetamol.
- NSAIDs help while awaiting hospital assessment. High-strength NSAIDs at night may reduce early morning stiffness and pain. Consider a proton-pump inhibitor such as omeprazole 10 mg daily for gastroprotection from NSAIDs in the elderly.
- Acutely inflamed joints can be injected with steroids, e.g. methylprednisolone (see p. 247).

Disease-modifying antirheumatic drug (DMARD) monitoring. See p. 330.

Care of the chronic case

The level of help required by the patient depends on the activity of the disease. Not all patients with rheumatoid arthritis have active disease.

- Liaison with the rheumatologist is helpful for prescribing, advice and follow-up.
- Physiotherapy can improve joint mobility and muscle wasting.
- Occupational therapy can address problems with activities of daily living by modification of the home and the provision of walking aids.
- Provide leaflets and support group details.
- Ask the patient to contact Social Services for allowances and benefits, e.g. the disabled parking badge.
- Be aware of potential complications, e.g.:
  - septic arthritis
  - neutropenia
  - drug side-effects
  - dry eyes
  - nodules
  - leg ulcers
  - pulmonary fibrosis
  - peripheral neuropathy.
  - atlantoaxial subluxation and quadriplegia in cervical spine involvement.
- Watch for depression and carer stress (see p. 292).
- Consider pain clinic referral.
- Some patients find fish oils and evening primrose oil helpful.
- Advise patients against being overweight.

> **Tip**
> Try to avoid an unnecessarily gloomy outlook. Many cases follow a mild, remitting course with no long-term disability.

SHOULDER PAIN

Shoulder pain can be a symptom of problems in the neck, such as cervical spondylosis, but is usually caused by either adhesive capsulitis (frozen shoulder) or the rotator cuff syndrome (e.g. supraspinatus tendonitis). Consider cardiac ischaemia or diaphragmatic irritation as a possible cause, e.g. gallstones.

Diagnosis

History. Ask about:

- Any history of trauma, such as a fall on the arm.
- Previous episodes of similar problems.
- Neck pain.
- Occupation and handedness: repetitive use of the arm may account for shoulder problems.

Examination. Look for:

- Bruising, which may suggest a fractured neck of the humerus, especially in an elderly person following a fall.
- Limitation of movement of the glenohumeral joint, in frozen shoulder.
- The painful arc: pain increases as the shoulder is abducted to about 90°, but reduces again as the arm is raised further above the head. This is a feature of supraspinatus tendonitis.

Tip
Neck problems often present with shoulder pain.

Management

- Physiotherapy can be useful for some painful arc syndromes, but is of little value in the treatment of frozen shoulder.
- NSAIDs, if not contraindicated, are useful in reducing pain and inflammation.
- The injection of long-acting corticosteroids into the subacromial space is useful in the treatment of supraspinatus tendonitis, e.g. methylprednisolone 40 mg with 2% plain lidocaine 2 ml. Warn the patient the pain will get worse over the ensuing 24 hours. If improvement is partial, a second injection is useful.

Beware the fractured neck of humerus. This is usually more painful initially. Bruising develops over the first 48 hours. Some movement of the glenohumeral joint is often possible.

TENNIS ELBOW

Tennis elbow is the name usually given to lateral epicondylitis, inflammation of the insertion of the forearm extensor muscles at the elbow.

Diagnosis

History. Ask about pain on the outer side of the elbow, especially when gripping. The pain often radiates down the forearm.

Examination. Tenderness can be elicited at the point of insertion of the forearm extensor muscles into the lateral epicondyle.

Management

- Tennis elbow can settle spontaneously, but this usually takes several months.
- Avoid trigger movements as far as possible.
- A short course of NSAIDs can help.
- A sports support for tennis elbow may be purchased.
- An injection of e.g. hydrocortisone and local anaesthetic is usually helpful but the recurrence rate is relatively high. Using a blue needle inject hydrocortisone 100 mg with 1% lidocaine 1 ml deep into the tender point of the elbow. Warn the patient that the symptoms will worsen over the ensuing 24 hours.
- Ultrasound from the physiotherapist can be an effective alternative.

TENOSYNOVITIS

Tenosynovitis is inflammation of the tendons of the dorsum of the hand or foot. It commonly presents in general practice following repetitive overuse. Occasionally it can occur spontaneously.

Diagnosis

History. Ask about pain and tenderness over the tendons, usually of the hand, where they cross the wrist within a synovial sheath. The pain is worsened by movement of the tendon within the sheath.

Examination. Look for:

- Swelling. This is a common feature of De Quervain's tenosynovitis (thumb extensors).
- Tenderness and exacerbation of the pain on palpating the affected tendon.

Management

- Rest for 2–3 weeks with immobilisation is often all that is needed. A temporary change of use of the hand may help.

- A short course of NSAIDs can help.
- An injection of hydrocortisone with local anaesthetic may be useful, if the GP is confident in the technique. Refer to a rheumatologist otherwise.
- Referral for surgical decompression is occasionally required, particularly if the above measures are unhelpful and the patient is handicapped by the symptoms.

CARPAL TUNNEL SYNDROME

Carpal tunnel syndrome is the most common cause of paraesthesiae in general practice. The syndrome of pain and tingling in the hand should always raise this possibility.

Diagnosis

History. Ask about pain and tingling in the median nerve distribution of the hand (radial 3½ digits). It is usually worse in the mornings and can be relieved temporarily by shaking the hand vigorously.

Examination

> Wasting of the small muscles of the hand indicates severe nerve compression, and prompt orthopaedic referral for decompression of the carpal tunnel is advised.

A positive Tinel's sign is highly suggestive of carpal tunnel syndrome. The symptoms are exacerbated by tapping on the median nerve at the wrist.

Investigations. If the diagnosis is in doubt, electromyelographic studies are diagnostic.

Management

- Rest the affected hand. This advice can be supplemented by the provision of a Futura-type wrist splint, or just a plain sling.
- NSAIDs can be useful in mild cases.
- Injection of methylprednisolone 40 mg with local anaesthetic under the flexor retinaculum of the wrist, around the median nerve (situated between the radial artery and palmaris longus tendon) can be useful if the GP is confident in this technique. Refer to orthopaedics or rheumatology outpatients otherwise.
- Refer to orthopaedic outpatients for carpal tunnel release if there is no improvement or if there is wasting of the small muscles of the hand.

GANGLION

A ganglion is a firm, cystic swelling, usually around the dorsum of the wrist or hand. Ganglions can also be found around the ankle. The problem is usually a cosmetic one.

Management

Inform the patient that 50% of all ganglions disappear spontaneously in time. If discomfort or inconvenience is caused by the ganglion it can be treated in a number of ways:

- Aspirate the lump under local anaesthetic using a 21G needle.
- Pierce the ganglion several times with a fine hypodermic needle and press on it gently for several seconds while the contents disperse.

> **Tip**
> In both these cases recurrence is possible, so warn the patient of this.

- If the above methods fail, consider referral to orthopaedic outpatients for a formal excision if the patient is troubled by the ganglion.

PARONYCHIA

A paronychia, or whitlow, is a suppurative collection around a fingernail. The pus can easily be seen adjacent to a nail as a white, tense, tender swelling.

Management

- Spray the whitlow with ethyl chloride for 5–10 seconds or until a frost develops.
- Incise through the cuticle into the paronychia using a No. 11 scalpel blade. The pus should be let out and should be seen to drain freely.
- Gently squeeze below the nail bed to 'milk' the pus from the finger. A simple dressing is all that is required.

 If the whitlow has a number of heads it may be herpetic. Aciclovir cream may then be a more appropriate treatment.

- If surrounding cellulitis is a feature, treat with an oral antibiotic, e.g. flucloxacillin.

- If the infection is mild and localised, a topical antibiotic is often sufficient, e.g. fusidic acid.

LOW BACK PAIN

Low back pain is the commonest cause of days lost from work in the UK. Decide first whether the patient is presenting with a new, acute episode of back pain, or a chronic problem.

ACUTE PRESENTATION

The acute onset of lumbar back pain usually follows lifting, and often radiates to the buttock or leg.

Diagnosis

History. Ask about: bladder paralysis symptoms, muscle weakness in the lower limbs, paraesthesiae. The following features are significant:

- Age <20 and >55.
- Nocturnal pain.
- Thoracic pain.
- Patient on oral steroids.
- Weight loss.
- Past history of carcinoma.

Examination. Look for: neurological signs in the lower limbs. Look particularly for weakness of dorsiflexion of the ankle and extensor hallucis (L4–L5 prolapse), weakness of the peroneal muscles, toe flexors, calf and tibialis posterior (L5–S1). Check for power/sensory loss, reflexes (knee and ankle) and straight leg raising.

Investigations. In the elderly with acute back pain, consider ESR, and PSA in men. X-rays are unhelpful except to exclude ankylosing spondylitis in young people and vertebral collapse or malignancy in the elderly. Limited MRI should be considered if nerve root symptoms persist for >4 weeks.

Management

Indications for immediate orthopaedic referral are:

- bladder paralysis
- extensive muscle weakness
- objective neurological signs.

In the absence of neurological signs:

- Mild low back pain (e.g. sacroiliac joint discomfort) often requires reassurance only.
- Advise mobilisation. Encourage activity within the limits of pain. Frequent short episodes of activity are best.
- Prescribe analgesics, e.g. co-codamol, 1–2 tablets 4–6-hourly (max = 8 tabs/24 hours). A laxative helps if opiates are prescribed, e.g. lactulose 10 ml bd. Diazepam 5 mg tds is useful, as a muscle relaxant and an anxiolytic, in the short term.
- Follow up if symptoms do not settle in 2–3 weeks. Repeat the neurological examination if suspicious symptoms develop.
- For the prevention of further attacks, advise on correct posture, lifting and exercises, and enquire about work-related back strain. Consider referral to a physiotherapist, chiropractor or osteopath.

CHRONIC PRESENTATION

 Always think of the possibility of neurological involvement by looking for leg signs and asking about bladder symptoms.

If the acute episode has not settled or repeated acute episodes occur, consider the following:

- depression
- hidden agenda
- carer stress.

Management

- Physical therapy, e.g. physiotherapist, osteopath, chiropractor.
- Orthopaedic or neurosurgical referral:
  - MRI scan for prolapsed disc
  - surgery.
- Rheumatology referral: facet joint injection.
- Antidepressants.
- Local back pain sufferers' group.
- Physiotherapist's back school.

KNEE PAIN

After low back pain, knee pain is the second most common orthopaedic problem in general practice.

Diagnosis

History. It is useful to divide knee problems into those associated with some trauma to the knee and those of spontaneous onset.

Without trauma. If the pain has been present for some time consider e.g.:

- chondromalacia patellae in the young
- osteoarthritis in the elderly.

If the pain is acute think of:

- prepatellar bursitis
- septic arthritis
- gout.

Prepatellar bursitis can be difficult to distinguish from the rarer septic arthritis. Factors in favour of prepatellar bursitis include:

- an otherwise well patient
- no history of fever
- no limitation of movement of the knee
- the ability to weight-bear.

With trauma. If there is no limitation of movement, and the patient can weight-bear, the likely diagnosis is a simple sprain.

Symptoms that suggest damage to the internal structures of the knee include swelling, locking, giving way, inability to weight-bear and an inability to extend the knee fully. Often these symptoms follow a recurring and remitting course.

Examination. Watch as the patient climbs onto the examination couch. This will tell you a lot about the functioning of the knee.

Look for redness, heat and swelling. These suggest the presence of acute inflammation or infection, usually gout, prepatellar bursitis or, occasionally, septic arthritis.

The examination is often normal in e.g. chondromalacia patellae and minor sprains.

If there is a history of trauma, test the ligaments and cartilages. Holding the lower leg at mid-calf level and with the knee slightly flexed, attempt to bend the knee sideways in each direction in turn. A few degrees of movement is normal, as can be demonstrated on the patient's good knee. Excessive movement suggests a collateral ligament tear. Ask the patient to roll onto their front. With the knee flexed to 90°, push down on the foot and rotate the foot in each direction in turn while extending the knee. Acute pain suggests a torn meniscus (Apley's test).

Management

Chondromalacia patellae

- Conservative management with explanation, analgesics, rest and quadriceps exercises usually suffice.
- Referral for consideration for surgery is rarely needed.

Prepatellar bursitis

- If the inflammation is confined to the patellar area, rest, analgesia and Tubigrip will suffice.
- If there is considerable swelling in front of the knee, aspiration under local anaesthetic will ease the pain by reducing the pressure within the bursa.
- If there is evidence of inflammation extending beyond the area of the patella, antibiotics should be prescribed, e.g. flucloxacillin 250 mg qds.
- If aspiration of the bursa produces pus and there is evidence of cellulitis, consider admitting the patient for surgical drainage and splinting of the knee.

Septic arthritis. Admit immediately if this is suspected.

Gout. See p. 239.

 Acute knee injuries with swelling require X-rays to exclude a fracture, and aspiration to exclude a haemarthrosis or lipohaemarthrosis. Refer to casualty.

In the absence of swelling and if the patient can weight-bear, the acute knee injury can be treated by rest, analgesia, Tubigrip, ice-pack and quadriceps exercises.

Chronic knee pain

- Chronic traumatic knee pain in a sportsperson can often be helped by a change of footwear.
- Referral to a sports medicine, rheumatology or orthopaedic clinic depending on local specialist interest.
- If the history or examination suggests the presence of either ligament or cartilage damage, consider referral for arthroscopy, especially if quadriceps exercises have not helped.

Osteoarthritis. See p. 241.

SPRAINED ANKLE

This is a common soft-tissue injury in general practice, usually due to inversion of the ankle, damaging the lateral talofibular ligament. Nearly all soft-tissue sprains settle with rest, followed in severe cases by physiotherapy, but the fractured ankle should be excluded early.

Diagnosis

History. Ask about:

- falls from a height/down a hole
- previous fracture
- running/jumping injury
- occupation.

Examination. Look for:

- tenderness below the lateral malleolus
- tenderness of the fibula above the malleolus (associated with fracture).

> **Tip**
> Examine the base of the 5th metatarsal for signs of fracture, which is more common if the injury is due to a fall, e.g. off the edge of a kerb.

Management

- RICE: **r**est, **i**ce, **c**ompression (e.g. Tubigrip), **e**levation.
- Mobilise gently after 24 hours.
- Refer more severe sprains, e.g. sports injuries, for physiotherapy early.
- Complete resolution of swelling may take several months.

> **Tip**
> Pain, swelling and bruising get worse over the first 24 hours in the sprained ankle. Use ice for 10–15 minutes at a time.

Referral. Referral for an orthopaedic opinion is appropriate if the patient does not improve to the point of returning to work after physiotherapy.

PAINFUL HEEL (PLANTAR FASCIITIS)

Plantar fasciitis causes chronic pain under the heel, especially when taking the first steps in the morning, with no history of trauma. There is usually a tender point just in front of the bony part of the heel. The condition usually resolves spontaneously after several months.

Diagnosis

Differential diagnosis

- Plantar wart: can usually be seen.
- Fracture calcaneum: follows quite severe trauma.
- Sever's disease (osteochondritis of the calcaneum): tender at the Achilles tendon insertion.

Management

- Consider a short course of NSAIDs with rest.
- Footwear – advise soft heels and heel padding. Sorbothane heel cups may help and are available from chemists and sports shops.
- An injection of hydrocortisone with local anaesthetic can be performed. Warn the patie nt that the symptoms will get temporarily worse over the ensuing 24 hours. Using an orange needle on a 5-ml syringe, inject 1% plain lidocaine 2 ml with hydrocortisone 100 mg or methylprednisolone 40 mg deep into the tender point. This can be repeated two or three times at intervals of 3 weeks.

INGROWING TOENAIL

An ingrowing toenail is a spike of toenail growing into the nail-fold, causing pain and often infection.

Management

Conservative management. Show the patient how to elevate the nail edge. Recommend that this is done after a long soak in a warm bath. A nail file or other blunt instrument can be used. A pledget of cotton wool can be pushed under the elevated nail. This should be done daily for a week or so.

If the nail-fold looks infected, prescribe an antibiotic, e.g. oral flucloxacillin, for 5 days.

Surgical management

- Nail edge excision can be performed in general practice if the GP is confident in the technique. Otherwise, refer to a surgical podiatrist or orthopaedic outpatients.
- Consider Zadik's procedure (bilateral wedge excision) for recurrent cases.

Prevention

Encourage square nail-cutting, i.e. advise the patient to avoid trying to cut the nail with a curve at the edges. This allows the edges to grow free of the end of the toe without digging in.

HAEMATOLOGY

Anaemia   258
Haemoglobinopathies   260
Splenectomy   260

ANAEMIA

Patients with anaemia are diagnosed because they look anaemic, have the symptoms of anaemia or are found incidentally to be anaemic.

Diagnosis

History. Ask about:

- Bleeding: heavy periods are a common cause of iron-deficiency anaemia. Rectal bleeding is the other common cause.
- Diet: the elderly often take a diet low in iron. Vegetarians are also at risk.
- A past history of iron-deficiency anaemia, which raises the chance of another episode of the same.
- Symptoms of anaemia: tiredness, breathlessness, exhaustion and palpitations can all be caused by anaemia. Angina can be unmasked or exacerbated by becoming anaemic.
- Symptoms occasionally accompanying anaemias: bruising and infections suggest aplastic anaemia. Paraesthesia of the feet can occur in pernicious anaemia. Chronic disease can cause anaemia, e.g. renal failure, inflammatory bowel disease and rheumatoid arthritis. Cancer often causes anaemia.

Examination. In general practice there is usually little to add by examining the asymptomatic patient other than to look at the conjunctivae for pallor. The yellowish appearance of the face in pernicious anaemia is characteristic.

Investigations

- Full blood count: the first test is the FBC and film. This alone is sufficient to confirm the presence of anaemia, which is characterised by a Hb less than:
  - 12.5 g/dl for men
  - 11.5 g/dl for women.
- Iron-deficiency anaemia is characterised by a low mean cell volume (<76 fl) and a low mean cell Hb concentration (<30 g/dl), and should be confirmed by checking for a low serum iron (<15 μmol/l in men; 14 μmol/l in women).
- Transferrin: a high transferrin (>400 mg/dl) supports the diagnosis of iron-deficiency anaemia. A low transferrin (<200 mg/dl) suggests the anaemia of chronic disease.

Tip
Where there is no obvious cause for the anaemia (e.g. heavy periods), the patient should be referred, if appropriate, for investigation of the gastrointestinal tract. Occult malignancy occasionally comes to light after presenting with anaemia.

Management

Iron-deficiency anaemia

Mild anaemia (Hb >7 g/dl) can be treated with ferrous sulphate tablets 200 mg daily, rechecking the full blood count after 1 month. Attention should be given to the underlying cause, i.e. dietary advice or treatment of menorrhagia.

Some patients cannot tolerate ferrous sulphate tablets due to gastrointestinal side-effects. Try ferrous fumarate in these cases. If oral iron fails to correct the anaemia, or if tablets cannot be tolerated, use iron for injection. (See *Data Sheet Compendium*, published by Datapharm, at www.emc.medicines.org.uk/.)

> **Tip**
> Patients with severe anaemia (Hb <7 g/dl) who are symptomatic should be considered for blood transfusion in hospital.

Anaemia of chronic disease

Many chronic diseases are accompanied by a mild anaemia with an Hb of around 10 g/dl. These patients are usually asymptomatic from the anaemia and require no treatment as such. In fact, their anaemia is often refractory to treatment.

Macrocytic anaemia

Treatment is of the underlying cause, as identified above.

> **Macrocytosis**
>
> If there is a macrocytosis on the FBC (mean cell volume >96 fl) this can be due to:
>
> - Vitamin B_{12} or folate deficiency. (Check blood levels.)
> - Hypothyroidism. (Check TSH.)
> - Alcoholism. (Take alcohol history or check γ-GT.)
> - Pregnancy.
> - Rarely:
>   - malignancy (check ESR)
>   - radiotherapy
>   - liver disease (check LFTs).

Vitamin B_{12} deficiency is usually due to pernicious anaemia, malabsorption of B_{12} from the gut (due to e.g. inflammatory bowel disease) or dietary deficiency. Check with a blood test for the presence of intrinsic factor antibodies. A positive result is strongly suggestive of pernicious anaemia.

Treat with intramuscular hydroxocobalamin 1 mg every 3 days for 2 weeks, then once every 3 months for life. Check an FBC after 1 month to make sure the macrocytosis has gone and to exclude iron-deficiency anaemia, which may complicate B_{12} treatment.

Folate deficiency is usually caused by malabsorption due to bowel disease, but rarely it is caused by dietary deficiency. Treatment is with oral folic acid 5 mg daily. Vitamin B_{12} deficiency should be excluded prior to commencing treatment with folic acid, as peripheral neuropathy in B_{12} deficiency can be precipitated by the administration of folate.

Anaemia of pregnancy. See p. 30.

Other causes of anaemia. Other anaemias should be investigated and treated by referral to the haematology outpatient department.

HAEMOGLOBINOPATHIES

Screening. In general practice, patients with anaemia should be screened for thalassaemia and sickle cell traits if they are from Mediterranean, South-East Asian or Afro-Caribbean races.

Investigations. Blood should be sent for haemoglobin electrophoresis. Most results are normal, but mild abnormalities commonly demonstrate thalassaemia or sickle cell traits. These usually cause no more than a mild, asymptomatic anaemia and a slightly reduced mean cell volume and mean cell haemoglobin.

Counselling. Consider referral for genetic testing and counselling if the patient is contemplating starting a family. Refer to a department of clinical genetics.

Sickle cell disease
Homozygous sufferers should have specialist involvement from a haematology outpatient department.

Be alert for a sickle crisis:

- sepsis
- painful swelling of the hands and feet
- rapid enlargement of the spleen
- acute fall in haemoglobin.

If suspected, admit the patient.

SPLENECTOMY

Patients without a functioning spleen have a 12-fold increased risk of infection from *Pneumococcus, Haemophilus influenzae, Neisseria meningitidis* and malaria compared with people with a normal spleen.

Immunisation

Four vaccines should be given at the time of splenectomy or as soon as possible after surgery:

- pneumococcal vaccine (reimmunise every 5–10 years)
- Hib vaccine (single dose)
- meningococcal group C vaccine (single dose)
- influenza vaccine (reimmunise annually).

Antibiotics

To help prevent pneumococcal infection in asplenic patients, give penicillin V 500 mg od. Continue to the age of 16 years in children. For adults, some authorities recommend treatment for 2 years postsplenectomy (period of greatest risk); others advise lifelong prophylaxis.

Have a low threshold for prescribing antibiotics for infections. (Prescribe 'standby' amoxicillin to start at once if necessary.)

Malaria

Explain the importance of taking antimalarials in view of the increased risk (see p. 194).

CHAPTER 17

SURGERY

Paediatric problems 264

Breast lumps 265

Gallstones 266

Herniae in the groin 267

Scrotal swellings 268

Testicular pain 268

Anal fissure 268

Haemorrhoids 268

Prostatism 270

Varicose veins and ulceration 270

Appendicitis 270

Periods of incapacity after surgery 271

PAEDIATRIC PROBLEMS

HERNIA AND HYDROCELE

These usually present in the first year of life as a swelling in the groin. They may present after an episode of crying or coughing.

 An obstructed hernia is tender and it is impossible to palpate above it, unlike other causes of a groin swelling:

- hydrocele
- incompletely descended testicle
- inguinal lymphadenopathy
- groin abscess.

Referral to a paediatric surgeon is indicated. Admit to hospital any patient with a suspected obstructed hernia.

UNDESCENDED TESTES

Incompletely descended testes are seen in 0.5–0.7% of boys at 1 year of age.

Referral to a paediatric surgeon is indicated after age 1 at the first presentation, regardless of degree of maldescent.

PHIMOSIS

The foreskin is usually non-retractile until the age of 5 years. A tight meatus and spraying urinary stream may suggest the need for circumcision.

Recurrent balanitis is best treated with improved hygiene and intermittent oral antibiotics. Circumcision is indicated for persistent cases.

UMBILICAL GRANULOMA

Pyogenic granuloma of the umbilical remnant is a common problem at the 6–8-week check.

The application of silver nitrate, or alternatively ligation, are effective, simple measures.

UMBILICAL HERNIAE

The true umbilical hernia, or protruding umbilicus, usually resolves spontaneously and surgical referral should only be considered if it persists over the age of 2 years. Strangulation is very rare in these cases.

Supraumbilical and epigastric herniae should be referred, as trapping of bowel or omentum is more common.

INTUSSUSCEPTION

Intussusception is most common under the age of 2 years and presents as severe colic, vomiting and pallor, often with blood in the stool.

Admission to hospital is clearly indicated.

LEG PROBLEMS

Some normal conditions cause parental anxiety. These include: bow legs, flat feet, knock knees, in- and out-toeing and walking on tiptoes. As long as there is no pain or limp, and the examination reveals a full range of pain-free movement, the parents should be reassured that all is well.

LIMP

A persistent limp is usually pathological and referral to an orthopaedic surgeon is indicated. The acute onset of a limp with pain in the hip requires an urgent orthopaedic opinion to exclude septic arthritis and slipped femoral epiphysis.

BREAST LUMPS

All breast lumps cause anxiety in the patient until a firm diagnosis is made.

Management

> **Tip**
> Refer patients with breast lumps to a surgeon with an interest in treating breast cancer.

Examination of the patient may reveal a softish lump that is neither fixed nor tethered to muscle or skin. The patient can then be reassured that there are no obvious features to suggest malignancy, prior to referral.

Aspiration. If the lump feels soft or cystic it is worth attempting to aspirate it. This is easy.

- Fix the lump between finger and thumb of the left hand, having cleaned the skin with an alcohol wipe.
- Pierce the lump with a green needle on a 10-ml syringe and withdraw the plunger.

- If the breast lump contains fluid, the syringe will start to fill. When no more fluid can be aspirated, remove the needle. Send the aspirate for cytology.
- Referral is unnecessary if the lump disappears completely, the aspirate is not blood-stained and cytology reveals no malignant cells.

LUMPY BREASTS

Anxiety about cancer in a woman with lumpy or large breasts poses a difficult problem. If normal on clinical examination, mammography may be useful.

PAINFUL BREASTS

Cyclical mastalgia in the absence of lumps can be treated by:

- reassurance that there are no lumps
- evening primrose oil, 2–3 capsules tds (only available OTC)
- furosemide 40 mg daily for premenstrual fluid retention.

GALLSTONES

The symptoms of gallstones are often confused with gastric problems. Most gallstones are asymptomatic.

Diagnosis

History. Ask about:

- right hypochondrial pain
- anorexia
- nausea
- fat intolerance
- jaundice
- pale stools and dark urine.

Examination. Look for:

- tenderness in the right hypochondrium, which is worse on deep inspiration
- jaundice.

Investigations

- Upper abdominal ultrasound usually shows gallstones if present.
- Request LFTs if the patient is jaundiced, to determine whether obstruction of the common bile duct has occurred.

Differential diagnosis

- Upper abdominal pain: gastric causes, e.g. gastritis, duodenal ulcer, reflux.
- Severe pain with constitutional upset: e.g. acute pancreatitis, perforation.
- Obstructive jaundice: e.g. tumour.

Management

Acute

- Pain relief, e.g. diclofenac 75 mg im, followed by e.g. co-codamol, 1–2 tablets 4–6-hourly (max = 8 tabs/24 hours).
- Advise a low-fat diet.
- Arrange an ultrasound routinely.

> In the severe attack with constitutional upset (vomiting, pyrexia, tachycardia), acute admission to hospital is necessary.

- If jaundice is present, with obstructive LFT changes, discuss with the on-call surgeon regarding admission for urgent ERCP.

Chronic. In patients with recurrent attacks of acute pain and with ultrasound evidence of stones, referral for surgery is indicated.

HERNIAE IN THE GROIN

Inguinal herniae are usually found by the patient as a painless swelling in the groin. Occasionally they present in the early stages as groin pain. Femoral herniae tend to be more painful.

Diagnosis

Examination

- Examine the patient standing up.
- Look for a swelling with a cough impulse.
- Is the swelling reducible?
- Can it be controlled by pressure on the internal inguinal ring (above and lateral to the pubic tubercle)? If so, it is an indirect inguinal hernia.
- A femoral hernia is above and medial to the pubic tubercle. In practice this makes it feel as though it is sitting on the pubic bone.
- If a swelling in the groin is due to a hydrocele, it is usually possible to palpate above the swelling.

Management

Referral. Femoral herniae need referring for elective surgery.

◢ Femoral and indirect inguinal herniae can strangulate, causing abdominal pain, abdominal swelling, vomiting and absolute constipation (obstruction). Give iv pain relief and admit the patient directly to hospital.

Conservative management. If the hernia is an easily reducible inguinal hernia, some relief can be obtained by the provision of a truss (prescribable on the NHS). Surgery may not be necessary. Encourage the patient to avoid straining and to lose weight if appropriate.

SCROTAL SWELLINGS

See p. 77.

TESTICULAR PAIN

See p. 78.

ANAL FISSURE

Diagnosis

History and examination. The patient experiences sharp anal pain on defaecation. An anal fissure can mimic some of the symptoms of piles, but appears as a sore-looking crack in the skin at the anal margin. If present, an anal fissure often makes digital rectal examination extremely painful.

Management

- The patient should avoid constipation with a high-fibre diet ± a bulking laxative.
- Stool-softeners often allow the fissure to heal.
- Steroid/local anaesthetic suppositories, e.g. Scheriproct, inserted before passing a stool, will allow the bowels to be opened less painfully.
- Glyceryl trinitrate ointment applied to the anal margins helps relieve sphincter muscle spasm pain.
- The anal fissure that is severe, or will not heal with suppositories and laxatives, may require surgical referral for an anal stretch or partial internal sphincterotomy.

HAEMORRHOIDS

Piles, or haemorrhoids, are one of the commonest causes of rectal bleeding.

Diagnosis

History. Ask about:

- The nature of the rectal bleeding. With haemorrhoids this is usually bright red, painless and often drips into the toilet pan or is seen on the toilet paper. It is not mixed with the stool, but more often streaked on the surface of the stool.
- Anal irritation.
- Prolapsed or external piles, which can be felt by the patient as lumps outside the anus. These may be confused with anal skin tags.

Examination. Look for:

- External piles and skin tags, which are obvious on inspection of the anal margin. Thrombosed piles are acutely tender, hard, purple lumps.
- Internal piles, which can be seen on passing a proctoscope, and look like small purple bulges about 4 cm (1.5 in.) inside the anal margin.
- A mass higher up in the rectum, by performing a digital rectal examination.
- An abdominal mass, by palpating the abdomen.

Investigations. Investigations are unnecessary for piles.

> Caution is needed in attributing new rectal bleeding to piles in patients aged over 40. Consider referral for colonoscopy in all cases, as large bowel cancer and piles are both common and can coexist.

Management

- Advise the patient to avoid constipation, straining at stool and sitting for too long.
- A laxative and/or a bulking agent, e.g. ispaghula husk granules, often help to prevent the piles worsening.
- Steroid/local anaesthetic ointment or suppositories are useful for anal irritation or soreness, and also for healing an anal fissure.
- Injection of piles with oily phenol is easy and will symptomatically cure about 50% of cases. This can be done in general practice or by referral to surgical outpatients.
- Consider referral for haemorrhoidectomy for third-degree piles, painful piles, heavy bleeding or failure of phenol injection.

PROSTATISM

See p. 70.

VARICOSE VEINS AND ULCERATION

Varicose veins and ulcers are ubiquitous problems in general practice.

VARICOSE VEINS

Diagnosis

History. Ask about:

- pain and aching
- appearance
- phlebitis
- ulceration.

Examination. Look for signs of ulceration, varicose eczema, bleeding and thrombophlebitis.

Management

- Advise elevation of the legs, when possible.
- Advise weight loss if appropriate.
- Advise support stockings, e.g. class one or two thigh-length graduated stockings (available on prescription).
- Referral for ligation and multiple avulsion should be considered if the patient is considerably troubled or handicapped by the complications of varicose veins. Patients requesting 'cosmetic' varicose vein surgery should be referred privately.

VARICOSE ULCERATION

See p. 143.

APPENDICITIS

Appendicitis presents about two or three times a year to the GP with the average list of 2000 patients. Pain in the right iliac fossa due to other causes is far more frequent.

Diagnosis

History. Pain in the abdomen is often the first symptom. It is usually in the right iliac fossa, having moved there from the centre of the abdomen over the preceding 24 hours. In the early stages this is often the only symptom and can be quite severe before the other symptoms (e.g. vomiting, fever) arise.

A concomitant URTI with abdominal pain suggests mesenteric adenitis in a child.

> **Tip**
> Diarrhoea is unusual in appendicitis, and suggests gastroenteritis.

Examination. Patients with appendicitis requiring hospital treatment will be mildly pyrexial and tender in the right iliac fossa, with guarding and rebound tenderness and quiet bowel sounds. They will also usually have a tachycardia, halitosis and dry lips.

The milder case may only have slight tenderness in the abdomen and no other symptoms.

Rectal examination confirms tenderness high on the right.

Management

Admit as a surgical emergency with a view to appendicectomy. If there is doubt in the GP's mind as to the severity of the case, it should be discussed with the surgical registrar.

In mild cases it is acceptable to treat in general practice. If appendicitis is suspected but the patient is not unwell, it is reasonable to treat with metronidazole and a cephalosporin in conjunction with some mild analgesia. It is important to review the patient for signs of worsening over 24–48 hours.

Grumbling appendix. Repeated attacks of appendicitis that settle down with conservative measures are due to a 'grumbling appendix'. Referral to surgical outpatients is advised for consideration for an interval appendicectomy, i.e. between the attacks.

PERIODS OF INCAPACITY AFTER SURGERY

Times off work following surgery vary depending on surgical complications, patient health and fitness, and occupation, but as a rule of thumb the following advice can be given to patients:

- Vasectomy: 2 days.
- Cholecystectomy: 2 weeks.

- Hernia repair: 2 weeks.
- Hysterectomy: 6 weeks.
- Caesarean section: 6 weeks.
- Coronary bypass: 2 months.
- Hip replacement: 2 months.

NEUROLOGY

Dizziness   274

Headache   275

Facial pain   277

Bell's palsy   279

Cerebrovascular accident
(CVA)   280

Transient ischaemic attack
(TIA)   281

Tremor   282

Parkinson's disease   283

Falls   284

Epilepsy   285

Multiple sclerosis   288

Head injury   290

Many different sensations are described as dizziness. These include light-headedness, muzziness and faintness. First decide whether the patient is experiencing true vertigo, which is a subjective sensation of rotation, either of the patient or the surroundings. It is often accompanied by nausea, and nystagmus is a common finding.

Causes of true vertigo

- Common: labyrinthitis, benign positional vertigo.
- Rare:
  - brainstem stroke/TIA
  - vertebrobasilar insufficiency
  - Ménière's disease
  - acoustic neuroma
  - multiple sclerosis.

Causes of other types of dizziness

- Infections, e.g. flu-like illnesses and URTIs
- anxiety and depression (see pp. 294 and 292)
- syncope (see p. 163).

LABYRINTHITIS

Diagnosis

Labyrinthitis is the commonest cause of true vertigo in general practice.
Apart from nausea and vomiting and possible nystagmus, there are no other symptoms or signs. Features such as hearing loss or tinnitus suggest Ménière's disease or acoustic neuroma. Focal neurological signs suggest an intracerebral pathology.

Management

- Reassure the patient that the condition is not due to a tumour, is common and that it resolves completely.
- Explain that the symptoms will be severe for 2–3 days and tend to resolve within 2–3 weeks. Labyrinthitis is probably due to inflammation of the inner ear and it is often recurrent.
- If symptomatic treatment is required, prescribe prochlorperazine 5 mg po tds or give 12.5 mg im if the patient is vomiting.
- Advise patients not to drive until symptoms are adequately controlled. Group 2 license holders are banned from driving for at least a year after symptoms have been controlled if they have suffered uncontrolled, disabling giddiness.

> **Tip**
> Referral to a neurologist or ENT consultant is indicated if the diagnosis is in doubt, if other features suggest an alternative diagnosis or if symptoms do not settle within 6 weeks.

HEADACHE

Ninety per cent of headaches are tension headaches; 10 % of the population have migraines. It is estimated that 0.004% of headaches are due to serious pathology.

Diagnosis

Causes of headache

- Common:
  - tension headache
  - associated with URTI
  - migraine
  - depression.
- Rare:
  - tumour
  - subarachnoid haemorrhage
  - subdural haemorrhage
  - meningitis
  - giant cell arteritis.

> **Tip**
> Often the cause of a headache cannot be neatly classified. As long as there are no features of serious disease (see below), reassurance and a 'wait and see' approach are reasonable.

Indicators of more serious disease in headache

- Sudden onset.
- New, severe headache.
- Progressively worsening headache.
- Onset of headaches after the age of 50.
- Altered level of consciousness.
- Recent head injury.
- Abnormal physical findings, especially focal neurology.
- Meningism.
- Tender temporal arteries.

Examination

- BP
- fundi
- neck muscles
- cervical spine movements
- temporal arteries.

Management

Referral. Indications for referral are:

- any of the above serious features
- failure to improve with adequate treatment
- uncertain diagnosis if the headaches are disabling
- patient's insistence.

TENSION HEADACHE

The features of tension headaches are:

- chronic, frequent and recurrent
- moderately severe
- generalised
- described as a tight band of pressure
- absence of nausea generally
- scalp tenderness in places.

Examination is otherwise normal.

Management

Reassurance, relaxation and analgesics are often all that are necessary (see anxiety, p. 294).

MIGRAINE

Migraine affects 10 % of the population. It can cause significant disability.

Features of migraines

- Headache is usually unilateral, aching, pulsating and worse on activity.
- Possible occurrence of nausea, vomiting, photophobia and phonophobia.
- Last from 4 to 72 hours and are recurrent.
- Visual disturbance in 20%.

Examination should be normal.

Management

- Discuss trigger factors: dietary factors, e.g. missed meals, caffeine, chocolate, cheese, alcohol; tiredness and stress; unaccustomed exercise; hormonal factors, e.g. menstrual periods, contraceptive pill, menopause; environmental factors, e.g. noise and temperature variations, wind, bright or flickering lights, strong smells.
- Analgesics are the first line of treatment, e.g. paracetamol, codeine, dihydrocodeine and NSAIDs.
- Antiemetics are also often required, e.g. metoclopramide.
- Combinations of analgesics and antiemetics are available, e.g. Migraleve.
- For severe attacks consider a 5-HT agonist, e.g. sumatriptan 50–100 mg po or 20 mg (one spray) intranasally.

Prophylaxis

For the patient experiencing frequent repeat attacks, say ⩾2 attacks per month, consider the need for prophylaxis, e.g. propranolol 40 mg bd or tds or pizotifen 1.5–3 mg nocte or a tricyclic antidepressant (even when the patient is not obviously depressed).

FACIAL PAIN

The common causes of facial pain in general practice are:

- sinusitis
- temporomandibular joint dysfunction
- ear infections
- trigeminal neuralgia
- dental infection or impaction
- submandibular lymphadenopathy
- mumps
- migraine.

A rare, but important, cause of facial pain is temporal arteritis.

Tip

Often the cause of a patient's facial pain cannot be neatly categorised. Patients with depression can present with a facial pain that is probably psychosomatic (see p. 297).

TEMPOROMANDIBULAR JOINT DYSFUNCTION

Diagnosis

The patient complains of pain in front of the ear, exacerbated by eating and often accompanied by clicking.

Management

- Reassurance that the condition is benign and temporary is often all that is required.
- Advising patients to alter their bite by chewing on the other side of the mouth is useful.
- Advise patients to avoid very chewy food, e.g. hard crusts.
- NSAIDs are sometimes required for more painful episodes.
- Severe cases, involving locking of the jaw, may need referral to a dentist or faciomaxillary surgeon.

TRIGEMINAL NEURALGIA

Diagnosis

The patient complains of severe, stabbing or burning pain in the distribution of one or more of the three branches of the trigeminal nerve (V). It is unilateral and made worse even on lightly touching the skin or on exposure to cold wind.

Management

- Simple analgesics are often all that is required, as most cases get better within a few weeks.
- Carbamazepine 100 mg od, increased to 400 mg tds according to response, taken during the acute stages.
- Treatment of depression, if present, may be indicated (see p. 292).
- Referral to a neurologist may be indicated if the above measures fail. Some patients benefit from injection or surgical resection of the affected trigeminal nerve branch.

OTHER CAUSES

Sinusitis
See p. 217.

Earache
See p. 212.

Dental infection or impaction
Refer to the patient's dentist.

Cervical lymphadenopathy
See p. 219.

Mumps
See p. 206.

Migraine
See p. 276.

Giant cell arteritis
See p. 242.

BELL'S PALSY

Bell's palsy is the idiopathic palsy of the facial nerve (VII) resulting in a unilateral facial weakness or paralysis. It may be preceded by pain behind the ear, but usually presents as a painless facial paralysis.

Diagnosis

Examination

- The whole of one side of the face is affected and the patient has unilateral difficulty raising the eyebrows, showing the teeth and puffing out the cheeks.
- Exclude geniculate herpes (Ramsay Hunt syndrome) by looking for vesicles in the ear and mouth.
- Make sure that the patient can close the eye on the affected side, to avoid corneal abrasion (see below).
- Examination of the other cranial nerves should be normal.

> A CVA involving the upper motor neurone of the seventh cranial nerve can give a similar facial weakness. In this case, however, the patient should still be able to raise the eyebrow normally on the affected side. This is not possible in Bell's palsy.

Management

- Sixty-five per cent of cases recover completely within a few weeks, with or without treatment. Others take longer.
- Prednisolone 40 mg daily for 1 week, reducing to zero over a further 3 weeks, may speed the recovery.
- For patients unable to close the affected eye, prescribe an artificial tear solution, such as hypromellose eyedrops, and advise that they tape the eyelid down at night. This helps to prevent corneal scarring.

Tip
Partial improvement by day 10 and a young age at onset are good prognostic indicators.

- Consider referral to a neurologist if the diagnosis is in doubt.
- For patients with residual paresis, contractures or facial asymmetry, the opinion of a plastic surgeon should be offered.

CEREBROVASCULAR ACCIDENT (CVA)

Among a GP's average list of 2000 patients there will be 3–4 strokes per year and about one transient ischaemic attack (TIA). The majority are either thromboembolic (70%) or haemorrhagic (20%).

> **Tip**
> An acute stroke is defined as a rapid onset of clinically evident focal cerebral deficit lasting more than 24 hours, with no obvious cause.

Diagnosis

Examination

- Neurological examination, as appropriate.
- Check for cardiac arrhythmias (e.g. atrial fibrillation), heart murmurs and carotid bruits.
- BP.

Investigations

- Bloods for FBC, ESR, C&Es, glucose and cholesterol/lipids.
- CXR.
- ECG.

Management

Referral. In general, all patients with acute strokes should be admitted to hospital urgently. Early CT/MRI scanning, thrombolysis or anticoagulation and antiplatelet therapy can all help prevent further attacks.

However, patients whose quality of life is poor, such as some severely disabled nursing-home residents, may not need admitting if they stand to gain little or nothing from this action.

Prescribing. For non-haemorrhagic stroke start the patient on aspirin 75 mg od, consider e.g. an ACE inhibitor such as ramipril 2.5 mg increasing to 10 mg a day, and a statin (see p. 150). In addition to aspirin for antiplatelet activity, prescribe dipyridamole m/r 200 mg bd for the 2 years following each ischaemic event. If the patient is allergic to aspirin, prescribe clopidogrel 75 mg od instead.

Management of the patient with disability

- Check that Social Services support is adequate.
- Be alert for signs of depression (see p. 292) and carer stress.

- Check that Attendance Allowance is being claimed, that the Driver and Vehicle Licensing Agency has been informed and that a disabled parking permit has been applied for, if appropriate.
- Refer the patient for speech therapy, if needed.
- Rehabilitation may also be necessary, e.g. physiotherapy and occupational therapy. Consider domiciliary services.

Secondary prevention of stroke

Check:

- lifestyle factors (see p. 146)
- BP (see p. 147)
- smoking status (see p. 313)
- cholesterol (see p. 150)
- blood glucose (see p. 106).

Prognosis. There is a 10% annual risk of a serious vascular event after a stroke, e.g. a further stroke, MI or death. This risk is reduced by 25% with the use of aspirin.

> **Tip**
> Be encouraging and optimistic with stroke patients about their functional recovery, which can be slow. Little improvement at 6 weeks, however, carries a poor prognosis, with permanent disability likely.

Patients can resume driving after at least 1 month following a stroke if recovery is satisfactory. Patients should inform the Driver and Vehicle Licensing Agency after this time if there is anything more than minor limb dysfunction.

Administration

Quality and Outcomes Framework for Stroke/TIA

- Record the smoking status annually and offer cessation advice to smokers.
- Achieve a blood pressure of 150/90 or below.
- Achieve a cholesterol of 5 mmol/l or below.
- Prescribe aspirin or an alternative antiplatelet drug.
- Give an annual flu jab.

TRANSIENT ISCHAEMIC ATTACK (TIA)

- Full recovery of all the neurological signs should occur within 24 hours.
- Examine the patient for signs of cardiac arrhythmias (see p. 165), heart murmurs and carotid bruits.

- Check BP.
- Blood for FBC, ESR, C&Es, glucose and lipids.
- ECG.
- Prescribing – As for CVA (see p. 280).

 Patients with suspected TIAs should be referred urgently to the local stroke clinic for brain imaging, carotid Doppler or angiography and cardiac echo.

Administration

Quality and Outcomes Framework for TIA

As for stroke (CVA), above.

TREMOR

Benign essential tremor is very common in general practice. Other common causes of tremor in general practice are Parkinson's syndrome, anxiety and thyrotoxicosis. Rare causes include the cerebellar disorders.

Categories of tremor

There are essentially three:

- positional tremors, e.g. essential, anxiety and thyrotoxicosis tremors
- the resting tremor of Parkinson's syndrome
- the intention tremor of cerebellar disorders.

POSITIONAL TREMOR

An essential tremor is a fine, rapid tremor, especially of the hands, exacerbated by holding the arms outstretched. No other features of Parkinson's syndrome should be present (see p. 283).

> **Tip**
> Pathological causes of this type of tremor are extremely rare but can be excluded by taking a history and checking blood tests for:
>
> - alcohol excess
> - thyrotoxicosis
> - drugs, e.g. salbutamol
> - carbon monoxide poisoning.

Management

The main drug used in the treatment of benign essential tremor is propranolol 40 mg bd, increasing at weekly intervals, according to the response, up to 80–160 mg daily.

Referral to a neurologist is unlikely to be necessary, but should be considered if the symptoms are worsening despite adequate doses of a beta-blocker.

RESTING TREMOR

See Parkinson's syndrome, below.

INTENTION TREMOR

Refer all cases of intention tremor, in order to exclude a cerebellar tumour. Other features may include:

- nystagmus
- ataxia
- past-pointing
- falls.

PARKINSON'S DISEASE

One per cent of people over 60 years of age have Parkinson's disease.

Diagnosis

History. Ask about:

- shaking
- falls
- stiffness
- slowness
- decreased handwriting size
- drug history.

Examination. Look for the triad of:

- tremor
- rigidity
- bradykinesia.

Common features are:

- a resting, pill-rolling tremor
- reduced arm swinging when walking, with festinant (hesitating) gait
- decreased facial expression
- cog-wheel rigidity
- small handwriting.

> **Tip**
> In the early stages of Parkinson's disease the diagnosis can be difficult to make.

Management

- If possible, stop any drugs which may be causing Parkinsonism, e.g. phenothiazines and butyrophenones
- If Parkinson's disease is suspected, referral to a neurologist with an interest in the condition should be made as soon as possible. L-dopa with a dopa decarboxylase inhibitor, e.g. Madopar, is the main drug in the treatment of Parkinson's disease. It is best in patients with marked bradykinesia.
- General support can be usefully provided in general practice. Consider physiotherapy, speech therapy and occupational therapy, Social Services, Attendance Allowance and day hospital. Emotional support and carer support are also important.
- Look out for depression (see p. 292) and dementia (see p. 303), both of which are more common in Parkinson's disease.
- Alterations to specialist-initiated drug treatments should be by liaison with specialist services.

FALLS

Falls are common in the elderly and have a multitude of possible causes:

- Visual: cataract, macular degeneration, refractive error.
- Environmental: loose carpet, steps.
- Musculoskeletal: parkinsonism, arthritis.
- Drugs: postural hypotension.
- Cardiac: arrhythmia, heart block.

- Neurological: TIA, epilepsy.
- Circulatory: vertebrobasilar insufficiency.

Diagnosis

History. Ask patients to describe what happens during a fall:

- Do they remember falling?
- Do they get any warning that they are going to fall?
- Are there any associated symptoms, e.g. palpitations?
- Take a drug history.

Examination

- BP sitting and standing, to look for a postural drop.
- Observe the gait.
- Check for cardiac arrhythmias and heart murmurs.
- Look for any gross neurological signs.

Investigations. ECG, if heart block or other cardiac causes are suspected.

Management
If the cause can be categorised, refer to the specific page, as necessary, for:

- decreased vision (p. 233)
- osteoarthritis (p. 241)
- Parkinson's syndrome (p. 283)
- loss of consciousness (p. 163)
- dizziness (p. 274)
- epilepsy (see below).

Tip
Often the cause cannot immediately be found. Advise the patient to use a stick or frame if appropriate. Physiotherapy or day hospital referral may be helpful. Referral to a falls clinic or a physician with an interest in the elderly may be indicated in frequent, undiagnosed falls.

Consider the need for osteoporosis prevention (see p. 243).

EPILEPSY

The GP with the average list of 2000 patients might expect to have about eight patients with epilepsy.

Diagnosis

History

- Suspect epilepsy after a seizure, i.e. uncontrolled nervous activity, with or without a convulsion or loss of consciousness.
- Take a careful history, from witnesses if possible. Particular reference should be made to rigidity, shaking, loss of consciousness, incontinence, tongue-biting and postictal drowsiness.
- Focal seizures and absence attacks are also included in the diagnosis.

Differential diagnosis

- Syncope: preceding faintness, pallor, sweating, rapid and full recovery (see p. 163).
- TIA: dysphasia, paresis or other temporary loss of function (see p. 281).
- Others: psychogenic, tic, panic attack, migraine

Management

Initial management

> **Tip**
> All patients suspected of having epilepsy should be referred after a single seizure.

Refer to a neurologist with an interest in epilepsy, if possible, and suggest that the patient is accompanied by a witness to the attacks.

Management during a fit

- Ensure the airway is clear and that the patient is breathing.
- Check the pulse at the carotid.
- Put the patient in the left lateral position.
- Administer rectal diazepam, 10 mg (5 mg in children).

Admit the patient to hospital if:

- this is the first fit
- the cause is not yet known
- the fit is prolonged
- there are poor social circumstances
- the patient has a head injury
- there are any residual problems, e.g. paresis.

Counselling after a diagnosis of epilepsy has been made

Safety. Advise the patient to avoid heights, e.g. ladders, and to swim only under supervision in shallow water.

Driving. Epileptics are banned from driving on an ordinary licence for 1 year after their last fit. A licence is granted if the convulsions have been solely nocturnal for at least 3 years. There is a total ban on vocational licences. After the first suspected fit, advise the patient not to drive until seen by a neurologist.

First aid and seizure control. Give advice to relatives about first aid during a seizure and prescribe rectal diazepam 10 mg to be used in the event of further fits.

Medic Alert bracelet. This is advisable for all epileptics.

Anticonvulsant drug interactions. Check whether the patient is taking any drugs that may interfere with anticonvulsants, especially the contraceptive pill. The effectiveness of both combined oral contraceptives and progestogen-only pills is reduced by carbamazepine, phenytoin, phenobarbital and primidone. Use 50 μg oestrogen pills or an alternative method (see p. 6).

Drug side-effects

- Carbamazepine: drowsiness, dizziness, headache, gastrointestinal upset.
- Phenytoin: acne, hirsutism, gum hyperplasia.
- Sodium valproate: weight gain, hair loss, nausea, ataxia, tremor.

Preconception counselling. Advise female patients that they will need to be referred to their neurologist if they are contemplating getting pregnant.

Breast-feeding. All anticonvulsants, except barbiturates, can be prescribed to breast-feeding mothers.

Prescription charge exemption. Patients with epilepsy are exempt from prescription charges.

Avoidance of triggers. Alcohol, tiredness and flashing lights are the common triggers for seizures in susceptible patients.

Disease monitoring

- If fits are still occurring, increase the dose of the first-line anticonvulsant until the fits are controlled without unwanted side-effects.
- Aim for therapeutic drug levels with:
  - carbamazepine 20–50 μmol/l
  - phenytoin 40–80 μmol/l.
- If the fits are not controlled with the maximum dose of the first-line drug, refer patients back to their consultant.
- If the fits are controlled, see the patient 12-monthly. Consider:
  - side-effects
  - drug levels, if appropriate (fits, side-effects, change of dose or starting a drug which interacts)
  - counselling, as above.

Administration

Quality and Outcomes Framework for Epilepsy

- Annual review of epilepsy medication.
- Record date of last fit.
- Record fit frequency.

MULTIPLE SCLEROSIS

The average GP's list of 2000 patients will contain one or two patients with multiple sclerosis.

The mean age of onset is 35 years, with a range, commonly, of between 20 and 40 years of age.

Diagnosis

History. There is a wide variety of presenting symptoms in multiple sclerosis. These are due to acute episodes of demyelination, and common examples are:

- optic neuritis: partial or complete loss of vision, with or without pain
- diplopia
- nystagmus
- vertigo
- weakness or paraesthesia in a limb (see dermatomes, p. 353)
- ataxia
- an extensor plantar reflex
- diminished vibration sense
- loss of abdominal reflexes.

The symptoms commonly develop in a matter of hours or days and disappear over weeks.

> **Tip**
> A careful history of past symptoms may reveal a previous episode of possible demyelination, making the diagnosis more likely.

Examination. Examination of the relevant part of the nervous system may reveal objective signs. A full neurological examination would be very time-consuming for a GP, but may demonstrate further signs of demyelination.

> **Tip**
> Physical examination is often normal in the initial stages of multiple
> sclerosis. It is a sad but well-recognised phenomenon that patients with
> their first episode of demyelination are often labelled as hysterical.

Management

All suspected cases should be referred for a neurological opinion.

Prognosis. Fifteen years from presentation, approximately one-third of patients
with multiple sclerosis will be severely disabled, but another third will be
unrestricted by disability.

The average life expectancy is 25 years from presentation.

Long-term care

- Close communication with the patient's neurologist is important, especially if
  the patient relapses or deteriorates.
- Physiotherapy is useful for contractures, immobility and poor posture.
- Occupational therapy helps with the activities of daily living.
- A social worker can help with employment matters, allowances and re-
  housing.
- For the treatment of spasticity, consider physiotherapy. Treatment with
  baclofen or dantrolene may be useful.
- Flexion deformities also may be helped by physiotherapy. Consider an
  orthopaedic referral if the patient is handicapped by deformities.
- Paroxysmal pain can be a problem in neuritis. Consider the use of
  carbamazepine, phenytoin or gabapentin.
- Constipation can be helped by ensuring an adequate fluid intake, bulking
  agents, suppositories or enemas.
- Obesity can be a problem for any patient with prolonged immobility. Consider
  referral to a dietician.
- Urinary problems are common in multiple sclerosis. Antibiotics for urinary
  tract infections may be needed. Try anticholinergics for bladder instability,
  e.g. oxybutynin 5 mg tds. An opinion from a urology specialist may be needed.
  Catheterisation is occasionally required.
- Sexual dysfunction is common in multiple sclerosis. Consider sildenafil, or
  referral for counselling or a urology opinion.
- The Driver and Vehicle Licensing Agency should be informed by the patient.
  A disabled parking permit should be applied for if appropriate.
- Depression is almost inevitable at some point in the life of every patient with
  multiple sclerosis (see p. 292). Stress in the carer is also common and is often
  overlooked.

HEAD INJURY

Patients with mild head injuries present commonly to GPs, often out of hours, and usually, initially, over the telephone. The decisions of whether to visit and whether to refer to A&E depend on the risk of the missed skull fracture.

Features requiring assessment

History

- Motor vehicle accident.
- Fall from a height.
- Striking head on hard surface, e.g. concrete.
- Striking side of head (temple).
- Loss of consciousness.
- Retrograde amnesia.
- Severe headache.
- Drunk.

Examination. Look for:

- altered consciousness level
- focal neurological signs
- bruising/haematoma, including around eyes and ears
- blood/CSF from ears or nose
- drunkenness
- bulging fontanelle
- irritability.

Management

- For analgesia use paracetamol, ibuprofen or codeine phosphate.
- If the patient is not admitted, give standard head injury advice to contact the doctor if the following develop over the next 24 hours:
  - severe headache
  - vomiting
  - drowsiness
  - confusion.
- If any of the above symptoms do develop within 24 hours of a head injury the patient should be seen in an A&E department.
- Head injury in the elderly may present several days or weeks later, with symptoms and signs of a subdural haemorrhage: confusion, falls, loss of balance, memory loss. Arrange urgent admission if suspected.

Head injury under 1 year of age=?Non-accidental injury.
Drunk with head injury=skull fracture until proven otherwise.

PSYCHIATRY

Depression   292

Anxiety   294

Obsessive–compulsive disorder   295

Insomnia   296

Psychosomatic illness   297

Fatigue   298

Suicide   300

Eating disorders   301

Dementia   303

Disturbed behaviour   305

Violence   306

Sectioning   307

Benzodiazepine addiction   308

Opiate addiction   308

Alcohol abuse   310

Smoking   313

DEPRESSION

Depression is the most common psychiatric problem of general practice. There are well over 5000 suicides in the UK each year, three-quarters of them among men.

Diagnosis

History. Ask about:

- low self-esteem
- low mood
- anhedonia
- poor concentration
- thought of suicide
- poor sleep and appetite
- loss of libido
- guilt
- irritability
- weight change.

Examination. Look for:

- tearfulness
- slowed thinking and speech
- indecisiveness
- sighing
- anxiety.

Questionnaires such as PHQ-9 can help assess the severity of depression and are now a requirement of the new GMS contract in the UK.

In children behavioural problems, school refusal and phobias may represent depression, and in the elderly, complaining, confusion and forgetfulness may be signs of depression.

When to suspect depression

Have a high index of suspicion of depression in the following:

- major illness
- chronic illness
- major life event (e.g. bereavement, unemployment, marital breakdown)
- previous mental illness
- alcohol or drug abuse
- frequent attendances
- carers.

Management

- Assess the risk of suicide (see p. 300).
- Explain the diagnosis to the patient:
  - depression is an illness
  - one might liken it to a deficiency state of chemical in the brain
  - the prognosis is excellent.

Non-drug treatment

- Continued GP support (offer follow-up with the same doctor).
- Family and friends, self-help groups.
- Counselling (e.g. with marital problems).
- Psychologist (e.g. for cognitive behavioural therapy).
- Community psychiatric nurse.

Prescribing

- Negotiate the use of drugs with the patient:
  - antidepressants are not addictive
  - they correct the chemical imbalance that is causing the patient's symptoms.
- Prescribe a selective serotonin reuptake inhibitor (SSRI), e.g. fluoxetine 20 mg od or citalopram 20 mg od. SSRIs should be used with caution in children and adolescents. Paediatric prescribing should only be initiated by a specialist child psychiatrist.
  - Warn the patient that the therapeutic benefit will not be felt for the first 10–14 days.
  - Side-effects: common side-effects which usually settle within the first 2 weeks include nausea, nervousness and insomnia.
  - Contraindications: avoid if the patient enters a manic phase.
- If response is poor, consider second-line antidepressants, e.g. venlafaxine, trazodone.
- Duration of treatment with antidepressants: 4 months to 2 years. After the patient is feeling well, continue treatment for 3 or 4 months. Treatment should not be discontinued if the patient is approaching an emotionally challenging time. Abrupt withdrawal of SSRIs should be avoided by reducing the dose to one tablet or capsule on alternate days for 1 month before stopping completely.

Referral. Referral to a psychiatrist is indicated with:

- uncertain diagnosis
- poor response to treatment at adequate doses
- suicide risk (immediate admission, see below)
- psychotic features
- behaviour disturbance, e.g. psychomotor retardation.

Special cases

- Postnatal depression (see p. 33).
- Manic depression: this is recognised by depressive episodes alternating with prolonged periods of euphoria. The latter are characterised by pressured speech, delusions of grandeur and loss of social inhibitions. Refer if the diagnosis is suspected. Admit if the patient is in danger.
- Bereavement (see p. 327).

Administration

> **Quality and Outcomes Framework for Depression**
>
> - Screen for depression annually in all patients with diabetes or coronary heart disease.
> - Assess the severity of new cases of depression using a questionnaire such as PHQ-9.

ANXIETY

True anxiety neurosis interferes with the patient's normal daily activities. Milder forms of anxiety are extremely common, may accompany physical illness and can cause a variety of symptoms.

Diagnosis

History. Patients most likely to suffer from anxiety are those with depression, stress, a major life event, somatisation symptoms, avoidance behaviour and dementia, and those who are frequent attenders.

Anxiety is a common cause of some typical complaints:

- tiredness
- headache
- low back pain
- dizziness
- dysmenorrhoea.

> **Tip**
> Thyrotoxicosis can present with anxiety. It is often accompanied by weight loss, agitation, tachycardia and tremor.

Panic attacks involve the patient in a vicious circle of self-sustaining physical symptoms caused by anxiety.

In phobias the anxiety state is generated by a specific trigger.

Management

- Exclude physical disease at the initial consultation. Thereafter avoid overinvestigating, as this reinforces anxiety rather than relieving it.
- Treat any underlying depression (see p. 292).
- Symptomatic hyperventilation may be relieved by rebreathing expired air via a paper bag.

Non-drug treatment. For chronic anxiety neurosis the treatment is mainly psychotherapeutic:

- Explain the condition to the patient.
- Reassure about the absence of physical disease.
- Explain symptoms in terms of autonomic stimulation.
- Try relaxation techniques: tapes, groups, yoga.
- Encourage regular exercise.
- Offer counselling.
- Self-help leaflets.
- Discuss complementary therapies.
- Offer cognitive behavioural therapy by referral to a psychologist, if available.
- Involve the psychiatric services if the patient's life is affected to any significant degree:
  - psychiatric social worker
  - community psychiatric nurse
  - consultant referral.

Prescribing

- For the acute, short-term relief of severe anxiety, e.g. in panic attacks, use diazepam 2–5 mg tds, as required. The maximum duration of treatment should be 14 days. Alternatively, prescribe propranolol 10–40 mg tds, as required.
- For chronic anxiety consider an SSRI, e.g. citalopram 20 mg od, or a tricyclic, e.g. clomipramine 10–75 mg od.
- For chronic agitation, e.g. in dementia, chlorpromazine 25–50 mg nocte is more appropriate.

OBSESSIVE–COMPULSIVE DISORDER

Obsessive–compulsive disorder (OCD) is a neurobiological condition that causes the patient to feel compelled repeatedly to think, speak or act-out irrational rituals, such as hand washing, touching objects or chanting mantras. The spectrum of severity is wide, with the mildest form almost going unnoticed by the patient and family. The most severe cases are disablingly time-consuming and can provoke extreme anxiety.

> **Tip**
> - OCD affects about 1% of children and adolescents.
> - It tends to run in families.
> - Children often keep their symptoms a secret.

Diagnosis

History. Ask about:

- unwanted thoughts or ideas that keep coming into the mind
- the need to perform rituals
- anxiety at the thought of not completing the rituals
- how long it takes to perform the ritual each time
- how many times a day the ritual has to be repeated
- interference with daily life, schoolwork, sleep
- other mental illness, e.g. brain injury, tics, Tourette syndrome.

Management
In mild cases the patient and family need reassurance that the condition is usually self-limiting.

Referral

- Patients who are upset by the OCD.
- Patients who take more than an hour a day to perform their rituals.
- Patients in whom the rituals interfere with everyday life.

Treatment. The SSRI group of antidepressants are the most useful, e.g. fluoxetine 20–60 mg od. The other effective treatment for OCD is cognitive behavioural therapy. A combination of the two is usually offered by the psychiatrists.

INSOMNIA

Insomnia can be divided into acute and chronic. The chronic variety is more common in the elderly.

Diagnosis

History. Take a careful history and try to decide if the problem is long-term or of recent onset.

The causes of acute insomnia include:

- trauma, physical or psychological
- jet lag
- change of environment, e.g. admission to a nursing home.

The causes of chronic insomnia include:

- day-time sleeping, e.g. in the elderly
- stimulants, e.g. caffeine
- drugs, e.g. SSRIs
- physical symptoms, e.g. pain, cough, nasal obstruction
- anxiety/depression (see pp. 294 and 292).

Explore patients' expectations: are they looking for a cure or short-term relief?

Management

- Explain that insomnia is not a disease.
- Treat the underlying cause, if any (see above).
- Try to avoid prescribing for chronic insomnia.
- Offer self-help leaflet.
- Advise a regular bedtime routine.
- Advise avoidance of stimulants, e.g. caffeine, alcohol.
- Are the patient's expectations unrealistic?
- For short-term treatment requiring rapid relief of symptoms, i.e. no longer than 2 weeks, prescribe, e.g.:
  - temazepam 10–20 mg nocte, or
  - zopiclone 7.5–15 mg nocte.

Addiction to benzodiazepines

Explain the addiction potential of benzodiazepines to the patient and record in the notes that this has been discussed. A number of successful litigation cases against doctors over the prescribing of benzodiazepines have hinged on the fact that the patients were not informed of the addiction potential of these drugs. State the maximum safe duration of treatment (2 weeks) to the patient and explain that drugs are not a long-term cure.

PSYCHOSOMATIC ILLNESS

Patients with psychosomatic illnesses all share the belief that they are physically unwell. The frequent attender, chronic somatiser and heartsink patient may all come under this heading.

Tip
The GP may have negative feelings towards such patients. Recognising this is an important step in coping.

Diagnosis

History. Psychosomatic illnesses may be difficult to distinguish from organic disease initially. The patient with globus hystericus, for example, may present with a straightforward sore throat.

However, a number of suspicious features make the possibility of a psychosomatic illness increasingly likely: multiple, unconnected physical symptoms; 'vague' symptoms such as spasms, churning or pressure; impossible symptoms, such as pain all over; and symptoms that defy treatment, such as wind, bloating and electric shocks.

Examination. Satisfy yourself that the physical symptoms have been adequately explored by examination, investigation and referral, if indicated.

Management

- Gently, but firmly, inform patients that their symptoms, while real, are not due to physical disease. Many patients are difficult to reassure, but an unwavering message is important. The slightest doubt in the doctor's mind is soon picked up by patients and used to reinforce their neurosis.
- Many patients will have emotional, social or family problems. Some may be clinically depressed (see p. 292). Some patients may have a justifiable phobia, e.g. after losing a close friend to cancer. Attempt to explore these areas.
- Encourage the patient to expect less of the doctor's abilities to cure the physical symptoms.
- Encourage the patient to lead a normal life despite the symptoms, rather than be dominated by them.

> **Tip**
> The above process is often spread over many consultations and may be repeated as patients 'relapse'.

Referral. Referral to a specialist to exclude organic disease can be a useful way of reassuring patients that they are not physically unwell.

Referral to a psychiatrist is sometimes necessary to lighten the load on the GP. Some psychiatrists have an interest in hypochondriasis. The community psychiatric nurse or social worker can help explore emotional, social and family problems. The clinical psychologist may be able to provide the patient with training in behavioural methods of coping with physical and mental symptoms.

FATIGUE

Fatigue is a common presenting symptom in general practice. It is often described as: tired all the time, exhausted, lacking energy, sleepy, worn out.

Physical causes of fatigue:

- acute infection (e.g. flu-like illness)
- postviral
- alcohol abuse
- heart failure
- malignancy (e.g. lung, breast, bowel, lymphoma)
- diabetes
- hypothyroidism
- degenerative neurological disease (usually described as weakness)
- chronic infection (e.g. TB, bronchiectasis)
- anaemia.

Diagnosis

Physical causes should be excluded largely on the history, supported by examination of the relevant system(s).

Investigations should be directed towards suspected physical illnesses, although normal FBC, ESR and TFTs help to reassure both patient and doctor.

Chronic fatigue syndrome. This is characterised by a history of fatigue lasting 6 months or more, accompanied by widespread muscle pains and profound weakness. Investigations fail to reveal a physical cause. The condition lasts from a few months to several years. Depression may coexist with chronic fatigue.

Management

- If the history suggests depression, explore and treat (see p. 292).
- Explain to the patient that a physical cause has not been found. Acknowledge the patient's problem of fatigue.

- If family or social problems emerge, it may be helpful to pursue these over time.
- It may be necessary to correct the patient's expectations of the doctor, e.g. 'I need a tonic, Doctor.'
- Chronic fatigue is best managed with empathy and encouragement. The ME Society is a valuable source of support. Medical certificates should be issued to the patient who claims to be too fatigued to work. The Benefits Agency generally takes a sympathetic view of this condition.

Referral. Referral is indicated if:

- a physical disease is suggested but cannot be ruled out (e.g. a suspicion of bowel cancer)
- depression proves difficult to treat (see p. 292)
- help is needed with psychosocial problems (e.g. family therapy)
- anxiety cannot be treated successfully in general practice.

SUICIDE

There are over 5000 deaths per year in the UK due to suicide. The majority of victims have consulted a GP shortly before death.

> **Tip**
> Most suicide patients suffer from a mental illness:
> - depression (most common)
> - alcoholism
> - schizophrenia.

Premorbid diagnosis

History. A number of factors in the history are associated with a higher risk of suicide:

- age 25–44
- male sex
- divorced/separated/living alone
- psychiatric illness
- alcoholism
- economic stress
- family history of alcoholism/mental illness/suicide.

Among women, suicide has also been associated with:

- loss of mother by death or separation before age 12
- three or more children under 3 years old
- lack of job/close relationship.

Also ask about:

- preoccupation with suicide
- active plans made for suicide
- fear of irresistible urge to commit suicide
- delusions of persecution
- auditory hallucinations instructing suicide.

Management

- Consider the possibility of suicide when dealing with mental illness.
- An open discussion with the patient of the risk of suicide is very useful, e.g. 'Do you ever think life is not worth going on with?' Most suicidal patients are grateful for this.
- Consider risk factors (see above).
- Try to establish the level of risk.
- Try to achieve a psychiatric diagnosis in simple terms: depression, psychosis, alcoholism, etc.
- Treat the underlying disorder:
  - depression (see p. 292)
  - alcoholism (see p. 310)
  - psychosis (see p. 305).
- Avoid overprescribing large quantities of drugs when seeing patients in a depressed state. Drug overdose with recently dispensed antidepressants is common.
- Consider admission to hospital:
  - via A&E if the patient has taken a drug overdose
  - via a psychiatric unit, by voluntary or compulsory admission (see p. 307).
- Frequent follow-up of depressed or disturbed patients enables smaller quantities of drugs to be dispensed, is good clinical practice, and enables the GP more accurately to assess a rising suicide risk.

EATING DISORDERS

ANOREXIA NERVOSA

Anorexia nervosa is most common in upper social class women, between the ages of 15 and 25. It affects up to 2% in this group. The mortality is 5–10%.

Diagnosis

History. Ask about:

- progressive weight loss
- reduction in food intake
- distorted body image

- morbid fear of getting fat
- indifference to food intake.

In other causes of weight loss, such as malignancy, thyrotoxicosis and malabsorption, patients usually acknowledge they are losing weight.

The patient with anorexia nervosa is at increased risk of:

- confusional states
- depression
- suicide
- electrolyte imbalance
- dehydration
- fitting
- death (5–10%)
- amenorrhoea.

> **Tip**
> Ordinary dieting can easily be distinguished from anorexia nervosa by a normal response to food in the former, e.g. a craving for high-calorie foods.

Management

Admit the patient to hospital if:
- severe depression is present (see p. 292)
- weight loss has been rapid and persistent
- the weight is below 60% of normal for sex and height.
Compulsory admission may be necessary (see p. 307).

Ask about emotional difficulties with e.g. parents, peers, sexual partner. Discuss aspects of adolescence such as sexual maturation, leaving home, adult responsibilities.

Frequent follow-up is important if the patient is to be managed in general practice. Check C&Es. Consultations should include weight, BP and pulse, food intake and attitudes to food and weight gain. If amenorrhoea is prolonged, consider arranging bone densitometry (increased risk of osteoporosis). Less severe cases commonly resolve with time, encouragement and support. Consider referral to a psychiatric department or specialist eating disorder unit (if available).

BULIMIA NERVOSA

Bulimia nervosa is characterised by avoidance of calorie intake by vomiting or purgation after overeating in binges. It is difficult to diagnose as the weight is often normal and the behaviour secretive. Half of patients with bulimia have previously suffered anorexia nervosa.

Management
Management is as for anorexia nervosa (see p. 302).

DEMENTIA

About 5% of people over 65 have moderate to severe dementia. The majority of cases are due to Alzheimer's-type or multi-infarct dementia. The prevalence increases with age.

Seventy-five per cent of patients with Alzheimer's disease die within 2–4 years of diagnosis.

Diagnosis

History. Dementia is characterised by slowly progressive deterioration in cognitive function:

- memory difficulties (particularly short-term)
- speech difficulties
- personality changes
- uncharacteristic behaviour
- loss of abstract reasoning.

These are often noticed first by a relative or neighbour.
There should be no change in conscious level.

Examination. The abbreviated mental test is helpful:

1. Age.
2. Time.
3. Remember address: '42 West Street'.
4. Year.
5. 'Where are we now?'
6. 'Do you know who I am?'
7. Date of birth.
8. Year of First World War.
9. Name of present Prime Minister.
10. Count backwards from 20 to 1.

A score of less than 8 is abnormal.
To exclude secondary causes look for:

- depression
- Parkinsonism

- hypothyroidism
- deafness
- stigmata of alcoholism
- acute steroid withdrawal.

Neurological examination should be normal. Focal signs prompt urgent referral.

Investigations (dementia screen)

- FBC and ESR
- C&Es, LFTs and glucose
- TFTs
- vitamin B_{12} and folate
- VDRL (or equivalent).

Management

All new cases should be referred to a neurologist if the diagnosis is uncertain or unusual (for a CT brain), or to a psychogeriatrician, if available. The patient should be accompanied by a relative.

Long-term problems

- Depression: treat in the usual way (see p. 292).
- Aggression (see p. 305).
- Loss of driving licence: advise patient/relative to inform the Driver and Vehicle Licensing Agency.
- Wandering and other safety aspects: Medic Alert bracelet.
- Financial difficulties: suggest early application for enduring power of attorney (see solicitor).

Prescribing. Treatment with major tranquillisers reduces the risk of self-harm:

- Agitation at night: e.g. promazine (Sparine) 25–75 mg on.
- Aggression: e.g. risperidone 1 mg od or bd.
- Nocturnal wakefulness: haloperidol 2 mg bd.
- Depression: (see p. 292).
- Sexual disinhibition: benperidol 0.25 mg od to 0.5 mg tds.
- Anticholinesterase inhibitors, e.g. donepezil or galantamine, may slow the progression of the disease and can be used in selected patients with moderate Alzheimer's disease on specialist advice.

Support

- Community psychiatric nurse.
- District nurse.
- Incontinence advisor.
- Social Services and benefits.

- Day centre.
- Respite admission.
- Residential/nursing-home care.
- Alzheimer's Society (see p. 355).

Administration

Quality and Outcomes Framework for Dementia

- Review the care of the patient with dementia once every year.

DISTURBED BEHAVIOUR

The GP may be called to attend a patient whose behaviour or speech is abnormal and characterised by delusions, hallucinations or acute confusion.

This behaviour may have:

- Psychiatric causes: e.g. schizophrenia, mania, depressive psychosis.
- Organic causes: e.g. acute infection, hypoglycaemia, head injury, brain tumour, encephalitis, drug side-effects, septicaemia, alcoholism.

Management

> The first priority is to gain control of the situation. The patient may already be calm and willing to try and answer questions, but some patients may be aggressive or give the impression of being frightened and ready to strike out at the doctor. (For violent behaviour, see below.)

Sedation. If sedation is necessary to gain control, the patient should be given haloperidol 10 mg im. The dose may be repeated up to three times if necessary.

Gain as much information as possible about the patient from a relative, the medical records, other health professionals, the community psychiatric nurse or receptionist, and obtain details of current medication.

Admission to hospital? Consider admission if the patient is likely to self-harm or is a danger to others, or there is serious physical illness or an undiagnosed acute mental disorder.

The patient may not need admitting if there has been a gradual deterioration in mental function (e.g. dementia) or there is a minor physical illness (e.g. delirium due to fever of UTI).

Medical or psychiatric admission? A patient with an acute psychiatric emergency should look generally well physically. There should be no suggestion of an acute medical problem and the predominant features of the illness should be a disturbance of thought or behaviour.

If the patient is unwilling to go into hospital, consider compulsory admission (p. 307).

Disturbed behaviour after psychiatric discharge from hospital may remain within socially acceptable limits. The community psychiatric nurse should review the patient regularly. Acute worsening of the patient's condition will probably warrant readmission.

Administration

Quality and Outcomes Framework for Schizophrenia, Bipolar Disorder and Other Psychoses

- Review general health once a year.
- Achieve therapeutic lithium levels every 6 months.
- Check TSH and creatinine annually in lithium patients.
- Document an agreed care plan.
- Follow up non-compliers for annual review within 14 days.

VIOLENCE

Violence against doctors is increasing. It can be verbal as well as physical. Some violence is due to psychiatric illness, e.g. schizophrenia, or organic diseases, e.g. hypoglycaemia and cerebral events. Some patients are simply violent people.

Some hints for preventing violence

- Have a written procedure for dealing with complaints.
- Listen sympathetically. Do not get defensive.
- Avoid physical confrontation. Talk to the person firmly but calmly, and do not provoke them.

> **Tip**
> If violence is threatened in the surgery and the situation seems likely to escalate, call for help and telephone the police on 999.

If violence appears likely while on a visit, leave immediately. Call by telephone and tell the person you will only return to the house with a police escort.

After an episode of threatened or actual violence

- Record the details of the episode accurately in the notes.
- Discuss the events with your colleagues. Similar episodes with the same patient may be revealed.

- Removing a person from the practice's list is the only way of guaranteeing safety for doctors and staff in the future. Inform the primary care organisation of your decision; they will contact the patient.
- Before removing a patient from the list, ensure there are no reasonable grounds to suspect an underlying illness to account for the behaviour.
- If a complaint was involved, inform your defence organisation.
- Consider criminal proceedings in cases of assault.

SECTIONING

The compulsory admission of a patient to hospital is most often used for suicide risk and acute psychosis. It allows the GP to admit a person, against their will, to a psychiatric unit under the Mental Health Act 1983.

Before seeing the patient

- Prior knowledge of the patient is useful. Obtain the GP records.
- Consider your own safety. Call the police if in doubt. See violence, p. 306.
- The patient may need sedating. Check you have a major tranquilliser, e.g. haloperidol 30 mg im.

Requirements of the Act

- The patient must be suffering from a mental illness, e.g. depression or psychosis, and not just be antisocial, drunk, etc.
- Admission is in the interest of the patient's health or safety or to protect others, e.g. if there is a high risk of suicide or the patient is dangerous.
- Voluntary admission is preferred if possible.

How to organise a compulsory admission

- Telephone the duty psychiatrist to discuss the case and request formal admission.
- A psychiatrist, an approved social worker (ASW) and a doctor who knows the patient (usually the GP) each need to assess the patient in order to admit under Section 2 (28-day compulsory admission for assessment and treatment). Arrangements are usually coordinated by the ASW. If the GP is unable to attend, the ASW will ask for a Section 2-approved doctor.
- On the patient's discharge from hospital, ensure that a suitable follow-up plan is in place.

Mental Health Act (MHA) 1983

Section 2: Admission for assessment and treatment up to 28 days.
Section 3: Admission for treatment for up to 6 months initially.
Section 4: Emergency admission for up to 72 hours.
Section 136: Removal from a public place to a place of safety by the police.

Administration

Complete the appropriate MHA form as arranging compulsory admission attracts a fee.

BENZODIAZEPINE ADDICTION

Many patients in general practice, especially the elderly, may have been on long-term repeat prescriptions for benzodiazepines.

Management

Patients who want to stop taking benzodiazepines

- Offer continuing support, including the prescribing of drugs if necessary.
- Explain the effect of benzodiazepines on memory and judgement and the effects of tolerance and dependence.
- Change to a short-acting drug, such as diazepam or temazepam, if the patient is not already taking one.
- Agree with the patient the timetable for withdrawal. This may need to be as slow as a quarter of a tablet a month.
- Address the psychiatric needs of the patient, e.g. depression (see p. 292), anxiety (see p. 294).
- Allow the patient to keep a small supply of tablets in the house, 'in case of emergency'.
- Suggest counselling or self-help groups.

Patients who do not want to stop

- A patient's commitment to stopping may fluctuate.
- Explain the risks as above and record the discussion in the notes. (Recent cases of litigation have made this more important.)
- Offer help with psychiatric problems.
- Try at a future date to encourage patients to stop, e.g. by including with their repeat prescription an invitation to discuss the issue with the doctor.

OPIATE ADDICTION

There are two new cases of opiate addiction per GP per year in the UK on average. The trend is increasing and there are higher rates in city practices. Opiate addiction is associated with a 20-fold excess mortality for age.

Diagnosis

History. Opiate addiction presents in a variety of ways to the GP, but most commonly:

- The patient admits to drug abuse and wants help.

- The patient wants a prescription to prevent or treat withdrawal symptoms.
- Drug abuse complicates or leads to other medical conditions: pain, hepatitis, HIV, depression and suicide, sepsis, overdose.

Tip
Some addicts present with withdrawal symptoms in an attempt to gain a prescription for opiates or benzodiazepines. It is wise to resist, especially if they are not known to the GP and if this is the first consultation.

Take a history of drug use to distinguish between the intermittent drug misuser and the physically dependent addict. Validate the history, as necessary, by telephoning the patient's usual GP and consultant psychiatrist.

Examination. Examine for evidence of injection, hepatitis, sepsis.

Investigations

- Urine sample for drug screen.
- Blood tests for hepatitis B and C and HIV status.

Management

- Deal with any urgent medical problems not requiring a prescription for opiates or other psychotropic medication, e.g. sepsis.
- Offer a longer consultation within the next 2–3 days, to provide a more thorough evaluation of the problem, before deciding on long-term management.
- Patients requesting opiates may become aggressive if refused. The management of the aggressive patient is dealt with on p. 306.
- Counsel for HIV testing if appropriate (see p. 201). Offer hepatitis B immunisation (see p. 342).
- The occasional drug misuser may only need advice, support and referral to the local drug counselling service or self-help groups.
- Patients with a short history of drug abuse may require the above, but with prescriptions and advice on the treatment of withdrawal symptoms: Imodium for diarrhoea, clonidine for sweating and propranolol for anxiety.

Advice

- Offer continuing medical support for general health matters.
- Advise about not sharing needles, safe injection techniques and needle-exchange programmes.
- Advocate smoking rather than injecting.

> **Tip**
> For the established opiate addict a withdrawal programme should be devised, based on the gradual reduction of methadone. This should be provided by the local specialist in drug addiction, who determines the prescribing and follow-up schedule for the patient. Writing out the prescriptions can be shared with the GP.

Prescribing controlled drugs. (For the main rules, see p. 319.)
   Additional rules for addicts include:

* There should be a written contract from the specialist outlining the duration of treatment and rate of withdrawal. No extra drugs should be given. Lost drugs are the patient's responsibility. The commonest drug used for controlled withdrawal is methadone.
* Discuss with the pharmacist or dispenser. Daily dispensing of the daily ration helps prevent the patient taking it all at once or from selling it. The prescription should be marked 'daily supervised consumption'. This ensures that the patient has to consume each daily ration in front of the pharmacist and should be continued for the first 3 months of treatment or until compliance is assured. It is easier to use a blue FP10, as there is space for the pharmacist to record up to 14 daily doses dispensed. Dispense 2-days' supply on Saturday if the chemist closes on the Sunday.
* Write 'Methadone mixture 1 mg/ml' on the prescription.
* Inform other GPs in the practice. Aim for care by one GP.
* Ongoing support from the drug counsellor is vital.

> **Tip**
> Dealing with drug abusers can be very difficult and specialist help should be sought early in most cases. As with tobacco and alcohol abuse, relapse is common.

ALCOHOL ABUSE

Alcohol abuse affects women as well as men, the elderly as well as the young, and all social classes. On a national basis the average GP will probably have 5–10 alcoholic patients per 2000 population per year.
   High-risk groups include:

* publicans
* caterers
* members of the armed forces
* business executives.

Diagnosis

Alcohol abuse presents in a number of ways:

- a complaint from a relative or friend
- a request from the patient for help with drinking
- memory loss
- stress
- poor performance
- fatigue
- depression
- gastritis
- an incidental finding.

History. The first task is to establish a diagnosis of alcohol abuse. Ask about:

- the level of alcohol consumption (answers from patients are notoriously understated and should be confirmed with the patient's partner if possible)
- memory gaps or amnesia
- any preoccupation with alcohol
- guilt about drinking
- a feeling they should cut down
- annoyance about criticism of drinking habit
- needing a drink early in the day to feel normal.

Examination. If appropriate, look for:

- hypertension
- obesity/malnourishment
- jaundice
- hepatomegaly
- cardiomegaly
- arrhythmias
- encephalopathy (tremor)
- polyneuropathy.

Investigations. Investigations are not always necessary. However, the following are useful:

- FBC for the macrocytosis of chronic alcohol excess
- γ-GT
- LFTs
- urine to screen for other drugs.

Management

Crisis intervention. Occasionally the patient presents with an acute medical or psychiatric problem due to alcohol abuse:

- Severe depression: there is a high risk of suicide in this group of patients. Admit to a psychiatric unit, by compulsory admission if necessary (see p. 307).
- Acute withdrawal complications, such as fitting, atrial fibrillation and delirium tremens: admit under the medical team.
- Acute complications of chronic alcohol abuse: these include pancreatitis, hepatitis, bleeding oesophageal varices and encephalopathy. Admit under the medical team.

Planned intervention

> **Tip**
> As alcoholism is not considered to be a psychiatric disease by itself, any treatment given must be with the consent of the patient. Often the cry for help comes from the spouse, in which case try to support the spouse also.

Detoxification

- Establish the patient's motivation to detoxify.
- Underline to patients that they are responsible for their drinking and for the success of the detoxification.
- Refer for inpatient detoxification if any of the following applies:
  - history of withdrawal fits or delirium tremens
  - there are coexisting medical problems
  - any psychiatric condition
  - inadequate domestic support
  - misuser of other drugs.

Home detoxification regimen. Prescribe:

- chlordiazepoxide (Librium) orally 5 mg and 10 mg tablets:
  - 20 mg qds for 1 day
  - 20 mg tds for 1 day
  - 15 mg tds for 1 day
  - 10 mg tds for 1 day
  - 10 mg bd for 1 day
  - 5 mg bd for 1 day
- vitamin B complex 1 tablet daily
- vitamin C tablet 1 daily.

Ask the pharmacist to dispense the drugs on a daily basis if the patient is likely to comply poorly with medication or become dependent on benzodiazepines.

> **Tip**
> Help and advice from the District Drug and Alcohol Team is useful, if it is available.

Long-term management

- Reiterate to patients that the responsibility for drinking is theirs.
- Encourage contact with self-help groups:
  - Alcoholics Anonymous (see p. 355)
  - Al-Anon Family Groups (for relatives) (see p. 355).
- Treat any contributory illness, such as depression (see p. 292).

SMOKING

Smoking is now recognised as an addiction treatable at the expense of the NHS.

Treatment should be offered to smokers who express a desire to quit, and should form part of an advice and encouragement programme.

NRT (nicotine replacement therapy) and bupropion are two forms of treatment available on the NHS.

Formulations

- Nicotine skin-patches, gum, lozenges, sublingual tablets, inhalators or nasal spray.
- Bupropion tablets. Generally, patients should be prescribed bupropion only after unsuccessful attempts at quitting with NRT.

Contraindications

- Age under 15 years.
- Unstable cardiovascular disease.

NRT patch

Choosing a patch. Smokers of over 20 cigarettes a day need the strongest patch to start with; smokers of 10 cigarettes or less a day can start with the medium-strength patch. Smokers who start smoking first thing in the morning need a 24-hour patch (e.g. Nicotinell or NiQuitin); later starters can use a 16-hour patch (Nicorette).

Using the patches. Prescribe 3 weeks supply on an NHS prescription and get the patient to set a quit date. The patient stops smoking on the quit date and uses one patch every day. If they are still abstinent after 3 weeks then a further prescription for 3 weeks can be issued. Each brand of patch has its own schedule for dose reduction and total duration of use.

Bupropion

Bupropion is prescribed on the NHS for 4 weeks initially and a further 4 weeks if abstinence is maintained. The patient's quit date is set for 2 weeks after the medication is started. The starting dose is 150 mg a day, increased to 150 mg bd after the first 6 days. Avoid bupropion if there are risk factors for seizure.

Further attempts to quit using NRT or bupropion should not be funded by the NHS within 6 months.

Each practice should have access to a lead person in smoking who can offer support to patients attempting to quit. Practice nurses and health visitors are valuable resources in this role.

CHAPTER 20

TERMINAL CARE

Breaking bad news 316
Pain 316
Controlled drugs 319
Vomiting 320
Anorexia 321
Anxiety 322
Constipation 323
Cough 323
Depression 324
Dyspnoea 324
Death 325
Bereavement 327

BREAKING BAD NEWS

Telling patients or their relatives about a terminal condition is never an easy job, but the GP, with a prior knowledge of the patient and family, is often the best person to break the bad news.

Before seeing the patient
Get all the facts beforehand, allow plenty of time and ensure there will be no interruptions.

Facts often needed include:

* prognosis
* symptoms to be expected
* treatment and side-effects.

What to say and how to say it

* Tell the truth.
* Recap on knowledge already gained, e.g. 'What did they tell you in hospital?'
* Stick to the terms used by the patient, e.g. 'growth', 'tumour'.
* Give factual knowledge in simple terms.
* Allow the patient to be defensive.
* Do not give more information than the patient wants.
* Try to discover the patient's fears.
* Give positive aspects, e.g. professional support, effective analgesia.

Follow-up. Make a further appointment to see the patient, who may feel isolated. Offer telephone access in the meantime. Suggest district nurse involvement.

> **Tip**
> The patient may come to terms with the realities of the illness only after several discussions along the above lines.

Administration
All patients with less than 6 months' life expectancy are eligible for Attendance Allowance, irrespective of their need for care. Apply with form DS1500 (available from Social Services). The reverse side of the form is for the GP to claim a fee for this service from the Benefits Agency.

PAIN

The thought of being in pain due to a terminal illness frightens many patients. This fear is sometimes not stated.

> **Tip**
> Pain and anxiety reinforce one another. Anxiolytics can help control pain.

Ask patients if they have pain, rather than waiting for them to volunteer it.

Management of pain relief in palliative care

- Diagnose the cause of pain if possible, e.g. tumour mass, bone metastases, nerve compression, abdominal distension.
- Think of non-drug methods of pain relief, e.g. radiotherapy, surgery, relief of constipation, draining ascites, psychosocial support.
- Do not forget to treat anxiety as an adjunct to pain relief (see p. 294).
- Always bear in mind the potential side-effects of drugs (see constipation, p. 323, and vomiting, p. 320).

> **Tip**
> Using combinations of analgesics early, rather than increasing the dose of one drug, is often useful. The resulting effect is often greater than the sum of the individual drugs.

Examples of useful analgesics
(See controlled drugs, p. 319.)

Mild analgesics

- Paracetamol 500 mg, 1–2 tablets 4–6-hourly prn.
- Ibuprofen 400 mg, 1 tablet tds prn.

Moderate analgesics

- Co-codamol 30/500, 1–2 tablets 4–6-hourly (max = 8 tabs/24 hours) prn.
- Dihydrocodeine 30 mg, 1–2 tablets 4–6-hourly prn.
- Diclofenac 50 mg tds prn.

Strong analgesics

- Morphine sulphate elixir 10 mg/5 ml (Oramorph).
- Morphine sulphate solution 20 mg/ml.
- Morphine sulphate Continus tablets (MST) 5, 10, 30, 60, 100 and 200 mg tablets.
- Morphine sulphate suppositories 10, 20 and 30 mg.
- Diamorphine injection 5, 10, 30, 100 and 500 mg.

How to achieve the correct dose of opiate

- Once it becomes apparent that mild and moderate analgesics are inadequate, substitute oral morphine 5 mg 4-hourly. Regular 4-hourly dosage is preferable, as the aim is total analgesia, without breakthrough pain.
- Increase the dose if necessary by titrating against the pain and giving more morphine, but at the same 4-hourly intervals.

Converting oral morphine solution to MST

- Once satisfactory pain control has been achieved, divide the total 24-hourly dose of morphine by 2 and give this dose as MST at 12-hour intervals, e.g. 10 ml of morphine sulphate elixir every 4 hours at 10 mg/5 ml equates to 60 mg bd of MST.
- As time goes on and the patient develops a tolerance to opiates, the dose of morphine will need to be increased. Use additional morphine sulphate elixir as a top-up initially, and when pain control is again achieved, divide the total 24-hourly dose by 2 and convert to the new dose of MST.
- Giving an NSAID such as diclofenac tablets 50 mg tds as well as the morphine can improve pain control, avoiding the side-effects of increased doses of opiates.

> **Tip**
> Morphine sulphate suppositories are useful if a patient whose pain is well controlled on oral medication starts vomiting (unless the vomiting is due to too high a dose of morphine).

Converting oral morphine to diamorphine

- Diamorphine injections are useful for short-term relief of severe pain in e.g. MI. In terminal care, however, diamorphine can be given by subcutaneous infusion via a syringe driver. For practical purposes, injected diamorphine is about three times as powerful as oral morphine on a dose-for-dose basis. For example, the patient requiring MST 90 mg bd would need 60 mg diamorphine over 24 hours.
- Common side-effects of opiates include:
    - constipation
    - nausea and vomiting, particularly in the initial stages of treatment
    - drowsiness
    - anorexia
    - confusion.

Specific types of pain

Gastrointestinal pain

- Gastric distension pain. Try an antacid with simeticone (e.g. Asilone) or domperidone, 10 mg tds.

- Bowel colic. Try loperimide 2–4 mg qds or hyoscine hydrobromide sublingually 300 μg tds.

Nerve pain, e.g. due to compression by a tumour mass or lymphadenopathy. Dexamethasone tablets 4–8 mg bd may reduce oedema around a tumour in the short term. Radiotherapy often provides relief for longer.

Muscle spasm. This may be helped by the muscle relaxant baclofen 5–10 mg tds. Alternatively, try diazepam 5–10 mg daily.

Bone pain, e.g. due to metastases. Opiate analgesics are the mainstay of treatment (see above). Radiotherapy and NSAIDs provide useful additional relief.

CONTROLLED DRUGS

For choices of drugs and dosages, see pain, p. 317.

Legal aspects

For prescribing opiates on the prescription form FP10 a few simple rules have to be followed:

- The form, strength and dose of the drug must be stated, e.g. morphine sulphate elixir 10 mg/5 ml, 10 mg 4-hourly.
- The total amount of drug must be stated in words and figures, e.g. one hundred millilitres 100 ml.

For carrying controlled drugs in the black bag there are a few legal requirements:

- Keep a bound ledger to record the acquisition and administration of all controlled drugs. Use a different page for each form of drug. Record the amount, form and concentration of each drug and the dates acquired and used. Any difference between acquired and used drugs should equal what is left in the bag.
- If the black bag is left in the car it should be locked and the car should also be locked. Alternatively, controlled drugs can be kept in a separate locked container if left in a locked car.
- If stock goes out of date it can either be returned to the chemist or destroyed. Officially, the destroying of controlled drugs should be witnessed by an appointed official of the PCT.

Ethical considerations

- In terminal care, the fear of addiction to opiates should not deter the doctor from adequately prescribing for pain relief.
- Addiction is unlikely to occur if the dose of opiate is adequate and given regularly.
- In the dying patient, pain and distress can prolong life by their stimulating effect on respiratory rate and arousal. Opiates relieve this distress and can

allow patients to die peacefully, if somewhat earlier than they would otherwise have done. This should not be considered a form of euthanasia. The dose of an opiate required to suppress the respiratory centre is much greater than that needed for pain relief.

VOMITING

Causes of vomiting in the terminally ill patient

- Drug side-effects, particularly chemotherapy drugs and opiates.
- Intestinal obstruction.
- Pain.
- Raised intracranial pressure, e.g. from cerebral metastases.
- Uraemia.
- Anxiety.
- Hypercalcaemia.

Nausea and vomiting are common symptoms in terminal care.

Diagnosis

History. Ask about:

- pain control
- drug regimen
- bowel/stoma function
- headache
- micturition.

Examination. Look for:

- abdominal signs of obstruction
- papilloedema if raised intracranial pressure is suspected.

Investigations

- C&Es
- calcium.

> **Tip**
> Treat the underlying cause if possible. Hospital/hospice admission is indicated if the cause of vomiting remains undiagnosed.

Management

Reassure patients that their nausea can be treated.

Prescribing. (e.g. for nausea associated with opiate analgesics):

- Prochlorperazine:
  - oral 5–10 mg tds
  - buccal 3–6 mg bd
  - suppository 5 and 25 mg
  - injection 12.5 mg.
- Metoclopramide: tablets and injection 10 mg tds.
- Domperidone:
  - tablets 10–20 mg 4–8-hourly
  - suppository 30–60 mg tds.
- Cyclizine: injection 50 mg tds. Cyclizine is useful when mixed with diamorphine in a syringe-driver as it can be given by subcutaneous infusion.

Side-effects

- Prochlorperazine and metoclopramide cause drowsiness and can cause acute dystonic reactions in younger patients.
- Domperidone is less sedating. Dystonia has been reported but is uncommon.
- Cyclizine can cause drowsiness, dry mouth and blurred vision.

Haematemesis. This may be the final event in the course of a terminal illness. Diamorphine by im injection can help relieve the acute distress to the patient. A red blanket on the bed helps to disguise the amount of blood being lost.

ANOREXIA

Anorexia is an inevitable feature of terminal care, as the appetite wanes and eating becomes too much of an effort.

> **Tip**
> Anorexia is very common in the final few days of life and is often of more concern to the carers than to the patient. It may require no treatment, although attempting to improve the appetite may improve morale.

Management

- Exclude treatable causes:
  - drug side-effects
  - nausea
  - depression
  - abdominal obstruction
  - sore mouth, e.g. due to thrush.

- Simple measures:
  - give small helpings of food
  - use a small plate
  - suggest alcohol as an aperitif.
- Drug treatment:
  - prednisolone E/C tablets 5 mg tds
  - alternatively, dexamethasone 2–4 mg daily.

Tip
It is rarely justifiable to use steroids simply to boost appetite, although steroids prescribed for other indications will improve overall well-being, including the appetite.

ANXIETY

Anxiety in the terminally ill may manifest itself as restlessness, confusion, agitation, depression or anger.

Diagnosis

History. Ask about:

- symptoms common to terminal care, e.g. pain, vomiting, dyspnoea, constipation, anorexia
- psychosocial problems, e.g. distressed relatives, fear of dying or suffering, fear of hospitalisation
- free-floating anxiety; also pre-existing anxiety states
- drug side-effects.

Management

- Treat the underlying cause if possible.
- Give regular support and reassurance.
- Recognise anxiety and depression.
- Involve the district nurse, Marie Curie nurse, Macmillan nurse and hospice or social worker, if appropriate, at an early stage.

Prescribing

- Antidepressants, e.g. citalopram 20 mg daily.
- Anxiolytics, e.g. chlorpromazine tablets or syrup 25 mg tds, increasing by 25 mg daily at weekly intervals until control is achieved.

Alternatively, use haloperidol 1–3 mg tds, which is less sedating.
    For short-term use in acute anxiety, use diazepam 2 or 5 mg up to tds.

> **Tip**
> Midazolam 40 mg can be given via a syringe-driver and can be mixed with diamorphine in the same syringe.

CONSTIPATION

Aim to prevent constipation in terminal care by prescribing laxatives in conjunction with opiate analgesics.

Causes of constipation in the terminally ill include:

- opiate analgesics
- decreased mobility
- decreased fluid intake
- anorexia
- obstruction, e.g. due to tumour.

> **Tip**
> The overloaded colon may present with overflow diarrhoea. In this case liquefied stool bypasses a constipated segment of bowel. This possibility is worth bearing in mind when a patient on morphine presents with diarrhoea.

Management
(See also p. 124.)

- Always prescribe a laxative when giving opiate analgesics, e.g. the faecal softener and peristaltic stimulant co-danthramer 5–10 ml bd.
- Exclude obstruction (absolute constipation, vomiting and distension, abdominal pain).
- If constipation occurs, consider an osmotic laxative e.g. lactulose 10 ml bd and a stimulant laxative, e.g. senna 2 tablets nocte.
- Stronger treatments may be necessary if the above measures fail, e.g. Movicol 1–3 sachets daily in divided doses or bisacodyl suppositories 10 mg (work within 20–30 minutes; may cause griping abdominal pains). Alternatively, glycerol suppositories, docusate sodium or phosphate enemas may be useful.

COUGH

Cough is a common symptom in carcinoma of the bronchus.

> **Tip**
> Some consequences of cough include insomnia and breathlessness. Carers may be disturbed at night.

Management

- Steam inhalations.
- Pholcodine linctus 10 ml 4-hourly.
- Morphine linctus 5 mg 4-hourly, increased until effective.

DEPRESSION

All terminally ill patients manifest depression at some stage of their illness. For depression in general, see p. 292.

Features of depression peculiar to terminal illness

- Ask about symptoms and look for signs of depression. The patient or carers may not volunteer these, leading to delayed diagnosis.
- Carer stress and depression are also common and should be sought.
- Features of depression may be masked by drugs used in terminal care, e.g. opiates and phenothiazines.
- Drug side-effects and interactions may complicate treatment, e.g. tricyclics and morphine both exacerbate constipation.
- District nurses, Macmillan nurses and Marie Curie nurses are an invaluable resource in the management of depression, both for identifying the condition and for supporting patients.

 The recently bereaved are at increased risk of suicide.

- The regular, close observation of the terminally ill patient by the GP should provide adequate opportunity for the detection and treatment of depression.

DYSPNOEA

Respiratory distress is common in terminal emphysema and carcinoma of the bronchus and may become a problem long before the patient is dying. Cheyne–Stokes breathing, on the other hand, is an almost universal feature of the last few hours of life, in anyone dying of malignant disease.

Management

Management of respiratory distress

- Exclude chest infection, pleural effusion and bronchospasm.
- Relieve the distress of dyspnoea with oral morphine 5 mg 4-hourly, increasing as necessary.
- Alternatively, use diazepam 5–10 mg daily.

Management of excessive respiratory secretions. These are the cause of the 'death rattle' heard during the last few hours of the dying patient's life.

Give hyoscine or atropine injection (sc or im) 600 μg tds. Hyoscine hydrobromide may be given in a subcutaneous infusion 0.6–2.4 mg/24 hours, and may be mixed with diamorphine.

DEATH

Most GPs will be involved in confirming or certifying a death approximately every 2 months, more frequently in the winter.

Talking to relatives
See p. 327.

Confirming death
When called to attend a patient who has died, the first task is usually to confirm death. Examine for:

- carotid pulse
- heart sounds
- general appearance
- fixed, dilated pupils.

> **Tip**
> If the death occurs in the middle of the night, but was expected by the relatives or nursing-home staff, the examination to confirm death can be performed by a nurse or undertaker. The GP will still need to see the body of the deceased if a cremation certificate is required, but this can be done in normal hours.

Who to inform
At the time of confirming death it may only be necessary to inform those present – usually the relatives, especially if the death was expected.

Other people may need informing under the following circumstances:

- Relatives: if requested by those present at death.
- Undertaker: if requested by relatives.

- Coroner, if:
  - the death is sudden or unexplained
  - a doctor has not attended within the preceding 14 days
  - the death may be due to industrial disease, or related to the deceased's employment
  - the death was violent, unnatural or suspicious
  - the death may be due to an accident
  - the death may be due to self-neglect or neglect by others
  - the death may be due to an abortion
  - the death occurred during an operation or before recovery from the effects of an anaesthetic
  - the death may be a suicide
  - the death occurred during or shortly after detention in police or prison custody
- Out-of-hours the coroner may not be available, in which case call the police.

Other people may need informing, but this can be done from the surgery during the next working day if necessary:

- a doctor from another practice if a Cremation Form Part B is required
- the patient's usual doctor
- primary healthcare team members, if involved
- practice receptionist, to de-register the patient and cancel appointment reminders.

Administration

Forms

Death certificate. The death certificate can be completed if the cause of death is known and the patient has been seen within the preceding 14 days by the doctor. If more than 14 days have elapsed, discuss the case with the coroner, who will probably 'pass' it if the cause of death is known. If in doubt, phone the coroner. Indicate on the back of the death certificate that the coroner has been informed.

   The death certificate, if completed, can be given to the relatives, who use it to register the death at the Registrar's Office. If the death is made a coroner's case, the coroner issues the death certificate.

Cremation form. The cremation certificate can be filled in only by doctors who have seen the dead body. Two doctors are required. The Part B doctor must have been fully registered for 5 years or more, must be from a different practice and must have discussed the death with the Part A doctor. The doctor completing Part B must also discuss the circumstances of the patient's death with either a relative or a member of the nursing team who was involved in the patient's final illness. The cremation form should be given to the undertaker.

Fees. A fee is paid by the undertaker for completing Part A or Part B of a cremation certificate. No fee can be claimed for completing a death certificate.

BEREAVEMENT

See also breaking bad news, p. 316.

See also breaking bad news, p. 316.

Tip
Anniversaries can rekindle various stages of bereavement.

Bereavement can be experienced following a loss other than a death, e.g. loss of marriage, job, pregnancy, limb.

The stages of bereavement

1. Shock.
2. Denial.
3. Anger.
4. Acceptance.

As a rule of thumb, the first two stages should last no longer than a few days. Any significant lengthening of these stages should alert the GP to the possibility of an abnormal bereavement. Stages three and four can take longer, sometimes months, to complete.

Management

Most patients appreciate continued support at this time. Encouraging patients to talk about their loss helps the grieving process.

Inform the patient about support groups, e.g. CRUSE (see p. 356).

Enlist the help of others. The district nurse, social worker or a bereavement counsellor (e.g. from the hospice) may be useful.

There is an increased suicide risk in the recently bereaved. Involve the psychiatric team early in suspected abnormal grief or severe depression.

Administration

Quality and Outcomes Framework for Palliative Care and Cancer

- Hold multidisciplinary case review meetings at least 3-monthly where all patients on the palliative care register are discussed.
- Review the care of each new cancer patient within 6 months of confirmation of diagnosis.

APPENDICES

Drug monitoring   330

Immunisations   334

Private medical examinations   346

Patient reports   346

Notifiable diseases   347

Management of anaphylaxis   348

Standard growth charts   349

Dermatomes   353

Adult height versus weight chart   354

Useful addresses and telephone numbers   355

DRUG MONITORING

Several drugs used in general practice require long-term monitoring in addition to the routine clinical follow-up of patients.

WARFARIN

Measurement. INR (international normalised ratio) – the ratio of the patient's prothrombin time to the laboratory standard. Appropriate INR ranges:

- 2.0–2.5 for:
  - prophylaxis of deep-vein thrombosis.
- 2.5 for:
  - deep vein thrombosis
  - pulmonary embolus
  - mitral stenosis with embolism
  - atrial fibrillation
  - tissue prosthetic heart valves.
- 3.0–4.5 for:
  - recurrent deep vein thrombosis
  - recurrent pulmonary embolus
  - mechanical prosthetic heart valves.

Values are often recommended in hospital discharge letters, or see *British National Formulary*.

Duration of treatment. Life, for all conditions except pig heart valve replacements and single episodes of deep vein thrombosis or pulmonary embolus (3 months). Anticoagulation can also often be discontinued if haemorrhage occurs, e.g. from a bleeding peptic ulcer.

Starting dose. 10 mg daily for 2 days, then between 3 and 9 mg daily according to the INR.

Frequency of measurement

- Prior to starting treatment.
- Daily initially, until the desired range is achieved (usually 3 days), then every 2 or 3 days. Thus, if commencing warfarin treatment in general practice, start on a Monday. Intervals increase as a stable dose is achieved. Aim for INR testing every 4–6 weeks once stable. Test more frequently if the INR is too high or too low, or following a change of dose.

LITHIUM

Measurement. Serum drug level.

- Take blood 12 hours after the last dose.

Therapeutic range

- 0.8–1.2 mmol/l in acute mania.
- 0.4–1.0 mmol/l in manic depression.

Frequency of measurement

- 1 week after any change of dose.
- 3-monthly as a routine.
- More frequently if toxicity is suspected by:
  - nausea, vomiting, diarrhoea
  - muscle weakness, confusion
  - ataxia, dysarthria
  - arrhythmias, renal impairment.

Also measure C&Es and TFTs annually to exclude hypothyroidism and renal impairment.

THEOPHYLLINE

Measurement. Serum drug level.

- Measure 8 hours after the last dose (12 hours for modified release formulations).

Therapeutic range.

- 55–110 μmol/l.

Frequency of measurement

- 2–3 days after a change of dose.
- Routine measurements are unnecessary.
- Check levels if:
  - toxicity is suspected due to: nausea and diarrhoea, insomnia, tachycardia and arrhythmia
  - asthma control deteriorates
  - the patient gives up smoking
  - iv aminophylline is contemplated.

DIGOXIN

Measurement. Serum drug level.

- Take blood 12 hours after the last dose.

Therapeutic range

- 1.0–2.6 nmol/l.

Frequency of measurement

- 8 days after any change of dose.
- Routine serum drug levels are unnecessary.
- Aim to control the ventricular rate <100/minute without side-effects.
- Measure drug level if toxicity is suspected due to:
  - anorexia, nausea, vomiting
  - confusion
  - arrhythmia.

Also measure C&Es if toxicity is suspected as hypokalaemia potentiates the effect of digoxin.

THYROXINE

Measurement. TSH (thyroid stimulating hormone).

- The timing of the sample is not important.

Therapeutic range

- 0.5–5.0 mU/l.

Frequency of measurement

- 1 month after a change of dose.
- Annual testing now a contractual requirement in the UK
- Measure the TSH and T4 and T3 if under- or overtreatment is suspected.
- Aim to maintain a euthyroid status.
- Reduce the dose of thyroxine if the TSH is below 0.08 mU/l.

PHENYTOIN

Measurement. Serum drug level.

- The timing of the sample is not important.

Therapeutic range

- 40–80 μmol/l.

Frequency of measurement

- 7–10 days after each change of dose.
- Routine drug level measurement is unnecessary.
- Aim to control fits without side-effects. Therefore, measure levels if:
  - toxicity is suspected due to: nystagmus, ataxia or dysarthria
  - fits occur.

- If the serum drug level is <20 μmol/l, increase the daily dose by 100 mg.
- If the serum drug level is 20–40 μmol/l, increase the daily dose by 50 mg.
- Also measure FBC as appropriate (risk of agranulocytosis).

ACE INHIBITORS

Measurement. C&Es.

Frequency of measurement. Prior to treatment, at 2 weeks and at every increase of dose (there is a risk of hyperkalaemia), then annually.

STATINS

Measurement. LFTs.

Frequency of measurement. Before, and 2 weeks after starting treatment.

DIURETICS

C&Es annually (hypo- or hyperkalaemia).

METHOTREXATE

FBC and LFTs every 2 weeks for 2 months, then 3-monthly.

SULPHASALAZINE

2-weekly FBC for the first 3 months, thereafter 3-monthly. LFTs and C&Es at 0, 3 and 6 months.

AZATHIOPRINE

FBC weekly for 6 weeks, thereafter monthly. LFTs and C&Es monthly for 3 months, then 3-monthly.

GOLD

FBC and urinalysis for protein and blood before each injection. LFTs and C&Es 3-monthly.

PENICILLAMINE

FBC and urinalysis for protein 2-weekly for 2 months, thereafter monthly. LFTs and C&Es annually.

IMMUNISATIONS

Childhood immunisations

Every effort should be made to immunise all children, even if they are older than the recommended age range. A minor non-febrile illness should not be a reason for delaying vaccination.

The schedule for routine immunisation is as shown in the table below.

Routine childhood immunisations		
Vaccine	*Age*	*Comment*
DTP/IPV/Hib 1st dose + pneumococcal DTP/IPV/Hib 2nd dose + meningitis C DTP/IPV/Hib 3rd dose + meningitis C and pneumococcal	2 months 3 months 4 months	Primary course
Hib and meningitis C	12 months	
Measles/mumps/rubella (MMR) + pneumococcal	13 months	Can be given at any age over 12 months
Booster DTP/IPV and MMR (2nd dose)	3.5–5 years	3 years after completion of primary course
BCG	10–14 years	For tuberculin-negative children
Booster diphtheria (low dose)/tetanus and polio (dT/IPV)	13–18 years	
DTP, diphtheria/tetanus/acellular pertussis; *Hib*, Haemophilus influenza *type b; IPV*, inactivated polio vaccine.		

Neonates should receive BCG if at high risk (see p. 339) and/or hepatitis B vaccine if the mother is a carrier (see p. 199).

Adult vaccinations

Adults should receive the following vaccines:

- Non-pregnant women who are seronegative for rubella: MMR.
- Previously unimmunised individuals: polio, tetanus, diphtheria.
- Individuals in high-risk groups: hepatitis B, hepatitis A, influenza, pneumococcal vaccine.

Live vaccines

These include the following:

- rubella
- measles
- mumps
- oral typhoid
- BCG
- yellow fever.

Live vaccines should not be given to:

- Pregnant women. (The risk is theoretical, so live vaccine may be given if there is a significant risk of exposure.)
- The immunocompromised, e.g. treatment with high-dose corticosteroids (prednisolone 40 mg per day for 1 week or more in adults; 2 mg/kg per day in children) within the last 3 months, malignancy of the reticuloendothelial system, treatment with radiotherapy.

HIV-positive patients may be given most live vaccines, but should not be given BCG or yellow fever.

When two live vaccines are required, they should be given either simultaneously at different sites or with an interval of at least 3 weeks. If time constraints make this impossible, it is better to give them within 3 weeks of each other than to omit them.

Immunoglobulin may interfere with the development of active immunity from live vaccines. Live vaccines should therefore be given at least 3 weeks before or 3 months after immunoglobulin. If time constraints make this impossible, this advice may have to be ignored.

Passive immunisation

Normal immunoglobulin is available for prophylaxis of measles and hepatitis A. Specific immunoglobulins are available for tetanus, hepatitis B, rabies and varicella-zoster.

For more detailed information on immunisations, refer to *Immunisation against Infectious Disease*, published by the Department of Health and distributed free to every surgery or on-line at http://www.immunisation.nhs.uk/files/greenbook.pdf.

PERTUSSIS VACCINE

A reinforcing dose of acellular pertussis vaccine is necessary after the primary course of acellular pertussis and is given between 3.5 and 5 years of age.

Adverse reactions

- Local swelling and redness, fever and malaise are common.
- There is no conclusive evidence to show that brain damage has ever been caused by the vaccine; however, the vaccine may very rarely be associated with an acute severe neurological illness in previously normal children, from which recovery is full.

Contraindications

- Postpone immunisation if:
  - The child is suffering from an acute febrile illness.
  - There is an evolving neurological problem. Immunisation should be deferred until the condition is stable.
- Do not vaccinate children who have had a severe local or general reaction to a preceding dose:
  - A severe local reaction is swelling and induration involving most of the injected part of the limb.
  - A severe general reaction is a fever of >39.5°C, inconsolable screaming for >4 hours, or any more severe reaction.
- If there is a personal or family history of febrile convulsions, there is an increased risk of these occurring after pertussis immunisation. Immunisation should be given, but advice on fever prevention should be given at the time of vaccination.

DIPHTHERIA VACCINE

Immunisation is recommended for:

- All children.
- All non-immune adults.
- All contacts. Immune contacts require a booster. Non-immune contacts require a full course of three doses at monthly intervals and a prophylactic course of erythromycin.
- Travel, if appropriate.

The primary course is given routinely together with tetanus, pertussis, inactivated polio (IPV) and Hib as part of the pentavalent vaccine at 2, 3 and 4 months. A booster is given at 3.5–5 years together with tetanus, pertussis and IPV. A further reinforcing dose is now recommended at school-leaving (low-dose diphtheria, usually given with tetanus and IPV vaccine).

Low-dose diphtheria vaccine should be used in patients over 10 years because of the possibility of a serious reaction in a patient who is already immune.

The Schick test is used to ensure immunity to diphtheria in those who may be exposed to diphtheria in the course of their work.

Contraindications

- Postpone immunisation if the patient is suffering from an acute febrile illness.
- Do not vaccinate if there has been a severe local or general reaction to a preceding dose. (Reactions to the pertussis or tetanus components of the triple vaccine are more likely.)

TETANUS VACCINE

Children
Tetanus is given as part of the pentavalent vaccine at 2, 3 and 4 months of age and reinforced at ages 3.5–5 and 13–18 years. If a course is interrupted it may be resumed; there is no need to start again.

Adults
Elderly women are at highest risk of the disease.

Previously unimmunised adults should be given primary immunisation (three doses with intervals of 1 month between each dose). They will require two booster doses at 10-year intervals. After five doses, as above, immunity is likely to be lifelong.

A tetanus-prone wound
This is any wound or burn sustained more than 6 hours before surgical treatment that shows one of the following:

- a significant degree of devitalised tissue
- a puncture-type wound
- contact with soil or manure
- evidence of sepsis.

Patients with a tetanus-prone wound who are not immunised should receive a primary course. Those who had their last booster >10 years ago should receive a booster. Both groups should be given a dose of tetanus immunoglobulin.

Contraindications

- An acute febrile illness.
- Adverse reaction to a previous dose.

HAEMOPHILUS INFLUENZA B (HIB) VACCINE

Hib vaccine is recommended for all babies at 2, 3 and 4 months as part of the pentavalent vaccine. A booster is given with the meningitis C vaccine at 12 months.

Unimmunised household contacts of Hib disease under the age of 4 years should receive Hib vaccine. Independently of immunisation, rifampicin prophylaxis should be given.

POLIO VACCINE

Inactivated polio vaccine is given at 2, 3 and 4 months as part of the pentavalent vaccine. Two booster doses are given:

- before starting school at age 3.5 to 5 years with diphtheria, tetanus and IPV
- before leaving school at age 13–18 years with diphtheria and tetanus.

The primary immunisation of adults consists of three doses of inactivated polio vaccine at intervals of 4 weeks given as the combined DT/IPV vaccine. Booster doses for adults are unnecessary unless they are at special risk, e.g. travellers to epidemic or endemic areas, contacts of polio.

Contraindications

- An acute febrile illness.
- Vomiting or diarrhoea.
- Immunosuppression.
- Reticuloendothelial system malignancy.
- Extreme sensitivity to penicillin, streptomycin, neomycin or polymyxin.

MEASLES/MUMPS/RUBELLA VACCINE

MMR is recommended for all children aged 12–15 months. A second dose is given to preschool children at the age of 3.5–5 years. It should be given despite a previous history of measles, mumps or rubella. MMR can be given to children of any age whose parents request it, and should be encouraged, especially for children who have never been immunised against measles. All children aged under 5 years should receive two doses at least 3 months apart. It can also be given to non-immune adults.

MMR vaccine is used to protect non-immune measles contacts, and must be given within 3 days of exposure. Immunoglobulin is given for contacts in whom vaccine is contraindicated.

Side-effects

- Malaise, fever and/or a rash may occur 1 week after immunisation.
- Febrile convulsions occur in 1:1000 children at the same stage. Parotid swelling occurs in 1:100 children in the third week.
- Mumps meningoencephalitis occurs in 1:300 000 children.
- There is no convincing scientific evidence that the MMR vaccine causes Crohn's disease or autism.

Contraindications

- Acute febrile illness.
- Immunosuppression.
- Allergy to neomycin, kanamycin or polymyxin.

- As for other live vaccines (see p. 335).
- MMR should not be given within 3 months of an injection of immunoglobulin.
- Pregnancy.
- Women who have been given MMR should avoid pregnancy for 1 month.

MUMPS VACCINE

Unimmunised adults requiring mumps protection may be given the MMR vaccine. Single mumps vaccine is no longer licensed for use in the UK. There is no available protection for contacts.

RUBELLA VACCINE

Rubella is part of the MMR vaccine given at 12–15 months and again at 3.5–5 years of age. Single rubella vaccine is no longer licensed for use in the UK.

- All women of child-bearing age should be screened for rubella antibodies.
- Non-immune women should receive a single dose of MMR vaccine unless they are pregnant. An LMP of <4 weeks previously excludes pregnancy.
- Advise women against pregnancy for 1 month after immunisation (see p. 22).
- Seronegative pregnant women should be immunised after pregnancy.
- There is no adequate protection for contacts.

Contraindications
As for MMR.

BCG VACCINE

BCG is recommended for the following groups, provided the tuberculin skin test is negative.

- Those at normal risk:
    - all children aged 10–14 years, according to local policy
    - all students, according to local policy
    - babies, children or adults where the parents or the individuals themselves request BCG immunisation.
- Those at higher risk:
- health service and veterinary staff
- contacts of cases of active respiratory tuberculosis
- immigrants from countries with a high prevalence of tuberculosis, and their children, wherever born
- travellers to high-prevalence areas for >1 month.

BCG immunisation and tuberculin skin-testing are organised at local chest clinics.

Contraindications

- Positive tuberculin skin test.
- Pyrexia.
- Immunosuppression.
- Malignancy of the reticuloendothelial system.
- Pregnancy.
- Those who are HIV-positive.
- As for other live vaccines (see p. 335).

The tuberculin skin test (Mantoux or Heaf)

A tuberculin skin test must be carried out before BCG immunisation (except in infants up to 3 months old, who may be immunised without a prior test).
A positive test implies past infection or past successful immunisation and BCG should not then be given.

INFLUENZA VACCINE

Influenza vaccine is recommended for everyone aged over 65 years, and all adults and children with any of the following:

- Chronic respiratory disease, including severe asthma.
- Chronic heart disease.
- Chronic renal failure.
- Diabetes mellitus and other endocrine disorders.
- Immunosuppression, including asplenia.
- It is also recommended for residents of nursing homes, old people's homes and other long-stay establishments and their carers.

Adults require one injection annually. Children require a primary course of two injections 4–6 weeks apart, and then annual injections. The ideal time for immunisation is late October/early November.

Warn patients that they will still be susceptible to colds and sore throats due to other viruses. Patients being given influenza vaccine should be considered for pneumococcal vaccine (see below).

Contraindications

- Anaphylactic egg allergy.
- Pregnancy.

PNEUMOCOCCAL VACCINE

Pneumococcal vaccination is now given routinely in childhood at the ages of 2, 4 and 13 months. It should be considered for all those aged >2 years for whom the risk of contracting pneumococcal pneumonia is unusually high or dangerous, i.e. those with:

- asplenia
- homozygous sickle cell disease
- immunosuppression
- chronic renal failure (or nephrotic syndrome), heart, lung or liver disease
- diabetes mellitus.

A single dose only is needed.

Pneumococcal vaccine may be given with influenza vaccine at a different site. Reimmunisation is only considered in those at greatest risk, e.g. asplenia or nephrotic syndrome, after 5–10 years.

Contraindications

- Acute infection.
- Pregnancy.
- Within 3 years of a previous dose of pneumococcal vaccine (except childhood routine).

HEPATITIS A VACCINE

Hepatitis A vaccine is recommended for:

- Travellers: for those who frequently visit areas of high/moderately high risk, such as Africa or the Far East, or for those staying in such areas for >3 months. Testing for antibodies to hepatitis A is advised prior to immunisation in those who are already likely to be immune:
  – those >50 years old
  – those born in areas of high hepatitis A virus endemicity
  – those with a history of jaundice.
- Occupational exposure, e.g. sewage workers.
- Patients with chronic liver disease.
- Haemophiliacs.
- Homosexuals whose sexual behaviour is likely to put them at high risk.
- Community outbreaks.

A single dose confers immunity for 1 year. A booster dose at 6–12 months extends immunity for up to 10 years.

Give children under 15 years old Havrix Junior.

Immunoglobulin gives short-term protection against hepatitis A to travellers (if appropriate) and to contacts. It can be given at the same time as hepatitis A vaccine if protection is required within 10 days of the first dose of hepatitis A vaccine. One injection only is necessary. There are two dosage levels. Use the higher dose for contacts and for extended protection (i.e. those travelling abroad for 3–5 months).

Contraindications

- Pyrexia.
- Pregnancy. (It should not be given unless there is a definite risk of infection.)

HEPATITIS B VACCINE

Hepatitis B vaccination is recommended in those at risk of contracting the virus, e.g. healthcare workers, staff and residents of homes for those with severe learning difficulties, drug abusers, those who change sexual partners frequently, prisoners, chronic renal disease patients, haemophiliacs.

Vaccination is unnecessary in those who are hepatitis B surface antigen positive.

- Three doses at 0, 1 and 6-month intervals are given.
- Check the antibody levels 3–4 months after the last dose. Non-responders should receive a fourth dose.
- A single booster dose 5 years after the primary course may be sufficient to maintain immunity.

Specific hepatitis B immunoglobulin can be given for postexposure prophylaxis (passive protection), e.g. after accidental inoculation. It should be given within 48 hours of exposure, and is normally used in combination with hepatitis B vaccine.

MENINGOCOCCAL VACCINE

The major cause of meningococcal disease in the UK is group B, against which there is no available vaccine. There are two vaccines against the other types of bacterial meningitis: meningitis C vaccine and the combined meningitis A and C vaccine.

Meningitis C vaccine is recommended for:

- babies at ages 3, 4 and 12 months, along with other routine childhood immunisations
- previously unimmunised adults aged ≤24 years – single dose.

Meningitis A and C vaccination is recommended for:

- close contacts of cases of group A or group C meningitis, who should be given meningococcal vaccine in addition to chemoprophylaxis
- control of local outbreaks in close communities
- for travellers, as appropriate, even if they have already received meningitis C vaccine. The vaccine is effective for 3 years.

Contraindications

- Febrile illness.
- A severe previous reaction.
- Pregnancy.

CHICKENPOX AND HERPES ZOSTER IMMUNISATION

Passive immunisation is available in the UK in the form of human varicella-zoster immunoglobulin. Varicella-zoster immunoglobulin is recommended for contacts of chickenpox or herpes zoster in the following groups:

- Those who are immunosuppressed.
- Those with debilitating disease.
- Non-immune pregnant women. Varicella-zoster immunoglobulin will not prevent congenital varicella syndrome, but it may attenuate the disease in pregnant women.
- Infants up to 4 weeks old:
  - whose mothers develop chickenpox from 7 days before to 1 month after delivery
  - who are in contact with chickenpox or zoster when their mother has no antibody on testing.

The supply of varicella-zoster immunoglobulin is limited by the availability of suitable donors.

Aciclovir should be used in the treatment of severe disease (see p. 193).

RABIES VACCINE

Pre-exposure prophylaxis
This should be offered to:

- anyone who, by the nature of their work, is likely to have contact with rabies
- travellers to high-risk areas where medical treatment might not be immediately available.

Rabies vaccine is only free on the NHS for the first category of patient.

The course consists of three doses at days 0, 7 and 28. Give booster doses at 2–3-year intervals to those at continued risk.

Postexposure treatment

- Ask about the rabies risk in the country concerned.
- Cleanse the wound thoroughly.
- Give:
  - Six doses of rabies vaccine on days 0, 3, 7, 14, 30 and 90. If the biting animal is symptom-free after 10 days of observation, stop treatment.
  - Rabies-specific immunoglobulin.

Contraindications
There are no absolute contraindications to rabies vaccine.

CHOLERA VACCINE

Cholera vaccination should not be required of any traveller. However, local officials sometimes require it, and one injection is sufficient to provide a certificate.

Contraindications

- Acute febrile illness.
- Hypersensitivity to previous dose.
- Pregnancy.

TYPHOID VACCINE

Give typhoid vaccine to travellers, if appropriate.

Vi polysaccharide vaccine. A polysaccharide vaccine can be given as a single dose only, with a booster dose every 3 years on continued exposure.

Oral typhoid vaccine. A live attenuated vaccine requires three doses of one capsule on alternate days. Protection lasts for 1–3 years.

Hepatyrix combines typhoid with hepatitis A vaccine as a single injection.

Side-effects

Local reactions to polysaccharide vaccine are usually mild, and systemic reactions are uncommon.

Contraindications

- Acute febrile illness.
- Severe reaction to previous dose.
- Pregnancy.

YELLOW FEVER VACCINE

Yellow fever vaccine is recommended for:

- laboratory workers handling infected material
- persons aged 9 months and over, travelling through or living in infected areas
- travellers requiring an International Certificate of Vaccination for entry into a country.

A single dose confers immunity for 10 years. The vaccine can only be given at yellow fever vaccination centres.

Precautions against mosquito bites should be taken.

Adverse reactions

- Mild flu-like symptoms in 5–10% of recipients 5–10 days after immunisation.
- Rarely, anaphylaxis and encephalitis have been reported.

Contraindications

- The usual contraindications to a live vaccine (see p. 335).
- Those who are hypersensitive to neomycin or polymyxin or who have had an anaphylactic reaction to egg.
- HIV-positive individuals.

JAPANESE B ENCEPHALITIS VACCINE

Japanese B encephalitis is a mosquito-borne viral encephalitis.

Vaccination is recommended for travellers who will be staying for a month or longer in endemic areas, especially if travel will include rural areas.

The vaccine schedule is three doses on days 0, 7–14 and 28. Full immunity takes up to 1 month to develop. A booster is recommended after 2 years, if at risk. The vaccine must be given on a named-patient basis, as it is unlicensed in the UK. Precautions against mosquito bites should be taken.

Adverse reactions

- Local reaction.
- Allergic reactions and, occasionally, angioneurotic oedema occurring within minutes or up to 2 weeks after receiving the vaccine.

Contraindications

- Fever.
- History of anaphylactic hypersensitivity.
- Pregnancy.
- Cardiac, renal or hepatic disorders and generalised malignancy.

TICK-BORNE ENCEPHALITIS VACCINE

This is recommended for walkers and campers in late spring and summer, in forested areas of central and eastern Europe and Scandinavia.

Two doses are given 4–12 weeks apart, giving protection for 1 year. The vaccine is available on a named-patient basis.

Protection is afforded by covering arms, tucking long trousers into socks and using insect repellent on outer clothing.

Adverse reactions

- Very rarely, local and flu-like reactions occur.
- Rarely, neurological symptoms have occurred.

Contraindications

Allergy to egg protein.

PRIVATE MEDICAL EXAMINATIONS

Private medical examinations are often requested by either the patient or a third party. Examples include insurance company examinations, vocational driving licence examinations, sports examinations and examination of children in care.

Before agreeing to do the examination, decide the following:

- How long will it take?
- Who is requesting it?
- Who is going to pay for it and what is the fee?
- Will I need extra equipment such as ECG, colour vision charts?

Set aside enough time. The receptionist can ask the patient to produce a specimen of urine before the appointment, if necessary, to save time.

Read through the questionnaire first to establish exactly what needs examining. Leave no blank spaces.

It is acceptable to tell the patient relevant findings of the examination, especially if these have implications for health. However, refrain from committing yourself on their likely insurance/licence risk – that is for the company to decide.

HIV testing forms part of some insurance examinations and is paid for separately by the companies. Make sure the patient is prepared to receive the result from the company and that they have contemplated the consequences of a positive result.

Keep a record of all earnings from private examinations and include the date done, patient name, company name, date the payment was received and the fee. This is for chasing up late payments and also for tax purposes.

PATIENT REPORTS

When asked to write a report on a patient, e.g. for a solicitor or an insurance company, several things make the job easier.

- Has the patient given written consent for details of their medical history to be revealed to the third party? If not, return the request asking for written consent.
- Often a pro forma questionnaire will accompany the request. This specifies the information needed and will usually be brief.
- Look at the patient's notes and computer record. Is there a copy of a recently completed questionnaire in the notes? If so copy it, changing only those parts of the medical history that have occurred since the date of the last report.
- Summarised notes and computer summaries make writing reports easier. Many insurance companies accept computer-generated summaries in place of their pro formas, as long as the same information is provided. Hospital letters may be helpful.
- If the patient has asked to see the report before it is sent, keep it for 21 days before posting it.

- Personal medical attendants' reports for insurance companies attract a fee agreed with the BMA and this is usually paid on receipt of the report by the company. Solicitors' reports do not specify a fee, and an invoice should be sent with the report, asking for payment by return of post. The fee should be based on the time taken to prepare the report and the BMA hourly rate for GPs.
- For all types of private reports keep a record of the date sent, patient name, company, the date payment was received and the fee. This will give an indication of who to send a reminder to for non-payment and also a running total for tax purposes.
- In many practices, the majority of the above tasks are undertaken by secretarial staff.

NOTIFIABLE DISEASES

The following diseases are statutorily notifiable by the GP if suspected or proven:

- anthrax
- cholera
- diphtheria
- dysentery (amoebic or bacillary)
- encephalitis (acute)
- food poisoning (microbiological or chemical)
- leprosy
- leptospirosis
- malaria
- measles
- meningitis
- meningococcal septicaemia (without meningitis)
- mumps
- ophthalmia neonatorum
- paratyphoid fever
- plague
- poliomyelitis (acute)
- rabies
- relapsing fever
- rubella
- scarlet fever
- smallpox
- tetanus
- tuberculosis
- typhoid fever
- typhus
- viral haemorrhagic fever
- viral hepatitis

- whooping cough
- yellow fever.

The most common is food poisoning.

UK HIV reporting is voluntary and confidential to the Health Protection Agency (see p. 357).

Notification is made to the Local Authority Environmental Health Department. Complete the form provided by the Environmental Health Office.

Notification by telephone is essential in suspected cases of food poisoning as it allows the Environmental Health Officer to take samples of faeces, vomit and food before the infection has gone.

A small fee is payable for each notification.

MANAGEMENT OF ANAPHYLAXIS

- Lie patient in the left lateral position. If unconscious, insert an airway.
- Give adrenaline 1/1000 im unless the carotid pulse is strong and the patient's condition is good (see below).
- Give oxygen, if available, by face mask.
- Start cardiopulmonary resuscitation, if appropriate.
- The following drugs may also be given:
  - chlorphenamine maleate 5 mg iv
  - hydrocortisone 100 mg iv (to prevent further deterioration in severe cases).
- If there is no improvement in the patient's condition after 10 minutes, repeat the dose of adrenaline up to a maximum of three doses.
- Admit to hospital for observation.
- Report to the Committee on Safety of Medicines, if appropriate.

Adrenaline dosage
(Adrenaline 1/1000 = 1 mg/ml)

Adults	0.5–1.0 ml
<1 year	0.05 ml
1 year	0.1 ml
2 years	0.2 ml
3 years	0.3 ml
4 years	0.4 ml
5–10 years	0.5 ml

STANDARD GROWTH CHARTS

Data reproduced with permission of Castlemead Publications.

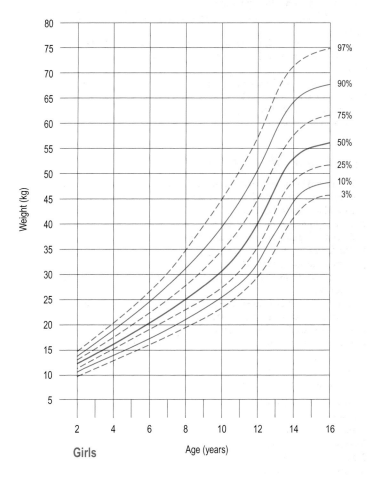

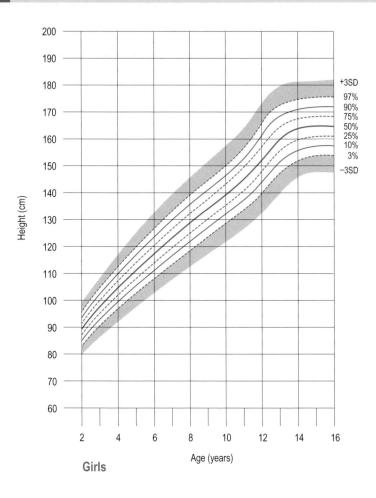

Girls

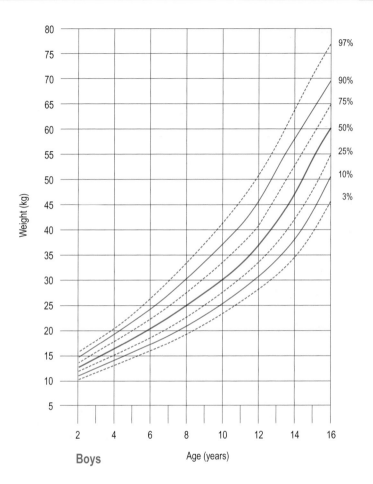

Boys

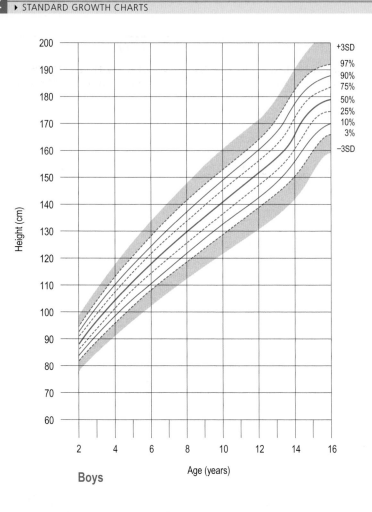

Boys

DERMATOMES

Reproduced with permission from Hayes PC, Mackay TW, Forrest EH 1996
Churchill's pocketbook of medicine, 2nd edn. Churchill Livingstone, Edinburgh

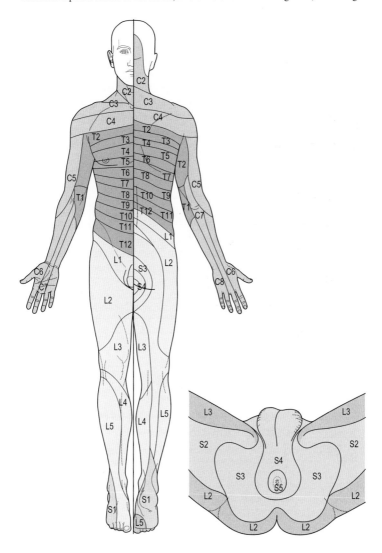

ADULT HEIGHT VERSUS WEIGHT CHART

Acknowledgements: Health Education Council, E Fullard, Oxford

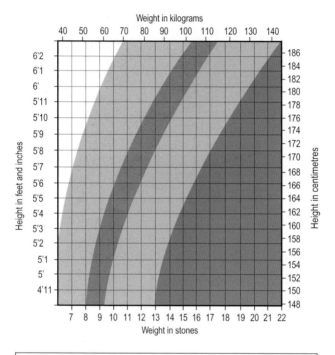

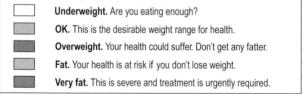

☐	**Underweight.** Are you eating enough?
▨	**OK.** This is the desirable weight range for health.
▨	**Overweight.** Your health could suffer. Don't get any fatter.
▨	**Fat.** Your health is at risk if you don't lose weight.
▨	**Very fat.** This is severe and treatment is urgently required.

USEFUL ADDRESSES AND TELEPHONE NUMBERS

Age Concern
Astral House
1268 London Road
London SW16 4ER
Tel. 020 8765 7200 (Administration)
Tel. 0800 009966 (Helpline)
www.ageconcern.org.uk

Alcoholics Anonymous (AA)
General Service Office
PO Box 1
10 Toft Green
York YO1 7ND
Tel. 01904 644026 (Administration)
Tel. 0845 769 7555 (Helpline)
www.alcoholics-anonymous.org.uk

Al-Anon Family Groups UK & Eire
61 Great Dover Street
London SE1 4YF
Tel. 020 7403 0888
www.al-anonuk.org.uk

Alzheimer's Society
Gordon House
10 Greencoat Place
London SW1P 1PH
Tel. 020 7306 0606
www.alzheimers.org.uk

beat (beating eating disorders)
103 Prince of Wales Road
Norwich NR1 1DW
Tel. 0870 770 3256 (Administration)
Tel. 0845 634 1414 (Helpline)
Tel. 0845 634 7650 (Youthline)
www.b-eat.co.uk

Breast Cancer Care
Kiln House
210 New Kings Road
London SW6 4NZ
Tel. 020 7384 2984 (Administration)
Tel. 0808 800 6000 (Helpline)
www.breastcancercare.org.uk

British Acupuncture Council
63 Jeddo Road
London W12 9HQ
Tel. 020 8735 0400
www.acupuncture.org.uk

British Association of
Psychotherapists
37 Mapesbury Road
London NW2 4HJ
Tel. 020 8452 9823
www.bap-psychotherapy.org

British Association for Counselling
and Psychotherapy
BACP House
15 St John's Business Park
Lutterworth LE17 4HB
Tel. 0870 443 5252
www.bacp.co.uk

British Heart Foundation
14 Fitzhardinge Street
London W1H 6DH
Tel. 020 7935 0185 (Administration)
Tel. 08450 708070 (Information
Line)
www.bhf.org.uk

British Homeopathic Association
Hahnemann House
29 Park Street West
Luton LU1 3BE
Tel. 0870 444 3950
www.trusthomeopathy.org

British Tinnitus Association
Ground Floor, Unit 5
Acorn Business Park
Woodseats Close
Sheffield S8 0TB
Tel. 0114 250 9922
Tel. 0800 018 0527
www.tinnitus.org.uk

Cancerbackup
3 Bath Place
Rivington Street
London EC2A 3JR
Tel. 020 7696 9003 (Administration)
Tel. 0808 800 1234 (Helpline)
www.cancerbackup.org.uk

Carers UK
20–25 Glasshouse Yard
London EC1A 4JT
Tel. 020 7490 8818 (Administration)
Tel. 0808 808 7777 (Helpline)
www.carersuk.org

Cervical Stitch Network
'Fairfield'
Wolverton Road
Norton Lindsey
Warwickshire CV35 8LA
Tel. 01926 843223

Child Death Helpline
Great Ormond Street Hospital
Great Ormond Street
London WC1N 3JH
Tel. 020 7813 8551 (Administration)
Tel. 0800 282986 (Helpline)
www.childdeathhelpline.org.uk

Childwatch
19 Spring Bank
Hull
East Yorkshire HU3 1AF
Tel. 01482 325552
www.childwatch.org.uk

CONI (Care of Next Infant)
Room C1
Stephenson Wing
Division of Child Health
The Children's Hospital
Western Bank
Sheffield S10 2TH
Tel. 0114 276 6452

CRUSE Bereavement Care
PO Box 800
Richmond
Surrey TW9 1RG
Tel. 020 8939 9530 (Administration)
Tel. 0844 477 9400 (Helpline)
www.crusebereavementcare.org.uk

Cry-sis
BM cry-sis
London WC1N 3XX
Tel. 08451 228 669 (Helpline)
www.cry-sis.org.uk

Diabetes UK
Macleod House
10 Parkway
London NW1 7AA
Tel. 020 7424 1000
www.diabetes.org.uk

Dyslexia Action
Park House
Wick Road
Egham
Surrey TW20 0HH
Tel. 01784 222300
www.dyslexiaaction.org.uk

ERIC (Education and Resources for Improving Childhood Continence)
34 Old School House
Britannia Road
Kingswood
Bristol BS15 8DB
Tel. 0845 370 8008
www.enuresis.org.uk

Foundation for the Study of Infant Deaths
Artillery House
11–19 Artillery Row
London SW1P 1RT
Tel. 020 7222 8001 (Administration)
Tel. 020 7233 2090 (Helpline)
www.fsid.org.uk

Health Protection Agency Centre for Infections
61 Colindale Avenue
London NW9 5EQ
Tel. 020 8200 4400
www.hpa.org.uk

Infertility Network UK
Charter House
43 St Leonards Road
Bexhill on Sea
East Sussex TN40 1JA
Tel. 08701 188088
www.infertilitynetworkuk.com

La Leche League (Great Britain)
PO Box 29
West Bridgford
Nottingham NG2 7NP
Tel. 0845 456 1855 (Enquiries)
Tel. 0845 120 2918 (Helpline)
www.laleche.org.uk

ME Association
4 Top Angel
Buckingham
Buckinghamshire MK18 1TH
Tel. 0870 744 8233 (Administration)
Tel. 0870 444 1836 (Helpline)
www.meassociation.org.uk

Medical Advisory Service for Travellers Abroad (MASTA)
Moorfield Road
Yeadon
Leeds
West Yorkshire LS19 7BN
Tel. 0113 238 7500 (Administration)
Tel. 0906 822 4100 (Helpline)

MedicAlert
1 Bridge Wharf
156 Caledonian Road
London N1 9UU
Tel. 020 7833 3034
Tel. 0800 581420 (Freephone)
www.medicalert.org.uk

Mencap
123 Golden Lane
London EC1Y 0RT
Tel. 020 7454 0454
www.mencap.org.uk

Miscarriage Association
c/o Clayton Hospital
Northgate
Wakefield
West Yorkshire WF1 3JS
Tel. 01924 200795 (Administration)
Tel. 01924 200799 (Helpline)
www.miscarriageassociation.org.uk

National Asthma Campaign
Summit House
70 Wilson Street
London EC2A 2DB
Tel. 020 7786 5000 (Administration)
Tel. 08457 010203 (Helpline)
www.asthma.org.uk

National Back Pain Association
– BackCare
16 Elmtree Road
Teddington
Middlesex TW11 8ST
Tel. 020 8977 5474 (Administration)
Tel. 0845 130 2704 (Helpline)
www.backcare.org.uk

National Childbirth Trust
Alexandra House
Oldham Terrace
London W3 6NH
Tel. 0870 444 8707 (Enquiries)
Tel. 0870 444 8708 (Breast-feeding
Helpline)
Tel. 0870 444 8709 (Pregnancy and
Birth Helpline)
www.nct.org.uk

National Eczema Society
Hill House
Highgate Hill
London N19 5NA
Tel. 020 7281 3553 (Administration)
Tel. 0870 241 3604 (Helpline)
www.eczema.org

NSPCC (National Society of the
Prevention of Cruelty to
 Children)
42 Curtain Road
London EC2A 3NH
Tel. 020 7825 2500 (Administration)
Tel. 0808 800 5000 (Helpline)
www.nspcc.org.uk

Parentline Plus
520 Highgate Studios
53–79 Highgate Road
London NW5 1TL
Tel. 020 7284 5536 (Administration)
Tel. 0808 800 2222 (Helpline)
(See telephone directory for regional
helplines)
www.parentlineplus.org.uk

Psoriasis Association
Milton House
7 Milton Street
Northampton NN2 7JG
Tel. 0845 676 0076
www.psoriasis-association.org.uk

Relate – National Marriage Guidance
Herbert Gray College
Little Church Street
Rugby
Warwickshire CV21 3AP
Tel. 01788 573241
Tel. 0845 456 1310
www.relate.org.uk

Release – The National Drugs and
Legal Helpline
388 Old Street
London EC1V 9LT
Tel. 020 7729 5255 (Administration)
Tel. 0845 4500 215 (Helpline)
www.release.org.uk

RNIB (Royal National Institute of
the Blind)
105 Judd Street
London WC1H 9NE
Tel. 020 7388 1266 (Administration)
Tel. 0845 766 9999 (Helpline)
www.rnib.org.uk

RNID (Royal National Institute for
Deaf People)
19–23 Featherstone Street
London EC1Y 8SL
Tel. 020 7296 8000 (Administration)
Tel. 0808 808 0123 (Helpline)
www.rnid.org.uk

The Samaritans
The Upper Mill
Kingston Road
Ewell
Surrey KT17 2AF
Tel. 020 8394 8300 (Administration)
Tel. 08457 909090 (National helpline)
(See telephone directory for local
24-hour helplines)
www.samaritans.org.uk

SANDS (Stillbirth and Neonatal
Death Society)
28 Portland Place
London W1B 1LY
Tel. 020 7436 7940 (Administration)
Tel. 020 7436 5881 (Helpline)
www.uk-sands.org

Terrence Higgins Trust
314–320 Grays Inn Road
London WC1X 8DP
Tel. 020 7812 1600 (Administration)
Tel. 0845 12 21 200 (Helpline)
www.tht.org.uk

Weight Watchers UK
Millennium House
Ludlow Road
Maidenhead
Berkshire SL6 2SL
Tel. 0845 345 1500
www.weightwatchers.co.uk

Index

AA (Alcoholics Anonymous), 355
Abdominal aortic aneurysm, 80–81
Abdominal examination
    appendicitis, 271
    neonate, 84
    postnatal, 34
Abortion, 60–61
    spontaneous (miscarriage),
        15, 23, 27–28
Absence seizures, 97–98
Abuse
    child abuse, 99–101
    sexual, 100
ACE inhibitors, 150, 160, 162, 333
Acetazolamide, 232
Aciclovir, 193, 197, 198, 230, 250
Acne, 131–133
Actinomyces-like organisms (ALOs), 58
Acupuncture: British Acupuncture Council,
        355
Adcortyl, 221
Adhesive capsulitis (frozen shoulder), 246
Adrenaline, 348
Age Concern, 355
Agranulocytosis, 112, 333
AIDS, 2, 201–202
Al-Anon Family Groups, 355
Alcoholics Anonymous (AA), 355
Alcohol intake
    Alcoholics Anonymous, 355
    alcohol abuse, 310–313
    as aperitif, 322
    epileptic trigger, 287
    gout, 239
Alendronic acid, 244
Allergies, skin, 143
Allopurinol, 240
Alopecia areata, 138
Alphosyl, 140, 141
Aluminium chloride hexahydrate, 138
Alzheimer's disease, 303–305

Alzheimer's Society, 355
Amenorrhoea, 9, 43–44
Amitriptyline, 123, 198
Amlodipine, 150, 157
Amniocentesis, 27
Amorolfine, 136
Amoxicillin, 33, 65, 118, 119, 261
    ENT, 212, 213, 217
    infectious diseases, 191, 205
    respiratory infections, 177, 179, 180,
        181, 185
    'standby', 261
Amphotericin, 136, 220
Ampicillin, 6
Anaemia, 258–260
    pregnancy, 30–31
Anal fissure, 268
Anaphylaxis, 348
Androgenic alopecia, 138
Aneurysm
    abdominal aortic, 80–81
    dissecting, 154, 155
Angina, 156–158
    anaemic, 258
Animal mites, 143
Ankles
    sprained, 254–255
    swollen, 29, 161
Anorexia
    anorexia nervosa, 301–302
    in the terminally ill, 321–322
    see also Bulimia nervosa
Antacids, 29, 117, 118, 318
Anticholinergics, 123, 184, 289
Anticonvulsants, 23, 287
Anti-D immunoglobin, 27, 28, 31
Antidepressants, 34, 75, 191, 277, 293, 296,
        322
Antihistamines, 137, 139, 143,
        215, 229
Antimalarials, 196, 261

Anxiety, 294–295
    in the terminally ill, 322–323
Appendicitis, 270–271
Arc eye, 230
Arrhythmias, 165–168
Arterial ulcers, 144
Arthritis *see* Osteoarthritis; Rheumatoid
        arthritis; Septic arthritis
Aspirin, 150, 157, 159, 160, 167, 176, 194
    CVA, 280
Asthma, 170–175
    in children, 94–97
    National Asthma Campaign, 357
Atenolol, 150, 157
Athlete's foot, 135–136
Atrial fibrillation, 167, 168
Atropine, 181
Azathioprine, 122, 333
Azelaic acid, 132

Babies *see* Infants; Neonates
Back pain, 251–252
    National Back Pain Association, 357
    pregnancy, 32
Baclofen, 319
Bacterial infections
    bacterial vaginosis (BV), 45, 46
    skin, 133–134
    staphylococcal, 134, 139, 199
    streptococcal, 133, 190, 218, 219
    vesicles, 198
Bad news, 316
Barium enema, 125
Basal body temperature, 17, 60
Basal cell carcinoma (rodent ulcer), 131
BCG vaccine, 339–340
Beat (beat eating disorders), 355
Beclometasone
    asthma, 95, 96, 97, 172, 173, 179
    COPD, 184
    hay fever, 215
    nasal blockage, 217, 222
    sinusitis, 217
Bed bugs, 143
Bed-wetting, 88–89
Behaviour
    disturbed, 305–306
    violent, 306–307
Bell's palsy, 279

Bendroflumethiazide, 150, 161
Benign superficial lumps, 130
Benperidol, 304
Benzodiazepine addiction, 297, 308
Benzoyl peroxide, 132
Benzydamine spray, 192, 221
Benzylpenicillin, 189
Bereavement, 327–328
    CRUSE Bereavement Care, 356
Beta-blockers, 150, 156, 157, 160, 162
    eyedrops, 235
Betamethasone (Betnovate), 139, 140
Billing's method, 17
BiNovum, 5
Birth control
    contraceptives *see* Contraception
    natural, 16–17
    sterilisation, 17–18
Bisacodyl, 323
Bladder
    instability, 289
    neuropathic, 88, 89
    paralysis, 251
    retraining, 69–70
Bleeding
    breakthrough, 4, 7, 10, 39
    haemoptysis, 181–182
    intermenstrual, 39–40
    irregular, 9, 40
    menstrual *see* Menstruation
    nose bleeds, 215–216
    occult, 126
    postcoital, 39–40
    postmenopausal, 40, 52
    postpartum, 30, 32–33
    pregnancy, 27–28
    rectal, 122, 125–126, 268–269
    STI risks, 2
    subconjunctival haemorrhage, 229
Blepharitis, 226
Blindness *see* Visual loss
Blood glucose
    diabetes, 106–108, 110–111
    glucose tolerance tests, 29–30, 107
    pregnancy, 22, 29–30
Blood pressure, 111, 147–148, 151, 158, 281
Blushing, 138
BMI (body mass index), 6, 11, 113, 114,
        152, 222
Body hair, 48–49

Boils, 198–199
  ears, 213
Bone density scans, 119
Bone pain, 319
Bottle-feeding, 85–86
Botulinum type A toxin injections (Botox), 138
Bowel colic (in terminal condition), 319
Bowel disease
  inflammatory bowel (Crohn's) disease, 122
  irritable bowel syndrome, 122–123
Bowel habit changes, 121
Breast Cancer Care, 355
Breast-feeding, 35–36, 85
  anticonvulsants, 287
Breasts
  blocked ducts, 35
  cancer, 18, 50, 51, 53
  engorgement, 35
  lumps, 35, 265–266
  mastitis, 35–36
  painful, 266
  screening, 50
  self-examination, 50
Brevinor, 5, 7
British Acupuncture Council, 355
British Association for Counselling and Psychotherapy, 355
British Association of Psychotherapists, 355
British Heart Foundation, 355
British Homeopathic Association, 356
British Tinnitus Association, 356
Bromocriptine, 36, 39
Bronchial carcinoma, 182
Bronchiectasis, 180, 183
Bronchiolitis, 94
Bronchitis, 182
Bronchodilators
  asthma, 95, 170–171, 173–174, 175
  COPD, 183, 184, 185
  hay fever, 215
Bronchopneumonia, 181, 194
Bulimia nervosa, 302–303
Bupropion, 314
Bursitis, prepatellar, 253, 254
Butyrophenones, 284

Calamine, 143, 193
Calcaneum, 255

Calcipotriol (Dovonex), 140, 141
Calcium-channel blockers, 150, 157
Calender method of birth control, 16–17
Campylobacter, 121
Cancer see specific cancers
Cancerbackup, 356
Candida infections, 136
  nappy rash, 91
  vaginal, 45–46
Carbamazepine, 278, 287
Carbimazole, 112, 219
Cardiovascular disease (CVD)
  lifestyle advice for prevention, 146
  risk factors, 146–149
Carers UK, 356
Carpel tunnel syndrome, 249
Carvedilol, 162
Cataract, 234
Cellulitis, 133
Cerazette, 5, 10
Cerebrovascular accident (CVA/stroke), 232, 280–281
Cervical cancer, 58–59
Cervical erosions, 40
Cervical lymphadenopathy, 219–220
Cervical polyps, 40
Cervical spondylosis, 240, 246
Cervical Stitch Network, 356
Cetirizine, 215
Chalazion, 226
Chest infection, 179–180
Chest pain, 154–159
Chickenpox, 193
  vaccination, 343
Child abuse, 99–101
  child protection procedures, 100–101
  NSPCC, 358
Child Death Helpline, 356
Childwatch, 356
Chlamydia, 15, 46–47, 76–77
  screening, 39
Chloramphenicol, 225, 228, 229, 230
Chlordiazepoxide, 312
Chlorhexadine
  cream, 138
  mouth rinse, 119, 221
Chloroquine, 196
Chlorpromazine, 295, 322
Cholera vaccine, 344
Cholesteatoma, 212

Cholesterol, 151–153
Chondromalacia patellae, 253, 254
Chorionic villus biopsy, 26
Chronic fatigue syndrome, 299–300
Chronic obstructive pulmonary disease
  (COPD), 183–185
Cilest, 5, 132
Cimetidine, 117
Ciprofloxacin, 47, 79, 120, 121, 177
Circumcision, 264
Citalopram, 293, 295, 322
Claudication, 153–154
Climacteric see Menopause
Clindamycin, 132
Clobetasol propionate (Dermovate), 139
Clobetasone butyrate (Eumovate), 139
Clomiphene, 44, 50, 60
Clomipramine, 295
Clonidine, 309
Clopidogrel, 280
Clotrimazole, 45, 46, 77, 136
Clubbing, 183
Coal tar, 139, 141
Co-amoxiclav, 33, 122, 177, 185
COC see Combined oral contraceptive
Co-codamol, 221, 252, 267, 317
Co-danthramer, 323
Codeine, 277
Codeine phosphate, 123, 290
Coeliac disease, 119–120
Coil see Intrauterine contraceptive device
  (IUCD)
Colchicine, 239
Cold sores, 197
Colds, 179, 212, 340
  infant coryza, 93–94
Colic
  babies, 35, 86–87, 265
  bowel colic (in terminal
    condition), 319
  ureteric, 66, 67
Colonic carcinoma, 121
Combined contraceptive transdermal
  patch, 8
Combined oral contraceptive (COC), 3–8
  acne, 132
  anticonvulsants with, 287
  menorrhagia, 43
  perimenopausal use, 18
  postpartum, 19

Compulsory admission, 307–308
Condoms, 13
Congestive cardiac failure, 161–163
CONI (Care of Next Infant), 356
Conjunctivitis, 215, 225,
  228–229
Consciousness, loss of, 163–165, 286
Constipation, 124–125
  acute, 87, 125
  chronic, 87, 124
  infants and children, 87–88
  irritable bowel syndrome, 122–123
  in the terminally ill, 323
Contraception, 2–19, 23
  anticonvulsants with, 287
  combined oral, 3–8, 18, 19, 43, 132
  combined transdermal patch, 8
  condoms, 13
  diaphragms, 13–14
  Fraser guidelines, 2–3
  injectable progestogens, 10–11
  intrauterine contraceptive device (IUCD),
    12–13, 14–16, 39, 58
  perimenopausal, 18
  postcoital, 11–13
  postpartum, 19
  progestogen-only pill (POP),
    8–10, 18, 19
  progestogen-releasing implant
    (Implanon), 11
  see also Birth control
Controlled drugs, 310, 319–320
Convulsions, 98–99
  see also Epilepsy; Seizures
COPD (chronic obstructive pulmonary
  disease), 183–185
Corneal abrasion, 229
Corneal foreign body, 230
Corneal light reflex, 226
Coronary heart disease, primary prevention,
  146–149
Corticosteroids, 122, 171, 174, 242, 247
Coryza, 93–94
Coughs
  acute, 176–178
  chronic, 178–179
  infants, 94
  terminal disease, 179, 323–324
  see also Whooping cough
Counselling

British Association for Counselling and Psychotherapy, 355
preconceptual, 22–23
Cover test, 226
Coxsackie viral infection, 192
Crab lice, 142–143
Cremation form, 325, 326–327
Crohn's disease, 122
Croup, 94
CRUSE Bereavement Care, 356
Cryotherapy, 47, 135
Cry-sis, 356
CVA (cerebrovascular accident), 232, 280–281
Cyclizine, 321
Cyproterone acetate, 49
Cystitis, 48, 79

Danazol, 42
De Quervain's tenosynovitis, 248
Deafness, 210–211
Death, 325–327
infants see SIDS (sudden death syndrome)
see also Bereavement
Decarboxylase inhibitor, dopa, 284
Deep-vein thrombosis, 330
Dementia, 303–305
Dental abscess, 213, 221
Depo-Provera, 11
Depression, 292–294
postnatal, 33–34
in the terminally ill, 324
Dermatitis
candida, 91, 136
eczema, 138–140
seborrhoeic, 137
Dermatomes, 353
Dervovate, 139
Desmopressin, 89
Desogestrel, 5, 6
Detrusor instability, 69–70
Dexamethasone, 319, 322
Diabetes, 106–111
gestational, 30
preconceptual counselling, 23
risk factors, 106
Diabetes UK, 356
Diamorphine, 159, 162, 317, 318, 321
Dianette, 7, 49, 50, 132, 133

Diaphragms, 13–14
Diarrhoea
infective, 120–121
irritable bowel syndrome, 122–123
Diazepam, 98, 182, 241, 252, 295
in the terminally ill, 319, 322
Diclofenac, 267, 317, 318
Diet
atopic eczema, 140
cholesterol control, 152
coeliac disease, 120
constipation, 88, 124
diabetes, 108, 109
gout, 239
obesity, 113
preconceptual, 22–23
vitamins see Vitamins
Digoxin, 167, 331–332
Dihydrocodeine, 277, 317
Dimethicone (Infacol), 87
Diprosalic scalp application, 141
Dipstick testing, 64, 66, 67, 69, 89, 90, 181
Diptheria vaccine, 336–337
Dipyridamole, 280
Dissecting aneurysm, 154, 155
Disturbed behaviour, 305–306
Dithranol, 140
Diuretic monitoring, 333
Diverticulitis, 121–122
Dizziness, 274
Docusate sodium, 323
Domperidone, 123, 321
Donepezil, 304
L-dopa, 284
Dovonex, 140, 141
Down's syndrome, 26, 27
Doxycycline, 45, 47, 77, 132, 205
Driving, 160, 234, 274, 287
DVLA notification, 109, 165, 281, 289
Drospirenone, 5, 6, 55
Drug addiction
benzodiazepines, 297, 308
opiates, 308–310
Release - The National Drugs and Legal Helpline, 358
Drug monitoring, 330–334
Dry eye, 225
Duchenne muscular dystrophy, 27
Dydrogesterone, 39, 55, 57
Dyslexia Action, 356

Dysmenorrhoea, 40–41
Dyspareunia, 41, 45, 58
Dyspepsia, 116–118
Dyspnoea
    COPD, 183–185
    in the terminally ill, 324–325

Ears
    discharge, 211–212
    earache, 212–213
    glue ear, 210, 217
    perforated drum, 212
    wax, 210, 213
Eating disorders, 301–303
    beat (beat eating disorders), 355
Econazole, 136
Ectopic pregnancy, 15, 44
Ectropion, 224, 225
Eczema, 138–140
    National Eczema Society, 358
Elbow, tennis, 248
Electrolysis, 49
Emergency contraception, 11–13
Emollients, 139
Emotional abuse, 100
Encephalitis vaccines, 345
Endometriosis, 41–42
Endometrium
    cancer, 54
    contraceptives and, 4, 14, 16
    hyperplasia, 54
    transcervical resection (TCRE), 43
Endoscopy, 116, 118, 125
Enemas, 88, 125, 289, 323
Entropion, 224–225
Enuresis, 88–89
Epicondylitis, lateral, 248
Epididymo-orchitis, 79
Epilepsy, 285–288
    children, 97–98
    during pregnancy, 23
    status epilepticus, 98
Epistaxis, 215–216
Erectile dysfunction, 74–75
ERIC (Education and Resources for
        Improving Childhood Continence),
        357
Erysipelas, 133
Erythrasma, 134

Erythromycin, 35, 47, 58, 121
    dermatological conditions, 132, 133, 134,
        139, 144
    ENT, 213, 218, 219
    infectious diseases, 188, 190
    respiratory infections, 177,
        180, 181
Ethinyloestradiol, 4, 8
Eugynon-30, 5, 7, 42
Eumovate, 139, 140
Eustachian tube dysfunction, 213
Evening primrose oil (gamolenic acid), 38,
        246, 266
Exorex, 140
Eyelids, 225–226
Eyes
    acute red eye, 227–230
    discharging eye, 224
    dry eye, 225
    floaters, 235
    painful eye, 230–231
    squints, 226–227

Facial pain, 277–279
Failure to thrive, 90, 92, 100
Fainting/faintness, 163, 164, 166, 274, 286
        see also Epilepsy
Falls, 284–285
Family planning see Birth control;
        Contraception
Fasciitis, plantar, 255–256
Fatigue, 119, 161, 191, 218, 298–300
    post-viral, 191
Febrile convulsions, 98–99
Femodene, 5, 7, 132
Femulen, 5
Ferrous fumarate, 259
Ferrous sulphate tablets, 259
Fifth disease, 192
Fish oils, 246
Fits, 99, 286–288
        see also Convulsions; Epilepsy;
        Seizures
Flea bites, 143
Floaters, 235
Flucloxacillin, 35, 250, 254, 256
    dermatological conditions, 133, 134,
        139, 144
    infectious diseases, 193, 194, 198, 199

Fluoride, 86
Fluorouracil, 131
Fluoxetine, 293, 296
Foetal abnormalities, 23, 26, 28
Folate, 30, 119, 260
    deficiency, 31, 259, 260
    prophylaxis, 31
Folic acid, 22, 23, 260
Folliculitis, 134
Foreign bodies
    ear, 211
    eye, 224, 230
    nose, 216
    vagina, 45
Formula milk, 85, 86
Foundation for the Study of Infant Deaths,
    357
Frozen shoulder, 246
FSH (follicle-stimulating hormone), 18, 42,
    44, 50, 52
Fucithalmic ointment, 226
Fungal infections, 135–137
    candida, see Candida infections
Funny turns, 163–165
Furosemide, 159, 162, 266
Fusidic acid, 134, 139, 193, 198, 225,
    229, 251

Gabapentin, 198
Galantamine, 304
Gallstones, 127, 266–267
Gamolenic acid (evening primrose oil), 38,
    246, 266
Ganglions, 250
Gardnerella, 45
Gastro-intestinal pain (in terminal
    condition), 318
Gastro-oesophageal reflux disease (GORD),
    118
Gaviscon, 117
Genital herpes, 47–48
Genital warts, 47
Gentamicin, 210
Gentisone HC eardrops, 213
Gestodene, 5, 6
Giant cell (temporal) arteritis,
    232, 242–243
Giardiasis, 121
Gingivitis, 221
Glandular fever, 190–191

Glaucoma
    acute angle closure, 232
    chronic open-angle, 234–235
Gliclazide, 110
Glucagon, 111
Glucosamine, 242
Glucose
    blood glucose see Blood glucose
    oral, 107, 111
Glucose tolerance test
    modified, 29–30
    oral, 107
Glue ear, 210, 217
Glycerol, 323
Glyceryl trinitrate ointment, 268
Glycosuria, 29–30
Goitre, 112, 113
Gold, 333
Gonorrhoea, 45, 47
GORD (gastro-oesophageal reflux disease),
    118
Gout, 239–240
Graves' disease, 112
Grief, 102
Griseofulvin, 6
Groin herniae, 267–268
Groin ringworm, 135
Growth charts, 349–352
Growth problems, 92–93
GTN (glyceril trinitrate), 156, 157, 162
Gum disease, 221
Guttate psoriasis, 141

H_2 receptor antagonists, 117, 118
Haematemesis, 321
Haematuria, 64, 65, 66, 90, 150
Haemoglobin, 30
    electrophoresis, 22
Haemoglobinopathies, 260
Haemophilia, 27
Haemophilus influenza B (Hib) vaccine,
    261, 334, 337
Haemophilus influenzae, 260
Haemoptysis, 181–182
Haemorrhage see Bleeding
Haemorrhoids, 125, 268–269
Hair
    hair loss, 138
    hirsutism, 48–49
Halitosis, 118–119

Haloperidol, 304, 305, 322
Hand, foot and mouth disease, 192
Hay fever, 214–215
    conjunctivitis, 229
Head growth, 93
Head injury, 290
Head lice, 141–142
Headache, 275–277
    migraine, 232–233, 276–277
Heaf test, 340
Health Protection Agency Centre for
        Infections, 357
Hearing tests, 210
Heart failure, 159, 161–163
Heart Foundation, British, 355
Heartburn
    pregnancy, 28–29
Heel, painful (plantar fasciitis), 255–256
Height, 93
    height versus weight chart, 354
Helicobacter pylori, 117–118
Hepatitis, 127, 199–201
    hepatitis A vaccine, 341–342
    hepatitis B vaccine, 342
Herniae
    groin, 267–268
    paediatric, 264–265
    umbilical, 264–265
Herpes simplex virus
    cold sores, 197
    genital, 47–48
Herpes zoster virus
    eye infection, 230
    vaccination, 343
Hidradenitis suppurativa, 133
Hirschsprung's disease, 87
Hirsutism, 48–49
HIV/AIDS, 2, 201–202
    private HIV testing, 346
Hoarseness, 220
Homeopathic Association, British, 356
Hormonal postcoital contraception, 11–12
Hormone replacement therapy (HRT),
        52–57, 244
HPV (human papilloma virus), 47
HRT (hormone replacement therapy),
        52–57, 244
Human papilloma virus (HPV), 47
Hydrocele, 264
Hydrocephalus, 84, 93

Hydrocortisone, 126, 139, 143, 175, 249, 256
Hydroxocobalamin, 259
Hyoscine, 181, 325
    hyoscine hydrobromide, 319, 325
Hyperhydrosis, 138
Hyperlipidaemia, 3, 149, 152, 239
Hypertension, 149–151
    pregnancy, 23
Hyperventilation, 295
Hypoglycaemia, 108, 110–111, 165, 305, 306
Hypotension, 159
    postural, 165
Hypothryroidism, 111–113
Hypromellose eyedrops, 225

IBS (irritable bowel syndrome), 122–123
Ibuprofen, 79, 181, 242, 290, 317
IHD *see* Ischaemic heart disease
Imidazoles, 45, 46, 91, 134, 136, 137
Immunisations, 334–345
    passive immunisation, 335
        see also Vaccinations
Immunoglobulin, 206, 335, 338, 339, 341
    anti-D, 27, 28, 31
    hepatitis B, 342
    rabies-specific, 343
    tetanus, 337
    varicella-zoster, 193, 343
Imodium, 309
Impetigo, 134, 193
Implanon, 11
Impotence (erectile dysfunction), 74–75
Incapacity after surgery, 271–272
Incontinence
    bed-wetting, 88–89
    ERIC (Education and Resources for
        Improving Childhood Continence),
        357
    faecal, 87–88
    urinary, 67–70, 88–89
Indometacin, 239
Infants
    6–8-week check, 84–85
    abuse *see* Child abuse
    babies with colic, 35, 86–87, 265
    bronchiolitis, 94
    Child Death Helpline, 356
    CONI (Care of Next Infant), 356
    constipation, 87

feeding, 85–86
Foundation for the Study of Infant Deaths, 357
growth problems, 92–93
nappy rash, 91
National Childbirth Trust, 358
obesity, 93
preschool check, 92
SANDS (Stillbirth and Neonatal Death Society), 359
seizures and convulsions, 97–99
sudden death, 101–103
urinary tract infection, 90
weaning, 86
  see also Neonates
Infertility, 59–60
Infertility Network UK, 357
Inflammatory bowel disease, 122
Influenza, 193–194
  vaccinations, 109, 184, 194, 261, 337, 340
Ingrowing toenail, 256
Inhalers, 171–175, 180, 184, 215, 220
Insomnia, 296–297
Interferon alfa, 201
Intertrigol angular stomatitisl chronic paronychia, 136
Intrauterine contraceptive device (IUCD), 14–16
  bleeding, 39
  infections, 58
  postcoital use, 12–13
  progestogen-only system (Mirena/IUS), 16
Intrauterine pregnancy, 15
Intussusception, 265
Iontophoresis, 138
Ipratropium bromide inhaler, 184
Iron prophylaxis, 30
Iron-deficiency anaemia, 30, 116, 126, 258–259
Irritable bowel syndrome (IBS), 122–123
Ischaemic heart disease (IHD), 50, 113, 153, 155–156
  angina, 156–158
  transient ischaemic attacks, 149, 165
Isosorbide mononitrate, 157
Isotretinoin, 133
Ispaghula husk, 123, 124, 269
Itraconazole, 46, 136, 137
IUCD *see* Intrauterine contraceptive device

Japanese B encephalitis vaccine, 345
Jaundice, 127
  gallstones, 266–267
  neonatal, 85
  Weil's disease, 204
Joint pain, 238–239

Kenalog, 215
Keratoses, solar, 131
Keratosis pilaris, 141
Ketoconazole, 137
Kliofem, 54, 56
Knee pain, 252–254
Koplik's spots, 205

La Leche League, 357
Labyrinthine disorder, 210
Labyrinthitis, 274–275
Lacrimal duct massage, 224
Lactation, suppression, 36
Lactulose, 252, 323
Lansoprazole, 117, 118, 179
Laparoscopic sterilisation, 17–18
Laparoscopy, 41
Laryngitis, viral, 220
Laryngotracheobronchitis (croup), 94
L-dopa, 284
La Leche League, 357
Left ventricular failure, 162
Leg problems, paediatric, 265
Leptospirosis, 204
Leukotriene receptor antagonists, 95, 96, 97, 172, 173
Levonorgestrel, 5–6, 12, 55, 57
Levothyroxine, 112
LH (luteinising hormone), 44, 50
  kits, 60
Lidocaine, 256
Limp, 265
Lisinopril, 162
Listeriosis, 22
Lithium, 330–331
Lochia, 32–33
Locorten-Vioform, 213
Loestrin, 5, 7
Lofepramine, 34
Logynon, 5, 7
Long-acting beta-agonists, 95, 97, 172, 173, 184

Loperimide, 120, 319
Loratadine, 143, 215, 229
Loss of consciousness, 163–165, 286
Lower respiratory tract infections (LRTIs), 177–178
Lumbar back pain, 251–252
Lung cancer, 183
Luteinising hormone *see* LH
Lyme disease, 205
Lymphadenopathy, cervical, 219–220

Maalox, 29
Macrocytic anaemia, 259–260
Macrocytosis, 259–260
Madopar, 284
Magnesium hydroxide, 124
Magnesium sulphate, 199
Magnesium trisilicate, 117
Malaria, 194–196, 261
Malathion, 142, 143
Malignant melanoma, 130–131
Mammography, 50, 51, 53, 266
Manic depression, 294
Mantoux test, 340
Marvelon, 5, 7, 132
Mastalgia, cyclical, 266
Mastitis, 35–36
Mastoiditis, 213
ME Association, 357
Measles, 205–206
    measles/mumps/rubella vaccine, 338–339
Mebendazole, 126
Mebeverine, 123
Medic Alert, 357
Medical Advisory Service for Travellers Abroad (MASTA), 357
Medroxyprogesterone, 55, 56, 57
Mefenamic acid, 41, 42
Mefloquine, 196
Meibomian cysts, 226
Melaena, 125
Melanoma, 130–131
Mencap, 357
Ménière's disease, 214, 274
Meningitis, 99, 188–189
    mumps meningitis, 206–207
    vaccine, 334, 342
Meningococcal vaccinations, 261, 342
Menopause

diagnosis, 51–52
    hormone replacement therapy, 52–57, 244
    perimenopausal contraception, 18
Menorrhagia, 41, 42–43
Menstruation, 40–43
    dysmenorrhoea, 40–41
    endometriosis, 41–42
    irregular bleeding, 9, 40
    menorrhagia, 42–43
    perimenopausal bleeds, 54
Mental Health Act, 307–308
Mercilon, 5, 7
Metformin, 50, 110
Methotrexate, 333
Methyldopa, 23
Methylprednisolone, 242, 246, 247, 249, 256
Metoclopramide, 123, 321
Metronidazole, 33, 45, 46, 118, 119, 121, 122, 133, 144, 191, 213, 221, 271
MI *see* Myocardial infarction
Miconazole, 134, 136
Microgynon 30, 5, 7
Micronor, 5, 57
Midazolam, 323
Mifepristone, 61
Migraine, 232–233, 276–277
Migraleve, 277
Minocycline, 132
Minoxidil, 138
Minulet, 5, 132
Mirena/IUS, 16
Miscarriage, 15, 23, 27–28
Miscarriage Association, 357
Mites, animal, 143
MMR (measles/mumps/rubella) vaccine, 338–339
Moles, 130
Molluscum contagiosum, 135
Mononucleosis, infectious (glandular fever), 190–191
Montelukast, 95, 173
Morphine, 159, 179, 318, 324
    diamorphine, 159, 162, 317, 318, 321
    morphine sulphate, 317, 318
Mouth ulcers, 221
Movicol, 323
Mucothermal method of birth control, 17
Multiple sclerosis, 288–289
Mumps, 206–207
    measles/mumps/rubella vaccine, 338–339

Muscle spasm, 319
Myeloma, 238, 243
Myocardial infarction (MI)
    acute, 158–160
    admission, 155, 158
    diagnosis, 154, 155
    emergency treatment of arrhythmias
        following, 167
    postmyocardial infarction, 160–161
Myocardial ischaemia, 155, 156
    see also Angina

Nappy rash, 91
Naproxen, 41, 239
Nasal blockage, 216–217, 222
Naseptin cream, 199
National Asthma Campaign, 357
National Back Pain Association, 357
National Childbirth Trust, 358
National Eczema Society, 358
National Society for the Prevention of
    Cruelty to Children, 358
Natural birth control, 16–17
Nausea
    pregnancy, 28
    in the terminally ill, 320–321
Neck pain, 240–241
Neglect
    child, 100
    death from, 326
Neisseria gonorrhoeae, 45
Neisseria meningitidis, 188, 260
Neonatal jaundice, 85
Neonates
    examination, 84–85
    immunisations, 85
    nappy rash, 91
Nerve pain (in terminal condition), 319
Neural tube defects, 22, 23, 26
Neuralgia
    postherpetic, 198
    trigeminal, 278
Neutropenia, 219
Nicotine replacement therapy (NRT),
    313–314
Nifedipine, 163
Nipples, sore/cracked, 35
Nitrate tablets/spray, 156, 157
Nitrofurantoin, 65, 90

Nits, 141–142
Nocturnal enuresis (bed-wetting), 88–89
Non-accidental injuries, 99–100, 290
Non-steroidal anti-inflammatory drugs see
    NSAIDs
Norelgestromin, 8
Norethisterone, 5–6, 38, 39, 42, 43, 55–57
Norgeston, 5
Noriday, 5
Norimin, 5
Norinyl, 5
Nose, blocked, 216–217, 222
Nose bleeds, 215–216
Notifiable diseases, 347–348
Nozovent, 222
NRT (nicotine replacement therapy),
    313–314
NSAIDs (non-steroidal anti-inflammatory
    drugs), 181, 241, 247, 248, 249, 256
    contraindications, 125, 126, 171
    dyspepsia, 116
    gout, 239–240
    migraine, 277
    osteoarthritis, 242
    palliative care, 318
    premenstrual syndrome, 38
    rheumatoid arthritis, 246
    temporomandibular joint dysfunction,
        278
    in the terminally ill, 319
    urinary stones, 67
NSPCC (National Society for the
    Prevention of Cruelty to Children),
    358
Nutrition see Diet
Nuvelle, 54
Nystatin, 91, 136, 220, 221

Obesity, 113–114
    infants, 93
Obsessive–compulsive disorder (OCD),
    295–296
Oedema
    angioneurotic, 345
    ankles, 29, 161
    cobblestone, 228
    pregnancy, 31
    pulmonary, 162
    scrotal, 79

Oedema (*cont'd*)
  tumours, 319
  venous ulcers, 143
Oesophagitis/reflux, 155, 156
Oestradiol, 38, 55–57
    see also Ethinyloestradiol
Oestrogens
  combined oral contraceptive, 4–5, 6, 7–8, 18, 19
  hormone replacement therapy, 53–57, 244
  premenstrual syndrome, 38
Omeprazole, 156, 242, 246
Opiate addiction, 308–310
Oral hygiene, 118–119
Orchitis, 79, 206, 207
Oseltamivir, 194
Osteoarthritis, 240, 241–242
Osteoporosis, 243–244
Otitis externa, 213
Otitis media, 213
Otosclerosis, 53
Otosporin, 213
Ovranette, 5
Ovulation, 60
Ovysmen, 5
Oxybutynin, 70, 289
Oxytetracycline, 132, 133

Paediatric surgery, 264–265
Pain control in terminal care, 316–319
Palliative care, 316–328
Palpitations, 165–168
Panic attacks, 294, 295
Paracetamol, 93, 94, 99, 176, 180, 193, 194
  earache, 213
  head injury, 290
  migraine, 277
  palliative care, 317
  rheumatoid arthritis, 246
Parentline Plus, 358
Parkinson's disease, 283–284
Paronychia, 136, 250–251
Patient reports, 346–347
PE (pulmonary embolus), 154, 155, 182
Peak flow measurement, 170–171, 173–174
Pelvic inflammatory disease (PID), 44–45
Pelvic pain, 44–45
Penicillamine, 334
Penicillin, 58, 133, 190

benzylpenicillin, 189
  penicillin V, 213, 218, 221, 261
Peppermint oil, 123
Perimenopausal contraception, 18
Perindopril, 150
Peripheral vascular disease, 107, 146, 149, 150, 152, 153
Permethrin, 142
Pernicious anaemia, 258, 259
Persona, 17
Pertussis (whooping cough), 188
  vaccine, 335–336
Pethidine, 67
Peyronie's disease, 74, 75–76
Phenobarbital, 287
Phenothiazines, 284, 324
Phenytoin, 287, 332–333
Phimosis, 264
Pholcodine, 179, 324
PID (pelvic inflammatory disease), 44–45
Piles (haemorrhoids), 125, 268–269
Pilocarpine drops, 232
Pityriasis rosea, 137, 141
Pityriasis versicolor, 137
Pizotifen, 277
Placental abruption, 28
Plantar fasciitis, 255–256
Plantar warts, 134–135
Plasmodium falciparum, 195
Pneumococcal vaccination, 109, 261, 340–341
Pneumococcus, 260
Pneumocystis jiroveci (formerly *carinii*), 202
Pneumocystis jiroveci (formerly *P. carinii*), 202
Pneumonia, 180–181, 182
  postinfluenza bronchopneumonia, 194
Podophyllin, 47
Polio vaccine, 338
Polycystic ovarian syndrome, 49–50
Polymylagia rheumatica (PMR), 242, 243
Polyps, cervical, 40
Postcoital emergency contraception, 11–13
Postmyocardial infarction, 160–161
Postnatal check, 34
Postnatal depression, 33–34
Postpartum period
  bleeding, 30, 32–33
  contraception, 19
  pyrexia, 33

Postural hypotension, 165
Postviral fatigue syndrome, 191, 299
Potassium citrate, 48, 65
Potassium permanganate, 138
Preconceptual counselling, 22–23
    epilepsy, 287
Prednisolone, 322
    anorexia, 322
    asthma, 96, 173, 175
    Bell's palsy, 279
    COPD, 185
    eczema, 140
    giant cell arteritis, 232
    glandular fever, 191
    inflammatory bowel disease, 122
    methylprednisolone, 242, 246, 247,
        249, 256
    mumps, 207
    polymyalgia rheumatica, 243
    urticaria, 143
    vaccine contraindication, 335
Pre-eclampsia, 31–32
Pregaday, 30
Pregnancy
    abnormal lie, 32
    anaemia, 30–31
    antenatal checkups, 25
    anxieties following previous infant death,
        102–103
    back pain, 32
    bleeding, 27–28
    booking visit, 23–25
    diagnostic tests, 26–27
    ectopic, 15, 44
    epilepsy, 23
    glycosuria, 29–30
    heartburn, 28–29
    high head, 32
    hypertension, 23
    intrauterine, 15
    miscarriage, 15, 23, 27–28
    National Childbirth Trust, 358
    nausea and vomiting, 28
    oedema, 31
    preconceptual counselling,
        22–23, 287
    pre-eclampsia, 31–32
    prenatal screening, 25–26
    proteinuria, 30
    swollen ankles, 29
    termination, 60–61
    varicose veins, 29
Premarin, 53, 56, 57
Premature ejaculation, 75
Premenstrual syndrome, 38–39
Premique, 54, 55, 56
Prempak-C, 54
Prenatal screening, 25–26, 31
Prepatellar bursitis, 253, 254
Preschool check, 92
Primodine, 287
Private medical examinations, 346
Procainamide, 203
Prochlorperazine, 159, 321
Proctoscopy, 125
Progesterone, 60
    medroxyprogesterone, 55, 56, 57
    premenstrual syndrome, 38–39
Progestogen contraceptives
    anticonvulsants with, 287
    injectable, 10–11
    intrauterine progestogen-only system
        (Mirena/IUS), 16
    progestogen-only pill (POP),
        8–10, 18, 19
    progestogen-releasing implant
        (Implanon), 11
Progestogens
    contraceptives see Progestogen
        contraceptives
    hormone replacement therapy, 54–57
    premenstrual syndrome, 38–39
Promazine, 304
Promethazine, 28, 91
Propranolol, 277, 283, 295, 309
Propylthiouracil, 203
Prostaglandin synthetase inhibitors, 41, 42
Prostaglandins, 61
Prostate cancer screening, 71
Prostatism, 70–71
Prostatitis, 66, 79
Proteinuria, 30, 31, 66, 109, 150, 151
Proton pump inhibitors (PPIs), 117, 118,
        156, 242, 246
Pruritus, generalised, 137
Pruritus ani, 126
Psoriasis, 140–141
Psoriasis Association, 358
Psychosomatic illness, 297–298
Psychotherapy

Psychotherapy (*cont'd*)
British Association for Counselling and Psychotherapy, 355
British Association of Psychotherapists, 355
Pulmonary embolus (PE), 154, 155, 182
PUVA (psoralens with UVA), 141
Pyrexia, 181, 204, 267, 340, 342
HIV, 202
meningitis, 188, 189
postpartum, 33
pyrexia of unknown origin (PUO), 202–204
Pyridoxine, 38

de Quervain's tenosynovitis, 248
Quinsy, 218

Rabies vaccine, 343
Ramipril, 280
Ranitidine, 117
Raynaud's phenomenon, 163
RBID (Royal National Institute for Deaf People), 358
Receptor antagonists
H_2, 117, 118
Receptor antagonists
leukotriene, 95, 96, 97, 172, 173
Rectal bleeding, 122, 125–126, 268–269
Red reflex, 227
Reflux/oesophagitis, 155, 156
Relate – National Marriage Guidance, 358
Release – The National Drugs and Legal Helpline, 358
Respiratory problems
children, 93–97
in the terminally ill, 324–325
Retinoids, 132, 141
Rhesus-negative mothers, 31
Rheumatoid arthritis, 244–246
Rifampicin, 189, 337
Ringworm, 135–136
Rinne's tuning fork test, 210
Risedronate, 244
Risperidone, 304
RNIB (Royal National Institute for the Blind), 358
Rodent ulcer, 131
Rosacea, 133

Rotator cuff syndrome (supraspinatus tendonitis), 247
Royal National Institute for Deaf People, 358
Royal National Institute for the Blind, 358
Rubella, 207–208
vaccination, 22, 334, 338–339

Safe sex, 2, 202
Salactol, 135
Salbutamol, 95, 173, 175, 179, 180, 183, 184, 215
Salicylic acid, 135, 141
Salmeterol, 95, 173, 184
Salmonella, 121
Samaritans, The, 358
SANDS (Stillbirth and Neonatal Death Society), 359
Scabies, 137, 142
Scalp psoriasis, 141
Scarlet fever, 190
Scheriproct, 268
Schick test, 336
Schirmer's test, 225
Screening
abdominal aortic aneurysm, 80–81
breast cancer, 50
cervical cancer, 58
chlamydia, 39
haemoglobinopathies, 260
hypothryroidism, 111
prenatal, 25–26, 31
prostate cancer, 71
self-examination for testicular cancer, 80
Scrotal swellings, 77–78
Seborrhoeic dermatitis, 137
Seborrhoeic warts, 130
Sectioning, 307–308
Seizures, 97–98
see also Convulsions; Epilepsy
Selenium sulphide, 137
Semen analysis, 59
Senna, 88, 124, 125, 323
Septic arthritis, 253, 254
Serum AFP test, 26
Sever's disease, 255
Sexual abuse, 100
Sexual problems
erectile dysfunction, 74–75

infertility, 59–60
Peyronie's disease, 75–76
premature ejaculation, 75
Sexual relations, 2
Sexually transmitted infections (STIs), 2,
46–48
chlamydia, 15, 39, 46–47, 76–77
HIV/AIDS, 2, 201–202
Shigella, 121
Shingles, 197–198
red eye with herpes zoster infection, 230
Shock wave therapy, extracorporeal, 76
Short stature, 93
Shoulder pain, 246–247
Sickle cell disease, 260
SIDS (sudden death syndrome), 101–103
Child Death Helpline, 356
Foundation for the Study of Infant
Deaths, 357
SANDS (Stillbirth and Neonatal Death
Society), 359
Sigmoidoscopy, 125, 269
Silver nitrate, 40, 216, 264
Simeticone, 318
Simvastatin, 107, 150, 153
Sinusitis, 178, 180, 217, 218, 231, 277
Skin
acne, 131–133
allergic rashes/urticaria, 143
bacterial infections, 133–134, 193
benign superficial lumps, 130
eczema, 138–140
fungal infections, 135–137
generalised pruritus, 137
hidradenitis suppurativa, 133
malignancies, 130–131
psoriasis, 140–141
rosacea, 133
viral infections, 134–135
Slapped cheek (fifth disease), 192
Sleep problems
children, 91
insomnia, 296–297
sleep apnoea, 217, 219, 222
Smoking, 313–314
breast cancer and, 51
cervical cancer and, 58
cessation advice, 22, 50, 74, 103, 108, 116,
151, 158, 184
claudication and, 153

coronary heart disease and, 4, 146, 158
postmenopausal hip fracture and, 244
pulmonary embolus and, 155
Snellen chart, 233
Snoring, 217, 219, 221–222
Snow blindness, 230
Sodium bicarbonate, 48, 65
Sodium cromoglycate eyedrops, 215, 229
Sodium phosphate enemas, 125, 323
Sodium valproate, 287
Soiling, 87–88
Solar keratoses, 131
Sore throat, 218–219
Spermicide, 13, 14
Spina bifida, 31
Splenectomy, 260–261
Squamous cell carcinoma, 131
Squints, 226–227
Staphylococcus, 134, 199
Statins, 109, 146, 152, 153, 157, 160, 280
monitoring, 333
nystatin, 91, 136, 220, 221
simvastatin, 107, 150, 153
Stature *see* Height
Status epilepticus, 98
Sterilisation, 17–18
Steroids
asthma, 95–97, 171–177
COPD, 184, 185
croup, 94
eczema, 139
nappy rash, 91
nasal blockage, 217
Still births, 23, 36
SANDS (Stillbirth and Neonatal Death
Society), 359
STIs *see* Sexually transmitted infections
Stomatitis, 136
Stones
gallstones, 127, 266–267
urinary, 66–67
Streptomycin, 210, 338
Stress incontinence, 68, 69
Stroke, 232, 280–281
Styes, 225
Subconjunctival haemorrhage, 229
Sudden death syndrome *see* SIDS
Suicide, 300–301
sectioning, 307–308
Sulphasalazine, 333

Sulphonylureas, 110
Sumatriptan, 277
Sun protection, 131
Support hosiery, 29
Supraspinatus tendonitis, 247
Supraventricular tachycardia, 167
Sweating, 138
  with opiate addiction, 309
Syncope, 163–165
Synphase, 5, 8
Syntometrine, 27

Tachycardia, 166, 167, 168, 267, 271, 294
Tall stature, 93
Tamoxifen, 76
Tay–Sachs disease, 27
TB see Tuberculosis
TCRE (transcervical resection of the
  endometrium), 43
Tear problems, 224
Temazepam, 297
Temporal arteritis, 232, 242–243, 277
Temporomandibular joint dysfunction, 213,
  277–278
Tennis elbow, 248
Tenosynovitis, 248
Terbinafine, 136
Terminal care, 316–328
Termination of pregnancy, 60–61
Terrence Higgins Trust, 359
Testes, undescended, 264
Testicular cancer, 80
Testicular pain, 78–79
Testosterone, 44, 49, 50, 74
Tetanus vaccine, 337
Tetanus-prone wounds, 337
Tetracaine drops, 229, 230
Tetracycline, 6, 18
    see also Oxytetracycline
Thalassaemia, 260
Theophylline, 331
Thiazides, 239
  bendroflumethiazide, 150, 161
Threadworms, 126
Throat, sore, 218–219
Thrush, 77, 91
Thyroid disorders, 111–113
Thyroid stimulating hormone (TSH),
  111, 112

Thyrotoxicosis, 282, 294, 302
Thyroxine, 332
  levothyroxine, 112
TIAs (transient ischaemic attacks), 149, 153,
  165, 280, 281–282
Tibolone, 53, 54, 56
Tick-borne encephalitis vaccine, 345
Tinea, 135–136
Tinnitus, 213–214
  British Tinnitus Association, 356
Tioconazole, 136
Tiotropium, 184
Toenail, ingrowing, 256
Tonsillitis, 182, 218
Toothache, 213
Torsion, testicular, 79
Torticollis, 240, 241
Toxoplasmosis, 22
Tranexamic acid, 42
Transcervical resection of the endometrium
  (TCRE), 43
Transient ischaemic attacks (TIAs), 149,
  153, 165, 280, 281–282
Trazodone, 293
Tremor, 282–283
  resting (Parkinson's syndrome), 283–284
Tretinoin, 132
  isotretinoin, 133
Triadene, 5
Trichomonas, 46
Tridestra, 55
Trigeminal neuralgia, 278
Trimethoprim, 48, 65, 66, 90, 121
Tri-minulet, 5
Trinordiol, 5, 7
TriNovum, 5
Triple blood test, 24, 25–26
Tuberculine skin test, 340
Tuberculosis (TB), 178, 182, 202,
  220, 299, 339
Typhoid vaccine, 344

Ulcers
  arterial, 144
  mouth, 221
  rodent, 131
  venous, 143–144
Ultrasound, 15, 42, 80, 113
  gallstones, 266, 267

jaundice, 127
neonate, 84
polycystic ovarian syndrome, 49–50
pregnancy, 24, 26, 27, 28, 32, 44
tennis elbow, 248
transrectal, 71
urinary stones, 67
UTI, 65, 90
venous ulcers, 144
Umbilical granuloma, 264
Umbilical heriae, 264–265
Upper respiratory tract infection (URTI), 176
Urethral syndrome, 48
Urge incontinence, 68, 69–70
Urinary incontinence, 67–70
bed-wetting, 88–89
Urinary stones, 66–67
Urinary tract infection (UTI), 64–66
children, 90
URTI (upper respiratory tract infection), 176
Urticaria, 143
UTI *see* Urinary tract infection

Vaccinations, 334–345
adult, 334–335
Hib, 261, 337
HPV, 58
influenza, 109, 184, 194, 261, 337, 340
live, 335
meningococcal, 261, 342
pneumococcal, 109, 261, 340–341
routine childhood, 334
splenectomy, 261
Vaginal discharge, 45
COC side-effect, 4, 7
lochia, 32–33
Vaginal oestrogen creams, 54
Valaciclovir, 48, 197
Valvular heart disease, 161, 165, 168
Varicella-zoster immunoglobulin, 193, 343
Varicella-zoster virus, 193, 197–198
Varicose ulcers, 143–144
Varicose veins, 29, 270
Vasectomy, 17–18, 271
Vasovagal faints, 163
Venlafaxine, 293
Venous ulcers, 143–144

Ventricular tachycardia, 166, 167, 168
Verapamil, 76
Verrucae (plantar warts), 134–135, 255
Vertebrobasilar insufficiency, 164, 165, 274, 285
Vertigo, 274–275
Violence, 306–307
Viral infections
Coxsackie virus, 192
glandular fever, 190–191
hand, foot and mouth disease, 192
hepatitis viruses, 127, 199–201
herpes simplex virus, 47–48, 197
herpes zoster virus, 230
HIV/AIDS, 2, 201–202
human papilloma virus, 47
respiratory syncitial virus, 94
skin, 134–135
throat, 218
varicella-zoster virus, 193, 197–198
Visual acuity, 106, 109, 227, 233
Visual loss
progressive, 233–235
sudden, 231–233
Vitamins
infants, 85, 86
vitamin A, 23, 85, 86
vitamin B complex, 312
vitamin B_6, 38
vitamin B_{12} deficiency, 259–260
vitamin C, 85, 86, 312
vitamin D, 85, 86, 140, 244
vitamin E, 76
vitamin K, 85
Voice loss, 220
Volmax, 173
Vomiting
pregnancy, 28
in the terminally ill, 320–321
Vulval pruritus, 45

Walking aids, 242
Warfarin, 167, 330
Warts, 134–135
genital, 47
plantar (verrucae), 134–135, 255
seborrhoeic, 130
Weaning, 86
Weber's tuning fork test, 210
Weight versus height chart, 354

Weight Watchers UK, 359
Weil's disease, 204
Wheezing
    asthmatic *see* Asthma
    hay fever, 215
Whiplash injuries, 240
Whitlow (paronychia), 136, 250–251
Whooping cough (pertussis), 188
    vaccine, 335–336
Wounds, tetanus-prone, 337

X-linked disorders, 27
Xylometazoline nose drops, 94, 217

Yasmin, 5, 132
Yellow fever vaccine, 344–345

Zanamivir, 194
Zinc paste and coal tar bandage, 139
Zinc paste and ichthammol bandage, 139
Zopiclone, 297